NATIONAL LEAGUE FOR NURSING

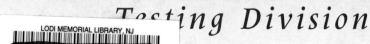
Testing Division

CHECK FOR ONE CD

REVIEW GUIDE FOR

LPN/LVN PRE-ENTRANCE

EXAM

THIRD EDITION

DISCARDED

World Headquarters

Jones and Bartlett Publishers
40 Tall Pine Drive
Sudbury, MA 01776
978-443-5000
info@jbpub.com
www.jbpub.com

Jones and Bartlett Publishers Canada
6339 Ormindale Way
Mississauga, Ontario L5V 1J2
Canada

Jones and Bartlett Publishers
  International
Barb House, Barb Mews
London W6 7PA
United Kingdom

Jones and Bartlett's books and products are available through most bookstores and online booksellers. To contact Jones and Bartlett Publishers directly, call 800-832-0034, fax 978-443-8000, or visit our website www.jbpub.com.

Substantial discounts on bulk quantities of Jones and Bartlett's publications are available to corporations, professional associations, and other qualified organizations. For details and specific discount information, contact the special sales department at Jones and Bartlett via the above contact information or send an email to specialsales@jbpub.com.

The authors, editor, and publisher have made every effort to provide accurate information. However, they are not responsible for errors, omissions, or for any outcomes related to the use of the contents of this book and take no responsibility for the use of the products and procedures described. Treatments and side effects described in this book may not be applicable to all people; likewise, some people may require a dose or experience a side effect that is not described herein. Drugs and medical devices are discussed that may have limited availability controlled by the Food and Drug Administration (FDA) for use only in a research study or clinical trial. Research, clinical practice, and government regulations often change the accepted standard in this field. When consideration is being given to use of any drug in the clinical setting, the health care provider or reader is responsible for determining FDA status of the drug, reading the package insert, and reviewing prescribing information for the most up-to-date recommendations on dose, precautions, and contraindications, and determining the appropriate usage for the product. This is especially important in the case of drugs that are new or seldom used.

Production Credits
Publisher: Kevin Sullivan
Acquisitions Editor: Emily Ekle
Acquisitions Editor: Amy Sibley
Associate Editor: Patricia Donnelly
Editorial Assistant: Rachel Shuster
Production Editor: Wendy Swanson
Associate Marketing Manager: Ilana Goddess
Manufacturing and Inventory Control Supervisor: Amy Bacus
Composition: diacriTech, Chennai, India
Text Design: diacriTech, Chennai, India
Cover Design: Brian Moore
Cover Images: from left to right © Photos.com; © PhotoCreate/ShutterStock, Inc.; © Photos.com; © Photodisc
Printing and Binding: Courier Stoughton
Cover Printing: Courier Stoughton

Library of Congress Cataloging-in-Publication Data
Review guide for LPN/LVN pre-entrance exam / National League for Nursing Testing Division.—3rd ed.
    p. ; cm.
  Includes bibliographical references.
  ISBN 978-0-7637-6270-4 (pbk.)
 1. Practical nursing—Examinations, questions, etc. I. National League for Nursing. II. National League for Nursing. Testing Division.
  [DNLM: 1. Nursing, Practical—Examination Questions. WY 18.2 R453 2009]
  RT62.R466 2009
  610.7306'93—dc22

2008030665

6048
Printed in the United States of America
12 11 10 09 08   10 9 8 7 6 5 4 3 2 1

Contents

Contents

SECTION C

SCIENCE CONTENT REVIEW   **163**

Preface

If you are applying for admission to a nursing program, you have found the reference book that will help you achieve your goal.

The first edition of this book was compiled in response to a large number of requests from applicants who were looking for a solid tool to guide them in preparing for nursing school entrance exams. The second edition was an update of that reference, which proved to be a valuable guide for admission test preparation. This third edition has expanded the subject matter reviews to bring them up to current curricula. The science section has been expanded to address topics in current science courses, not previously covered, such as modern genetics. Added to the Science Content Review is a vocabulary list for each science category and a review of health topics. This edition includes more than 100 new items.

You will find this book to be a valuable preparation tool for the NLN Pre-Admission Examination. Applicants who are preparing for the Psychological Services Bureau's PSB-Nursing School Aptitude Examination, the Educational Resources Nurse Entrance Test (NET), the Pre-Nursing Assessment Test from the Center for Nurse Education and Testing (CNET), or the Test of Essential Academic Skills (TEAS) from Assessment Technologies Incorporated will also find it to be a worthwhile study aide. In addition, if you are seeking admission to programs in various health-related fields, such as medical technology, dental hygiene, or dietician and physician's assistant programs, you can use this book to assist them in preparing for your entrance exams.

In addition to subject matter overviews for the verbal, math, and science content that is included on most pre-entrance examinations, this book contains more than *1000* practice questions from previous NLN Pre-Admission exams. Although these questions are no longer used in the current exams, they are actual questions that were used on previously administered NLN Pre-Admission exams.

The Introduction discusses career options in nursing and describes the types of nursing programs available. Helpful advice is offered to assist you to select the nursing program that is right for you. The Introduction also reviews the content of pre-admission exams and provides proven study strategies and test-taking skills to help you to maximize your score.

Section A provides a comprehensive review of the verbal and reading comprehension components of a nursing school pre-admission test. This section offers a number of practical methods to improve your vocabulary and reading skills. A detailed analysis of a reading comprehension passage is also offered. At the end of this section, three practice tests, each consisting of 60 questions, provide opportunities to test your ability with verbal and reading comprehension questions. Answer keys are provided for each of the practice tests, which can be used to analyze your strengths and weaknesses.

Section B offers an excellent overview of the math content that you will need to be familiar with for a nursing school pre-admission exam. Detailed examples are provided to help you solve the various problems and identify your strengths and weaknesses. Four math exams (40 questions each), with answer keys and explanations, are provided for practice at the end of the section. In many cases, multiple ways of solving these problems are provided.

Section C reviews the science content that is included on a nursing school pre-admission exam. Summaries of high school biology, anatomy and physiology, chemistry, physics, and health will guide your study in these areas. Three science exams (60 questions each), with answer keys and explanations, are provided for practice at the end of the section.

Three Comprehensive Practice Tests are provided in the final section. New questions have been substituted for previous questions throughout these tests. Each of these tests is compiled from questions that were included on actual NLN Pre-Admission Exams that are no longer in use. Each of the Comprehensive Practice Tests has 160 questions: 60 verbal, 40 math, and 60 science. Answer keys and explanations follow each exam.

The actual NLN Pre-Admission Exam contains 214 questions: 80 verbal, 54 math, and 80 science, with 1 hour allowed for completing each section. Therefore, if you want to simulate the real test experience, you should time yourself to finish each section of the Comprehensive Practice Tests in 45 minutes. If you are planning to take another pre-admission exam, it is important for you to find out how many questions you must answer in the allotted time.

Free CD-ROM Included with Book. The enclosed CD-ROM allows you to simulate a computer-based testing experience. As more and more schools are requiring students to take the pre-entrance exam on a computer, the enclosed CD-ROM should be an important part of your preparation. This CD allows you to customize your own practice tests and then review your results—an excellent way to study. Immediate feedback is also available for every question on the CD.

The NLN Review Guide for LPN/LVN Pre-Entrance Exam provides a sound basis for successful preparation for a nursing pre-admission exam. You will find it to be a useful tool to assist you to maximize your exam score and gain admission to the nursing program of your choice.

W. Michael Margolin, MA
Test Consultant
National League for Nursing

Contributors

Michael Daniel
BS Math/Physics Engineering:
    Washington Lee University
MEd Secondary Education: Xavier
    University, Ohio
High School Math Teacher
Colerain High School
Cincinnati, OH

James Halverson
AB American Literature: Brown
    University
MA English: New York University
High School English Teacher
Saint Ann's School
Brooklyn, NY

W. Michael Margolin
BS St. Lawrence University
MA New York University
Adjunct Instructor in Science Education
City College of New York

Mary E. McDonald
BSN Nursing: Boston College
MA Nursing Education: New York
    University
MA Applied Psychology-Measurement:
    New York University

Sean E. McDonald
BA Physics, Math-Economics
Wesleyan University, CT

Alexis Papageorge
BA Biology: University of Chicago
Biology Graduate Student: New York
    University
High School Chemistry and Anatomy &
    Physiology Teacher

John R. Smith
AB Psychology: Harvard
    University
High School Math Teacher
Saint Ann's School
Brooklyn, NY

George B. Stengren
BS American Studies: Central Michigan
    University
MA Science Education: Teachers
    College, Columbia University
Doctoral Student: Teachers College,
    Columbia University
Secondary Level Science Teacher
The Heritage School
New York, NY

Introduction

CAREER OPTIONS IN NURSING

You purchased this book because you have decided that you want to be a nurse. You have made *two* wise decisions. First, nursing is a rewarding and challenging career that allows you to make a meaningful difference in the lives of others. Second, this book is designed to assist you in succeeding in your initial step toward reaching your career goal—scoring your best on a nursing school entrance examination.

Despite the fact that more nurses are employed today than ever before, there is an alarming shortage of licensed practical nurses. The opportunities currently available in nursing are extensive, and education is the key to career advancement. You must carefully consider your professional goals before choosing a particular educational path. You should evaluate each of the three types of educational programs in nursing that are available in the United States before deciding which route to follow.

1. **Licensed practical nurse (LPN), licensed vocational nurse (LVN),** or **practical nurse (PN)** preparation focuses on technical skills and includes coursework in basic sciences, in addition to nursing courses in the care of adults, children, childbearing families, and individuals with mental illness. These programs vary in length from 12 to 24 months and are usually offered in state-approved vocational schools, community colleges, and hospitals. The practical nurse graduate is qualified to take the practical nurse (LPN/LVN/PN) state licensure exam and, once licensed, is prepared for immediate employment under the supervision of a registered nurse.

2. **Diploma programs** are the oldest type of educational programs for preparing both practical and registered nurses in the United States. The number of these programs is steadily declining because advanced degree nursing (ADN) programs have increased in popularity. State-approved diploma programs are affiliated with hospitals and last from 24 to 30 months, preparing their graduates to take the state licensing exam for either practical or registered nurses. In addition to nursing courses in the care of adults, children, childbearing families, and individuals with mental illness, diploma students are required to take prerequisite science courses. General education courses are not always required because diploma programs do

1

not grant a degree. Diploma graduates are intensively vocational prepared to provide individualized, direct care to hospitalized patients.

3. **Associate degree nursing** (ADN, AS) programs may also prepare their graduates to take the practical or the registered nurse (RN) state licensure examination. Most of these programs require 1 academic year of LPN/LVN/PN study or 2 academic years of RN study, and they are usually offered at community colleges. Following completion of the program, students are awarded an associate degree. Requirements include general education and basic science courses, as well as nursing theory and clinical experience in the care of adults, children, childbearing families, and individuals with mental illness. Associate degree graduates are equipped to solve healthcare problems, make decisions, and provide direct patient care.

4. **Baccalaureate programs** are at least 4 years in length and are offered in colleges and universities. Baccalaureate students take the general education requirements of their college in addition to prerequisite courses in the physical, biological, and behavioral sciences. The nursing major requires clinical coursework in the care of adults, children, childbearing families, and individuals with mental illness, with an emphasis on community health, leadership, and the role of the professional nurse as a manager. Nursing theory, professional ethics and issues, and nursing research are also included in the baccalaureate curriculum. The baccalaureate nurse is eligible to take the registered nurse state licensing exam and is prepared for positions in community health. The baccalaureate degree is considered a requirement for managerial and advanced nursing positions.

Nursing education at all levels provides a basis for career development. A large number of ADN programs offer upward mobility programs for diploma graduates. Many baccalaureate programs offer a completion track for registered nurses who are graduates of diploma and ADN programs. These programs often admit students with advanced standing based on their nursing experience and on their performance on an advanced standing exam, such as the National League for Nursing's Nurse Accelerated Completion Exam (NACE). In this way nurses are able to build on their experience to complete the requirements for the baccalaureate degree, which is required for entrance to graduate education. Graduate preparation at the master's and doctorate levels opens the door to even greater career opportunities in nursing, including teaching, administration, and nursing research.

WHICH NURSING PROGRAM IS RIGHT FOR YOU?

When selecting a nursing path to pursue, the first thing you should consider is your career goal. Do you want to work in a community health setting? Are you interested in providing direct patient care in a hospital? Do you envision yourself as a nursing administrator or in a nursing leadership position? Does your ultimate career goal require graduate nursing education? Should you choose another entry-level program to achieve your goals through career mobility programs? Or, should you choose a basic baccalaureate program to provide you with the foundation for an advanced nursing education? Your ultimate decision should be based on a careful consideration of your individual needs.

Nursing can be a satisfying career, both personally and financially. However, remember that, no matter what educational level you choose to pursue, nursing is a career that requires intelligence, self-discipline, and a lifelong dedication to learning. The nursing profession will provide you with many opportunities for continuing education and career advancement. It will be up to you to take full advantage of the opportunities to grow, both as a person and as a professional.

HOW WILL YOU FINANCE YOUR EDUCATION?

Nursing education can be expensive. Examine your individual situation before making a decision about which avenue to pursue. Several factors affect your school choice and nursing path. For example, baccalaureate programs are the most expensive because they require the most extensive coursework. Private colleges are more expensive than public institutions. Also, the demands of a full-time program may prevent you from working. Perhaps your financial situation obliges you to consider a part-time program that will allow you to continue to work. You may decide to obtain a diploma or pursue an associate degree in nursing. Each of these credentials enables you to pursue a satisfying nursing career and acts as a stepping-stone for you to advance your nursing education. Whatever program you choose, nursing is a profession that encourages career mobility and provides you with much opportunity to reach your ultimate career goal.

When considering your educational options, remember that financial assistance is available for all types of nursing programs. Aid may be available in the form of scholarships and grants that do not need to be repaid. Educational loans that carry a low interest rate and that are repaid after graduation are also available. The amount and type of aid you receive depend on your need and on the amount of the financial aid available at the institution you attend. There is always competition for financial aid; so you have to find out early from the institutions that you are considering what aid is available, what the eligibility requirements are, and what the application procedure involves. Applying early to several programs that meet your criteria provides you with the best opportunities both for admission and for receiving the financial aid package you need. In addition, be sure to learn about financial aid available from the federal government at www.studentaid.ed.gov.

WHICH PROGRAMS DO YOU QUALIFY FOR?

Before you submit an application to a nursing program, you must honestly evaluate your credentials. Acceptance depends on several factors, including your grade point average (GPA), standardized pre-admission test scores, references, extracurricular activities, an interview, work experience, and writing ability. Admission is competitive, and schools establish their own criteria for admission.

Nursing programs are very rigorous. The coursework requires long hours of intense study, and nursing students are often scheduled for 8 to 16 hours a week of clinical practice. Schools are all looking for motivated students who will succeed. Schools accept the most qualified students who apply, and the number of admissions to each program is limited. Therefore, apply to several programs.

As a general rule, the higher the educational level of the program is, the higher the standards for admission will be. Your high school or community college grades are very important. The higher your GPA and pre-admission test score are, the better your chances will be, although schools consider the level of difficulty of the coursework you have taken.

Your GPA and pre-admission test score neither guarantee nor preclude your admission to a program. This is why your personal references and interview are so important. References from qualified teachers and employers can provide a school with a more complete picture of you. If a school offers you an interview, be sure to make the most of the opportunity; arrive early and dress professionally. Your personal interview gives you the opportunity to present yourself as a motivated and qualified applicant, as well as allowing you the chance to explain any weakness in your application.

SELECTING A PROGRAM TO MEET YOUR NEEDS

Once you have sorted out your career goals and identified the educational path that best suits you, the next step is to identify several schools that fit your criteria. In addition to financial aid availability and admission requirements, evaluate the quality of the programs you are interested in. There are several questions to ask.

Is the Program Approved by the State?

Each state's Board of Nurse Examiners grants permission for nursing graduates to take the National Council Licensure Exam for Practical Nurses (NCLEX-PN®). Nursing graduates who successfully pass this exam apply directly to their state to obtain licensure to practice as a practical nurse. For information on your state's licensing procedure, visit the National Council of State Boards of Nursing's Web site at www.ncsbn.org.

Is the Program Accredited?

Accreditation assures you of the quality of the educational program. If you plan to continue your education, many nursing programs will accept your credentials for advanced placement or graduate work only if your nursing program is accredited by the National League for Nursing Accrediting Commission (NLNAC). For information, visit the NLNAC's Web site at www.nlnac.org.

What Was the NCLEX-PN® Pass Rate for the Graduates of the Program Over the Last Five Years?

Determine how successful the school's graduates have been in passing the licensure exam. A high pass rate over the prior several years indicates that the graduates are well prepared to take the NCLEX® exam.

What Is the Reputation of the School's Graduates?

Are the graduates well respected in the healthcare community? A high employment rate for new graduates indicates that the program is preparing its students well for the work environment.

Is the Environment of the School Comfortable for You?

Some people prefer to attend a large institution that offers many extracurricular activities. Others prefer the close community atmosphere of a small institution. Are you interested in dormitory life, or would you prefer to commute to school? Examine the social experience that each school offers, and decide whether you are comfortable with it.

Also look seriously at all the available options. Once you identify the schools that meet your needs, you will probably find that these schools will consider you an attractive candidate. Admission to a nursing program is not dependent on one factor. Schools consider you as a whole package. Maximize your profile and be an informed applicant. There are many routes to your ultimate career goal in nursing.

NURSING SCHOOL ENTRANCE EXAMINATIONS

Most nursing programs require that you take an admissions test, such as the NLN's Pre-Admission Examination.

You will find this book to be an invaluable tool. The book contains actual questions from previous NLN Pre-Admission Examinations. The questions thoroughly cover the areas that are tested on all nursing school admission exams.

Each school of nursing that you are applying to will provide you with the necessary admission information, application form, and direction to register for National League for Nursing (NLN) Pre-Admission Examination at https://www.nlnonlinetesting.org. Although each school determines for itself how these test scores are used for admission, the higher your test score is, the better your chance will be for nursing school admission. Find out exactly how the test scores are used at the school to which you are applying; then use this book to maximize your pre-admission test score.

CONTENT OF THE NLN PRE-ADMISSION EXAMINATION

The purpose of this pre-admission examination is to evaluate academic ability in order to identify the most qualified applicants. Nursing entrance exams are carefully designed to measure an individual's ability in areas that provide a basis for nursing education. The exams provide the faculty of schools of nursing with a common criterion for evaluating the academic abilities of applicants for admission. All of the nursing pre-admission tests use four-option, multiple-choice questions to assess an applicant's verbal ability, reading comprehension, mathematic ability, and knowledge of physical and life sciences.

The practice examinations in this book consist of actual questions used in previously administered NLN Pre-Admission Examinations. These practice examinations provide you with an actual preadmission exam experience. Answer keys and rationales for every question give you important feedback to maximize test preparation.

1. The 60-question **verbal** test measures your word knowledge ability and reading comprehension. Word knowledge questions require you to identify the meaning of a word as it is used in a sentence. The reading comprehension section focuses on your reasoning and critical thinking ability. Five short passages in each test require you to analyze and interpret the material presented. The related questions assess your ability to determine the main ideas and supporting details, draw conclusions, make inferences, and apply information to new situations.

2. The 40-question **mathematics** test consists of straight calculations and word problems that cover basic operations (integers, decimals, fractions, and percentages), algebra, geometry, conversions, graphs, and concepts. Data interpretation, applied mathematics, and scientific notation are also included.

3. The 60-question **science** test measures high-school-level knowledge of science. Questions are included on general biology, chemistry, physics, and health.

The actual NLN Pre-Admission Examination contains 214 questions: 80 verbal, 54 math, and 80 science, with 1 hour allowed for completing each section. Therefore, if you want to simulate the real test experience, you should time yourself to finish each section of the Comprehensive Practice Tests in 45 minutes.

USE THIS BOOK TO MAXIMIZE YOUR SCORE

Step one for success on an exam is to keep your anxiety at a minimum. Being well prepared is the best antidote for test anxiety, and this book is designed to help you maximize your test score with thorough preparation. The guidelines are all here; it is up to you to commit the time necessary for your own success.

This book is divided into three review sections: verbal, math, and science. Each section begins with a comprehensive overview that summarizes the important facts and concepts of the subject. The review is meant to be a "refresher" for what you have already learned, not an introduction to the subject. If you have not completed a high school course in a subject, these reviews do not provide you with the knowledge that you need to be successful on a nursing entrance examination.

Carefully plan your study strategy. Start early, set a study schedule, and stick to it. Plan to finish your test preparation 3 to 4 days before the test. Cramming right before the test is not as helpful as a planned approach over time. Use each review section as a study guide to review the content summary for each subject carefully before you answer the practice questions. Study one section at a time, and then follow the Test-Taking Strategies (the next section) to answer the practice questions. Check your answers with the key, and review the rationales to identify your strengths and weakness.

Use your score as a guide for further study. Refer to the bibliography at the end of each review section for study references to improve your knowledge in the areas where you are weak.

After you have completed the verbal, math, and science sections following these guidelines, take the three comprehensive practice tests at the end of the book. Time yourself carefully, and use the answer sheet provided on pages 12 and 13 to "bubble in" one of the exams. Be very careful to fill in the circle that corresponds to your answer choice. Using these answer forms helps to familiarize you with the actual format used on the tests.

Score your exams, and carefully focus on the rationales provided for each question. For each answer that you missed, ask, "Why did I answer this question incorrectly?" Did you misread the question, or were you unfamiliar with the content? Analyzing your weaknesses gives direction to your review preparation. Decide which areas you need to focus on for your final review. Carefully following these guidelines to complete your review helps boost the confidence that you need to succeed on any of the nursing pre-admission exams.

SCORE REPORT

On page 11 is a sample of a report that you will receive after taking a pre-admission exam. This particular report is an NLN Pre-Admission performance report. Your test results are sent to you and to whichever schools you choose. Notice that a *Guide for Interpretation of the Test Report* comes with the results. Read the guide carefully. It explains how to interpret your scores and shows you how to determine where you rank among all the applicants who have taken the test. Find out how the nursing programs to which you are applying use these scores for making admission decisions. Remember, an informed applicant is a successful applicant. (See the sample score report on page 11, Figure 1.)

TEST-TAKING STRATEGIES

Nothing is more important to successful test taking than studying. A thorough understanding of the test material is essential to your success. While test-taking strategies are not a substitute for good study habits, these skills enhance your overall performance on a test, as long as you have a good grasp of the knowledge being measured. Follow the study plan guidelines presented in the previous section, and use these hints to increase your probability of choosing the correct answer. The correct answer is right there in front of you. Have confidence in yourself.

Plan Ahead

The night before the test is no time for cramming. Put your books away, and review the following test-taking strategies. Relax and get a good night's sleep. Plan to wear comfortable clothes. It is hard to predict the climate variations of most testing sites; so dress in layers and bring a sweater. Avoid confusion on the day of the test by being well prepared. Have your admission ticket, your photo identification, a watch, and several #2 pencils ready. Make sure you are familiar with the trip to the testing site, and allow yourself plenty of time. Arrive early and choose a seat where you feel comfortable. A little bit of anxiety is a positive force, and planning ahead helps keep your anxiety level at this positive level. Relaxation techniques, such as controlled breathing, help you feel calm and unhurried when the test begins.

Listen to Directions

Once the testing session begins, the proctor gives directions about filling in your identifying information and answer sheet. Pay close attention to the proctor, and read the written directions carefully. Completeness and neatness are important. Incorrect or stray marks on your answer sheet can cause your score to be delayed or, worse, negatively affect your final score. The proctor tells you how much time you have for each section and when breaks are allowed. When the proctor tells you to begin the test, note the time and jot down the time when you will have 10 minutes left to review your work.

Read Each Question Carefully

Read each question all the way through. Pay attention to detail; every word counts. Be alert for key words. Words such as "only," "never," "first," "last," "always," "except," or "never" are strong words that limit the choice of the correct answer. Ask yourself, "What is this question asking?" Consider the question *as it is written*. Do not read anything into it. No one is trying to trick you. Rephrase and answer the question in your own words.

Read Each Answer Choice Carefully

Even if the first or second answer choice looks good to you, read the other choices. Sometimes another choice provides a more precise answer or makes you realize that you misunderstood the question. Under the stress of taking a test, you may be tempted to select the first answer that looks right. Resist that temptation. Careful examination may reveal that your first choice does not answer the question at all.

Eliminate the obviously incorrect options quickly, and compare the plausible options for similarities or conflicts. Because there is only one correct answer to each question, similar options must be wrong. If two options are opposite, one of them is frequently correct. Eliminate wrong answer choices one by one. This process of elimination is completed quickly for simple recall questions, but it may take longer for more complex questions.

Although this method sounds time-consuming, it assists you in clarifying the question and selecting more correct answers. Practicing this method of eliminating answers on the sample tests included in this book helps you to develop the speed you need in the real exam.

Reread the Question and the Answer Choices

Choose your answer from the remaining choices based on the rereading. Spend time considering the plausible choices. Have confidence in your selection, but, if you are unable to answer the question after eliminating the obviously wrong choices, move on to the next one. Do not get bogged down on any one question; spending too much time on a difficult question could compromise your final test score. If you skip a question, remember to skip the corresponding number on the answer sheet. Check frequently to make sure that you are filling in the correct "bubble" on the answer sheet. Go through the whole test this way, answering only the questions that you are sure of.

Stay Focused

Keep yourself focused. Think only about the question in front of you. If stray thoughts distract you or if you find yourself wandering back to a previous question, turn your focus back to the question at hand. Congratulate yourself for being in control of the situation.

Pace Yourself

Do not puzzle over any question for more than a few seconds. On the other hand, do not race through the test so fast that you make careless errors. Pace yourself. Answer all the questions that you are sure of first, and then go back to the more difficult ones. Your objective is to consider all the questions at least once and some more than once. Plan your timing strategy in advance. The application materials tell you how many questions are in each section of the test that you are scheduled to take and how much time is allowed. Use the practice tests in this book to practice pacing yourself, and use all the allotted time. Rushing to finish a test does not benefit your score. Do not be distracted by other students who leave the testing room before you do. Everyone works at a different pace, and paying attention to what others are doing takes time away from your test. Use every minute of the allotted time to maximize your final score.

Take an Educated Guess

When you apply to take a test, read all the material provided. Be sure that you know whether there is a penalty for guessing. If there is, your score is reduced by the number of incorrect responses indicated. Do *not* guess. If your score not penalized for wrong answers, that is, if it is equal to the total number of correct answers, then take a guess for each question you are unsure of.

Wild guessing should always be avoided, but, even with a penalty for guessing, a guessing strategy can improve your score. Your chance of guessing the correct answer increases with every option that you can eliminate. You can probably spot one or two wrong choices in even the most difficult questions. If you eliminate the clearly wrong options and make an educated guess from the remaining choices, you are bound to pick up some extra points.

Obviously, the most effective way to eliminate wrong choices or to choose the correct one is to base your decision on your knowledge of the subject. You should guess only after you have tried your best to answer the question knowledgeably. However, here are some tips to help you to make an educated guess when you are unable to pick the correct answer. (Just remember that test developers are also very aware of these tips and attempt to eliminate them from their exams.)

- Watch for grammatical inconsistencies. If an answer is inconsistent with the question, it probably is an incorrect response.

- A word that is used in both the stem and one option is a clue that the option is the correct choice.

- There can only be one correct answer. When two answers are very similar, neither one is correct.

- Definitive words such as "always," "never," "only," or "all" in an option usually mean that the option is incorrect.

- Avoid looking for an answer pattern. It is not unusual for several consecutive questions to have the same answer letter.

- Do not assume that one letter is favored as the answer. Test developers are very cautious to equally distribute answers across all four-letter options; one letter is not chosen over another. Because an effort is made to equally distribute the answers randomly, each letter has an equal chance of being the correct response. First, make sure that there is no penalty for guessing. Then, if you have absolutely no idea of the correct answer or if you have run out of time, choose a letter and pick that letter consistently throughout the test. You will have a 25% chance of guessing correctly. Many times the correct answer is the longest one. Test developers are very cautious about keeping the choices of equal length, but, if you are in doubt, you may decide to choose the longest option as the correct one.

- Recall clues from other questions. Sometimes information in one question gives away the answer to another.

- Stay with your first answer unless you have a very specific reason to make a change. Do not change your answer on a whim, but you should be willing to change it for a good reason. When you score your practice tests, note whether your changed answers helped or hurt your score. If they helped, you have a tendency to improve your score by changing answers. If you find that you tend to change your answers to incorrect choices, stop changing your answers.

In addition, there are exceptions to every rule; so answer with caution and never let a hunch or a tip overrule an answer that you have decided on based on your knowledge. Have confidence in yourself because the best chance for successfully answering a question is based on a thorough understanding of the subject.

POSITIVE ATTITUDE

Having a positive attitude about yourself and your test-taking ability is fundamental to success on any exam. Getting down on yourself can rob you of your confidence. Think positive thoughts that keep your confidence up. You took the first step toward developing a positive attitude when you purchased this book. Follow the guidelines outlined in this introduction, and you will be well on your way to sharpening your positive attitude. Remember to keep the admission test in perspective. The test is only one factor in nursing school admission. Your grades, recommendations, and interview all play important roles in the admission decision. In addition, schools sometimes allow you to repeat the test if you do not do as well as you want.

You can increase self-confidence by studying effectively, and you can maximize your test-taking ability by utilizing the skills outlined in this book. If you follow the guidelines and practice your skills on the sample examinations in this book, you will develop the positive attitude that you need for success on a nursing school pre-admission examination.

NLN ASSESSMENT AND EVALUATION   61 BROADWAY   NEW YORK, NY 10006

Site #   **NATIONAL LEAGUE FOR NURSING**   Form   45
                          REPORT OF PERFORMANCE ON
                          Pre-Admission Examination -   RN

Applicant Name   **Identification Number**   Test Date   Report Date
                                                             04/03/99   04/12/99

                                 Program Code

| Test | Score | Percentile Norms* | | |
		DI	AD	All
Verbal Ability	40	82	69	73
Mathematics	31	94	94	94
Science	34	79	72	74
Composite	121	87	82	83

*PERCENTILE NORMS ARE BASED ON PERFORMANCE OF:	INDIV.	PROG.	STATES	
APPLICANTS TO DIPLOMA PROGRAMS ------------	641	39	13	1983
APPLICANTS TO ASSOCIATE DEGREE PROGRAMS----	1897	33	20	1983
ALL APPLICANTS TO BASIC NURSING PROGRAMS---	2615	75	25	1983

SCORES ON THIS EXAMINATION FORM WERE UPDATED USING A
PRE-EQUATING SAMPLE OF 22.962 EXAMINEES TESTED IN 1993-94.

A copy of this report was sent to:

GUIDE FOR THE INTERPRETATION OF THE TEST REPORT

SCORES The individual tests included in the examination are identified in the left-hand column of the report. Immediately to the right, in the column labeled "Score" is the **raw score** earned. This score is the number of test items you answered correctly. Each test contains some additional items that were included for test development purposes only. These items were not used to calculate the scores. The highest possible raw score in each test is as follows: Verbal Ability - 60; Mathematics - 40; Science - 60.

THE COMPOSITE SCORE is based on your performance on the total examination, but is not the sum of the items answered correctly. It is a standard score, i.e., a weighted combination of the scores on the individual tests. Composite scores may range from 0 to 200. The average is 100, and the standard deviation, a measure of variability around this average score, is 20. Most scores range between 50 and 150.

A PERCENTILE SCORE for each test and for the composite score is reported in the column labeled "Percentile Norms." Percentiles, which range from 0-99, indicate what portion of a reference group of applicants to similar nursing programs earned raw scores lower than yours. For example, if the report shows a percentile score of 84 for a raw score of 049 on the Verbal Ability test, it means that 84% of the norms group received a raw score of 49 or less. The percentile scores do NOT indicate the percentage of items that were answered correctly.

NORMS GROUP Each norms group used in preparing this report is identified at the top of the column labeled "Percentile Norms." For the Pre-Admission Examination-PN the norms group is comprised of all applicants to practical nursing programs who took this test during the period identified at the bottom of the report. For the Pre-Admission Examination-RN three sets of norms are provided: "DI" refers to applicants to diploma programs; "AD" refers to applicants to associate degree programs; and "ALL" refers to all applicants to any of the three types of programs preparing students for registered nurse practice. The most appropriate norms group to use is the group which matches or includes the type of program to which you are applying. This allows comparisons with other applicants to similar programs. Each norms group is described in the section following the test scores.

INTERPRETING THE SCORES Percentiles substantially above the 50th percentile indicate better than average performance, percentiles ranging from about 40-60 average, and those substantially below the 50th percentile poorer than average. Areas of strength or weakness may be identified by noting those parts of the examination for which the percentiles are high or low. It should be noted that equal differences in percentiles do not indicate equal differences in ability since examinees' test scores tend to group around the average score. The further one is from the average, in either direction, the greater is the degree of ability represented by each additional percentage point. The difference between percentiles of 80 and 89 is far greater in terms of ability than the difference between 50 and 59; similarly, the difference between percentiles 10 and 19 is greater that the difference between 50 and 59.

While no test score is an exact measure, the score should provide a very good estimate of your ability and achievement level at the time the examination was taken. The scores reported here are one source of information that can be used along with other information about an applicant, by nursing education programs when making admission decisions.

Figure 1. Sample Score Report

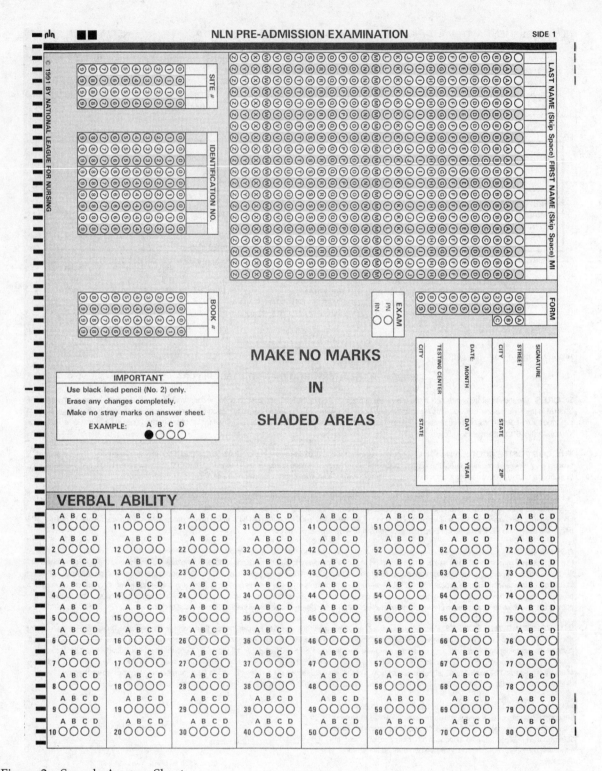

Figure 2a. Sample Answer Sheet

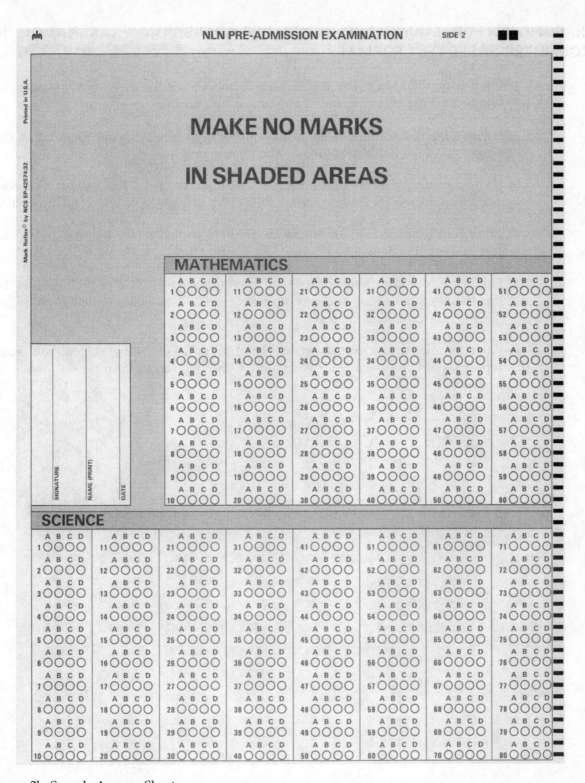

Figure 2b. Sample Answer Sheet

DIRECTIONS FOR TAKING THE NLN'S PRE-ADMISSION EXAMINATION IN COMPUTER-BASED TEST FORMAT

1. Launch the "NLN Online Testing" application from the desktop. This software will be on a computer provided by your testing facility.

2. If you already have an examinee account with NLN, enter your login name and password in the fields provided on the login screen.

3. If you do not have an account, click the "Create Account" button. Follow directions as they appear on the screen, ending with entry of your login name and password.

4. Enter your exam code in the "Exam Code" field and click the "Launch Exam" button. The exam code will be provided by the proctor.

5. Following your launching of the exam, the status screen will appear. It will display the status of the exam and any options available to you for that exam. Click "Begin" to start taking the test.

6. After completing the exam, you will be returned to the status screen. Your score report should be available for your review one-two weeks from the test date.

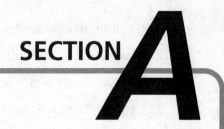

Verbal Content Review

Many smart and articulate people have trouble when taking a test on verbal skills. Fortunately, there are proven methods to help people overcome some of their test-taking problems and to maximize their performance on standardized tests. Some of these methods are long-term programs that students use to develop their verbal skills; some are very simple techniques that test takers use when answering specific kinds of questions.

In this guide you will find methods you can use to improve both your basic reading skills and your test-taking ability.

WAYS TO DEVELOP YOUR READING SKILLS

Building Your Vocabulary

You have probably noticed that almost every test of reading skills includes two types of questions: (1) those that ask you about the details, main ideas, and implications of readings, and (2) those that ask you the meanings of words, that is, vocabulary questions. Vocabulary is important because you cannot be a good reader—or a good writer or even a good thinker—if you don't know an ample number of words. Take this sentence, for instance:

Sandra grimaced when she tasted the brackish water.

The reader who knows the words "grimaced" and "brackish" will have a much better understanding of what Sandra did (made a sour face) and why she did it (because the water was slightly salty) than the reader who knows only one of those words or neither of them. One of your long-term goals, then, should be to improve your vocabulary, not just to score well on tests but also to become a better reader and a more effective communicator.

You can do five things to build your word power:

1. Make vocabulary study fun.

2. Read as much as possible.

3. Use a dictionary often.

4. Make word lists.

5. Break words down into roots and affixes.

Make Vocabulary Study Fun

No vocabulary development program is likely to succeed if you don't enjoy learning new words and have fun pursuing their meanings. Play word games, do crossword puzzles, and listen to effective speakers for new words that intrigue you, words that you want to make yours.

To remember new words, use memory devices that are fun and fanciful. For example, if you want to remember the meaning of "brackish," you might play with the word and make a sentence: "Brrrr! . . . Ack! . . . Ish! It's salty!" Sometimes the sillier the association is, the easier it is to remember the word.

Read as Much as Possible

When you converse with friends, go to movies, or watch television, you are exposed to many words—but not nearly as many as when you read. Some reading material can be daunting, with so many new words that you don't know where to begin. However, by using the context in which a word is used, you can often get a general indication of its meaning. Someone, for example, who knows the meaning of the word "grimaced" in our illustrative sentence but does not know "brackish" can still be quite sure that "brackish" describes something negative.

When you come across a new word in your reading, stop and see whether you can work out its meaning from the context. If cannot deduce the meaning, look it up in the dictionary. If you are reading something that requires you to look up words all the time, be reasonable and patient; look up only the ones that seem crucial to the meaning of a passage or that you find interesting. Do not try to learn impossible numbers of words from your reading, or you will likely give up on your program before it really gets started. With time, you will find yourself needing to check fewer and fewer words.

Use a Dictionary Often

When you read, have a dictionary nearby so that you can look up the meanings of words that you don't know or know only vaguely. A word whose meaning is hazy in your mind, one that you recognize but cannot exactly define, is probably the most important to look up, because that effort may be just the refresher you need to retain the word's definition clearly and permanently. (Most of us have a hard time remembering the meaning of a brand-new word that we have looked up only once.)

Make sure your dictionary is large enough to contain full definitions, pronunciation keys, and word origins. By checking the pronunciation of a word and saying it aloud, you burn its memory into different parts of your brain. And knowing the origin of a

SECTION A

SECTION B

SECTION C

COMPREHENSIVE PRACTICE Test 1

COMPREHENSIVE PRACTICE Test 2

COMPREHENSIVE PRACTICE Test 3

word—"grimace," for example, is related to the Old English word "grima," a mask— can also help you understand and retain its meaning.

Make Word Lists

Of course, you cannot always have a dictionary with you, but if you are in school or watching an educational program, you can have a pen and paper handy to jot down new and interesting words. (If you have time, write them in their context, in the phrase or sentence that the speaker used, because words often have more than one meaning.) Look up the words on your list later, and then use them in sentences of your own to make them easier to remember.

A second and more important word list is the one that you should keep in a study notebook (journal). After looking up a word, write it on this list with a short definition. The writing process itself helps you remember the word by putting it into still another area of your brain. Go over your list from time to time, testing yourself on the words, always saying them aloud to enhance retention. Then see if you can work the new words into your conversations or writing.

Another way of working with vocabulary is to make flash cards, with the vocabulary word on one side and the definition on the other. You can carry your stack of flash cards with you and study them whenever you have a free moment.

Break Words Down into Roots and Affixes

A shortcut to vocabulary development is to learn the meanings of word roots and affixes (word fragments that we add on to roots).

- The *root* of a word (sometimes called its *stem*) is its main part, its core meaning.

  EX: The root of brackish is "brack-," derived from the Dutch word "brac," which means salty.

- An *affix* is a letter combination that we add to a root to modify its meaning. A *prefix* is added on before a root and a *suffix* after it.

  EX: To the root "brack-" we add "-ish," a suffix that means "like" or "somewhat," and we get brackish, somewhat salty.

By learning word roots and knowing the meanings of common English affixes, you can easily learn whole groups of words. If you know, for example, that the root "fract" means break, then it is much easier to learn and remember words like "fracture" (a break), "fraction" (a portion—i.e., a breaking of the whole), "diffract" (break light apart), and "fractious" (unruly, irritable—i.e., breaking from propriety).

So when you look up a word in the dictionary, note its history (or etymology). Look for the root from which the word is derived, often a Latin, Greek, or German word, and try to think of other words that are derived from the same root. Later, when you encounter a new word, you will more likely be able to spot its root and, by putting the root together with its context, formulate a very close approximation of its definition without even consulting a dictionary.

The following sample list contains roots and affixes, along with some common words made from them. You can also find many vocabulary study books, some listed in the bibliography at the end of this section, that have sections devoted to roots and affixes.

Prefix	Meaning	Examples (Short Definition)
ante-	before	antecedent (preceding event or word)
anti-	against	antidote (something that acts against poison)
hyper	more than	hypertonic (containing more solute than environment)
hypo	less than	hypotension (low blood pressure)
hetero	different, unlike	heterozygote (having different alleles)
homo	same, like	homogeneous (evenly mixed, alike throughout)
bene-	good, well	beneficent (producing good, like charitable acts)
intra-	within	intravenous (within the veins)
mal-	ill, evil	malady (illness); malevolent (wishing evil)
mis-	incorrect	misconduct (incorrect behavior)
omni-	all	omnipotent (all powerful)
sub-	under	subcutaneous (under the skin)
trans-	across	transgress (go beyond the limits; violate)

Root	Meaning	Examples (Short Definition)
aqua	water	aquatic (living in or pertaining to water)
clude, clus	shut, close	preclude (shut beforehand; prevent)
cog, cogn	know, knowledge	cognizant (knowledgeable about; aware)
duce, duct	lead	induce (lead to; bring about)
fact, fect, fict	make, do	factory (place where things are made)
graph, gram	write, record, picture	graphic (creating a strong image)
hydr, hydro	water	dehydrate (remove water from)
ject, jac	throw, cast	interject (throw in between)
logue, logy	speech; science	eulogy (speech of praise); zoology (animal science)
man; manu	hand; by hand	manual (handbook)
meter	measure	thermometer (instrument to measure temperature)
ped, pod	foot	pedal (relating to the foot); podiatrist (foot doctor)
pend, pense	hang, weigh	impend (menace, as in "hanging overhead")
scribe, script	write	inscribe (write on, autograph); inscription (something written)
sec, sect	cut	bisect (cut in half)
spire, spirat	breath, breathe	expire (die, as in "breathe your last breath")
tract	draw, drag	extract (draw out)
vene, vent	come	convene (come together)

| vocat, voke | call | vocation (profession, as in your "calling"); evoke (call out) |
| volve, volu | roll, turn | evolve (develop, as in "roll forward"); revolution (a turn around) |

Suffix	Meaning	Examples (Short Definition)
-able, -ible	capable or worthy of	defensible (capable of being defended)
-ance, -ence	relating to, state of	despondence (state of being dejected, depression)
-ic	pertaining to	dramatic (pertaining to drama); aquatic (see above)
-ish	like, somewhat	mulish (like a mule); greenish (somewhat green)
-less	without	childless (without a child)
-ment	result; action	deferment (act of delaying)
-ness	condition, quality of	happiness (condition of being happy)

Becoming a Better Reader

Increase Your Reading Speed

Some people think that slow readers must be good readers, but slow reading can actually hinder your overall comprehension, especially your understanding of the main ideas. Getting "the big picture" is harder when you are stalled on every little detail along the way. Furthermore, slow readers are more likely to let their minds wander from the text. You can pick up courses and books that teach so-called speed reading, but you can also practice a few simple techniques on your own to make reading a quick and enjoyable process.

First, *avoid regression,* which is having to go back and reread a sentence—or a whole paragraph or more—because, even though our eyes have been traveling over the words on the page, our minds have been elsewhere. When you let your mind wander as you read, you not only cut your speed dramatically because you have to read some passages twice, but also because it is harder to connect ideas, to see the "big picture."

Regression can be a difficult habit to break, but there are several ways to combat it. First of all, learn to read with a purpose. If you are just enjoying a story and you want to review a deep idea or reread a beautiful sentence, that is fine; do not worry about regressing. But if you are reading something for comprehension, or if you want to get the main idea of a piece in a hurry, then tell yourself before you start that you are not going to look back and that you're going to get all the main ideas the first time. As a mechanical aid, take a postcard or a piece of paper and hold it above the line you are reading, dragging it down the page line by line as you read so that it covers the text you have just read. As you employ such a no regression policy, practicing at first for short durations and gradually extending your commitment, your reading will become increasingly efficient.

A second technique to increase your reading speed is quite simple and obvious: *practice pushing yourself.* You will be surprised at how just trying to read faster— telling yourself that you are going to concentrate and increase your speed for a short

SECTION A

SECTION B

SECTION C

COMPREHENSIVE PRACTICE Test 1

COMPREHENSIVE PRACTICE Test 2

COMPREHENSIVE PRACTICE Test 3

while—can increase your reading speed. And unless you choose a Shakespearean play, a tax instruction manual, or some other dense reading, you will be surprised to find that you understand the reading just as well as if you read at your normal speed.

Sometimes people read more slowly because they fear not catching every idea. Speed reading courses try to break through this anxiety by requiring only about 80% comprehension in their questions about reading passages. But if you know that you are more likely to grasp the main ideas if you push yourself and if you eliminate regression, you can increase your reading speed considerably and still achieve very high comprehension levels.

Finally, *avoid vocalization* (also known as lip reading), that is, moving your lips or pronouncing the words to yourself even though you are not supposed to be reading aloud. Your eyes can dart across a line of print much more quickly than you can say the words. Make sure that you are just taking ideas into your mind, not using your throat muscles even if your lips are still, not even hearing the words spoken in your head.

Find the Main Ideas Efficiently

Whether you are reading a passage on a test or a newspaper article, one of your primary goals is always to determine the main idea of the writing. In newspapers, main ideas are usually easy to spot because editors distill them into headlines, and reporters include their key points in the first few lines of their articles. But in most of your reading, it is up to you to cull out crucial ideas and controlling themes. Here are a few techniques that good readers use to find main ideas.

1. Scan before Reading   If you decide to drive to a new vacation spot, you do not get right into your car and begin driving. First, you consult a map. And when you look at the map, you do not start tracing your route until you have located your destination and have an overall idea of the kinds of roads you are going to take and the areas you will be passing through.

Readers who fail to get an overall view of the reading journey that they are about to embark on face the same problems as travelers who start without consulting a map. Not knowing where they are going, they are probably going to encounter unwanted surprises, get lost, and have to retrace their steps, that is, reread whole sections to find out where they are and why. So, to make your reading journey fast and efficient, you need to do preliminary "map reading" by using a technique that is called scanning. Scanning is really no more than looking over your reading material quickly before setting out to read it.

For a short article or test questions, first glance through the whole piece to see how it has been divided into paragraphs. Then very quickly read the first sentence of the piece, one or two of the sentences that begin paragraphs in the middle, and the last sentence of the work. Get a feel for the author's style and tone, and develop some expectations. Does the author intend to amuse you with a personal anecdote, instruct you about a new scientific discovery, convince you about the importance of a historical event? Now when you read the material, you already have an idea of where you are going and of the way the author is going to take you there.

2. Be Aware of Topic Sentences   *Most writers, in addition to stating the main idea of their whole book or article at the beginning of the work, start each paragraph with the main idea of that paragraph* (like this sentence, which is set in italic type). When you had to write essays in school, your teachers probably asked you to state the essay's thesis (or maybe

Ways to Develop Your Reading Skills 21

SECTION A
SECTION B
SECTION C
COMPREHENSIVE PRACTICE Test 1
COMPREHENSIVE PRACTICE Test 2
COMPREHENSIVE PRACTICE Test 3

they called it the theme or the purpose statement) in the first paragraph. However they expressed it, they were asking you to put the main idea of your writing into the opening paragraph, more often than not as the very first line.

Sentences that state the main ideas of paragraphs are called topic sentences, *and they often appear at the beginning of the paragraph.* Sometimes, though, writers organize their paragraphs by building up to the main idea with a series of details or examples. In that case, the topic sentence comes at the end of the paragraph. Or, as in this paragraph, in addition to a topic sentence at the opening, there may be a so-called clincher sentence at the end that provides a summary of the main idea. *As a reader, then, you should pay special attention to the beginnings and endings of paragraphs.*

Be advised, however, that not every paragraph contains a topic sentence, and not every article or book has a thesis statement. The author may have seen no need to state the main idea blatantly if it is already apparent in the details of the discussion. *Nevertheless, you will find the main ideas much faster if you look for and pay attention to topic sentences.*

As you have probably gathered, the topic sentences in this section have been set in italic type to illustrate not only the idea of topic sentences, but also the fact that they usually—but not always—appear at the beginning of a paragraph or a discussion. Notice that the second and third paragraphs stated new topics and then summarized the main ideas with clincher sentences. And the clincher sentence at the end of the preceding paragraph contained the main idea of the entire discussion: Be on the lookout for topic sentences because they help you find the main ideas more efficiently.

3. Separate Main Ideas from Supporting Material   Before you begin a reading comprehension test, you already know one of the questions that you are going to be asked: What is the main idea of this passage? It may not be phrased exactly that way. Perhaps you will be asked for the best title for the passage, or maybe the question will start with something like, "It is the author's belief that . . . ." Whatever the phrasing, because every author's purpose is to impart particular ideas, reading tests are always going to check to see whether you grasped them.

As the section on topic sentences explained, the main idea of an essay, an article, or even a book is very often found at the beginning of the piece. Sometimes, however, writers open with a provocative fact or incident and then, once they have caught your interest, move from the specific to the general, letting the main idea grow out of the example. It is important, therefore, to have an idea of the type of material you are reading. Does the supporting material illustrate or prove a main idea, or is the supporting material itself the main idea?

If reading can be likened to a journey, then the main idea should be seen as your destination. The supporting ideas, explanations, and examples are the roads that you must take to get there. As you read, then, you should keep track of what kind of road you are on—a main highway with signs providing key ideas and crucial facts, or a byway that offers interesting scenery but is not really essential to reaching your destination. You might want to practice this by choosing newspaper articles or textbook passages and finding the one most important idea in each paragraph.

4. Be Aware of Tone

"You look great today!" Marcia said _____.

How did Marcia say that? Spurred on by the exclamation point, you probably filled in the blank in your mind, not even knowing that you did so, by supplying the word "enthusiastically" or "admiringly." But Marcia may have used a very different tone.

What if the word should actually be "sarcastically"? In that case, Marcia meant just the opposite of what her words said. Without the blank filled in, we can't really know what Marcia meant. That missing word defines her *tone*.

Fiction writers can indicate a speaker's tone just by telling us—sarcastically, morosely, earnestly, sadly. But all writing has a tone, even if the writer, as is usually the case, never identifies it for us. We cannot communicate without, in some subtle way, indicating our underlying attitude—either about what we are saying or about the person who is hearing or reading what we are saying. In writing, tone is the author's attitude that you "hear" when you read. Is she being ironic? Is he being sentimental? Is the material objectively stated, passionately argued, cautiously optimistic, or quite nostalgic? To understand a person fully, we must hear not just what she says, but how she says it.

5. Be Objective   *Y*ou probably can remember occasions when parents or friends have not understood you because they were hearing what they thought you were saying rather than what you were really saying. They may already have decided what you were going to say before you ever opened your mouth and then did not really listen to you. Readers can be just as deaf to an author's ideas if they let their prior expectations influence their reading experience.

Such subjective misunderstandings are also caused by entrenched attitudes about a topic. In our desire to have our own ideas or values confirmed, we distort what a writer is actually saying. We do not have to agree with everything we read, but we should try to understand clearly and fairly the ideas on the printed page. Although we probably cannot eliminate subjectivity completely, we should make it a goal to approach texts with an open mind and a desire to be objective.

WAYS TO BECOME A BETTER TEST TAKER

There are two types of questions on these tests: ones that test your *word knowledge* and ones that test your *reading comprehension*. In this section are explanations of these types of questions and of techniques to help you answer them correctly.

THE WORD KNOWLEDGE TEST

Sample Questions

Vocabulary tests are not all alike. Some ask you to find synonyms, some ask you to choose antonyms, and some ask you to complete sentences in which words have been omitted, testing both reading comprehension and vocabulary at the same time. Another approach, which is used by the NLN tests, asks you to determine the meaning of words used in sentences, allowing you to see them in context.

Here are three sample questions of the type you will find on the NLN tests:

1. The athlete was famished after a long workout.
   Famished means
   a. exhausted.
   b. strained.
   c. hungry.
   d. well known.

The Word Knowledge Test   23

SECTION A

SECTION B

SECTION C

COMPREHENSIVE PRACTICE   Test 1

COMPREHENSIVE PRACTICE   Test 2

COMPREHENSIVE PRACTICE   Test 3

2. Dr. Stone showed great animosity toward his colleagues. He treated them with
   a. gratitude.
   b. respect.
   c. discernment.
   d. hatred.

3. To say that William Shakespeare typed his plays is an
   a. affinity.
   b. antithesis.
   c. anachronism.
   d. atrophy.

Before you check your answers (which follow), look again at the questions themselves. Notice that:

- The three questions are essentially alike because they all provide full sentences to give you a definition or a context.

- In the second sample, the word in question—"animosity"—has not been underlined or singled out in any way for you.

- The third question does not even provide a synonym, but asks you to complete the thought with the appropriate word.

Analysis of the Answers

Question 1: *The answer is c.* You might—unwisely—try to take a shortcut by looking only at the last part of the question: "**Famished** means ... ." As long as you know the meaning of "famished," you probably will get the answer right. When questions of this type get difficult, however, you are much more likely to choose an incorrect answer if you do not give yourself the benefit of seeing the word used correctly in a sentence. Also, you should read all the answer choices. If you jump at the first answer that sounds "about right," you may miss the right one that sounds even better or that makes you realize that you were confusing the word with another, similar word. Not reading the opening sentence and all the answers in this type of question may save a second or two, but those saved seconds are totally negated if you answer the question incorrectly.

Notice that all of the answer choices could fit into the context of the sentence. You are not, for example, given an answer choice, such as "cold," that would be easy to eliminate as wrong. But even if the sentence does not give away the answer, it can still help you make the correct choice by stimulating your memory about the kind of situation where you might have heard the word used. Even if you do not know that "famished" means hungry, you might get a feeling that it is a negative word, ruling out answer d, "well known."

The feeling of a word—whether it has a positive or a negative aura—is its *connotation*; its regular dictionary definition is its *denotation*. For example, the synonyms "fat" and "chubby" both mean overweight, but "chubby" has a more positive connotation. Often when we are not sure of a word's denotation, we know, from having heard the word before, that it has a positive or negative connotation. On word knowledge questions you should "check your feelings" even when you are not sure of a word's literal meaning, because your feelings can often lead you to the right answer.

Question 2: *The answer is d.* In this question, you cannot know which word you are to define without reading the first sentence. It is "animosity," but it might also have been "colleagues." In this type of question, you must first be sure to ascertain which word or idea you are being asked to define.

This question illustrates one of the pitfalls to avoid when you see the word in context. Like most people, you probably have positive feelings about doctors, and thus you are likely to expect Dr. Stone to be a fine fellow. If you do not know the meaning of "animosity" and take a guess, you are likely to choose a positive word like "respect." On the other hand, if you do not know the exact meaning of "animosity" but know that it is a negative word, you would guess right because the other three choices all have positive connotations.

Question 3: *The answer is c.* This third type of question provides no synonym. The question itself supplies a definition or, in this case, a situation that can be defined by one of the right words in the answers.

In this question, you can get some help if you know word roots. "Anachronism" has at its heart the root, "-chron-," which means time. The prefix *ana* means backward, and the suffix *ism* means something that is. If we put it all together, we get a word that indicates a situation where something is out of its proper place in time, the meaning of the word.

THE READING COMPREHENSION TEST AND ANALYSIS OF THE ANSWERS

Like all reading tests, this test asks you to read several short passages and determine the main ideas, pick out important details, draw conclusions, identify vocabulary, and infer ideas that are implied but not specifically stated. Since there are only six questions about each passage, you do not have to do all these things for every passage, but you can be sure that you will be asked each time for the main idea and key details.

The following sample reading comprehension passage is accompanied by an analysis of the questions and the answers.

Sample Reading Comprehension Test

Titles frequently fall into three different categories. It's your decision as the writer to choose the one that suits your purpose.

Summary titles are those that provide the most general information. By giving facts without details, they lure the reader into the paper if she or he would like to know more. Newspaper headlines are frequently good examples of these kinds of titles: "Hurricane Hits Florida Coast," "Sunset Concert Series Starts Saturday," and "Star Wars Breaks Box Office Records."

Preview or Give-a-Glimpse titles aim to create reader curiosity. They introduce the subject by attempting to grab a reader's attention with a question or thought-provoking statement like "If Shakespeare Were Alive Today," "Why Won't Disco Disappear?" or "Where Will You Be in 2001?"

Teasing or Whimsical titles leave your reader guessing about what's to come. They usually refer to the subject indirectly and make readers curious enough to read on. These titles can be fun for both the writer and the reader, although you might want to include a subtitle under the teaser to avoid any confusion. How about something like "Good Morning, Sunshine" (subtitled "Solar Energy in Our Town") or "Boiling Water and Opening Cans" (subtitled "My Turn to Cook").

A striking title, whatever the type, can only work in your favor. Just be certain that it is not misleading. A good title should honestly lure the reader into the rest of the paper and not promise more than it will actually deliver. (Several newspapers and magazines are noted for sensational-type headlines. This practice of selling a product by exaggerating what's in the copy only serves to anger and alienate readers and is not a recommended example to follow.) Here are some things to keep in mind when you're trying to think of a good title:

1. Consider the material. The title should be related to the central idea or thesis of your paper.

2. Consider the audience. Will your readers understand a serious, technical title? Will they appreciate a humorous or clever title?

3. Consider the words carefully, thinking of how they sound as well as what they mean.

(Copyright © 1980 by Diane Rubins. Reprinted by permission of Scholastic Books Service, a division of Scholastic, Inc.)

Question 1

1. The best title for this selection is
   a. "Three Categories of Writing."
   b. "Choosing a Good Title."
   c. "Leading and Misleading Titles."
   d. "Gaining the Reader's Attention."

This question asks you to formulate the main idea of the passage, and asking for a good title for the piece is a frequent way to pose this question. Here are several other ways in which main idea questions are worded:

- What is the main topic of the passage?

- The author's primary focus is . . . .

- What is the main idea of the selection?

The key to answering main idea questions correctly is finding the choice that is neither too broad nor too specific. Answer d is too broad because the article focuses on only one aspect of gaining the reader's attention: choosing a good title. Answer c is too narrow because, although this idea is mentioned in the fifth paragraph, it is not the main idea of the whole article. Answer a does not mention titles and is a distortion of the idea presented in the opening sentence. The correct answer is b.

Question 2

2. The end result of using the three types of titles mentioned in the passage is
   a. arousing the reader's curiosity.
   b. providing general information.
   c. amusing the writer and reader.
   d. selling a product.

This question asks you to generalize information found in the passage and to draw conclusions. Nowhere in the article is it explicitly stated that one purpose of each kind of title is to arouse reader curiosity, but each of the three discussions of title types mentions this idea: "lure the reader into the paper" in the second paragraph, "create reader curiosity" in the third paragraph, and "leave your reader guessing about what is to come" in the fourth paragraph. This suggests that a is the correct choice. On the other hand, answers b and c state the functions of some titles, but neither of them is true for all three kinds of titles mentioned in the passage. Be sure that your answer fits all of the requirements of the question. Selling a product (answer d) is not mentioned in the passage at all. The correct answer is a.

Question 3

3. For an article on the frustrations of losing weight, the title "Don't Be a Sore Loser" would be considered a
   a. sensational-type title.
   b. give-a-glimpse title.
   c. summary title.
   d. teasing title.

Sometimes questions ask you to take what is stated in a passage and apply it to a new situation. In this question, you have to see that the pun in "Don't Be a Sore Loser" puts it into the category of teasing or whimsical titles, like the examples at the end of the fourth paragraph—such as "Good Morning Sunshine" for an article on solar energy.

When you are asked about situations similar to, but not exactly the same as, what is in a passage, you need to make sure that they fit the main idea of the piece and that they are similar to the details or examples in the passage. The correct answer is d.

Question 4

4. Subtitles are recommended in order to
   a. provide additional details.
   b. amuse the reader.
   c. provoke thought.
   d. avoid confusion.

This question requires you to pick out a correct supporting idea based on the statements and details of the passage. The fourth paragraph contains text that points to the right answer: "you might want to include a subtitle under the teaser to avoid any confusion."

Be careful about answer choices that state ideas mentioned in the passage but that are not relevant to the question. Answer b—amuse the reader—states a purpose of teasing titles but not of the subtitles added to the teasers. Answer a—provide additional details—illustrates another possible pitfall. It completes a statement that is surely true for many subtitles but that, even if correct, is not the one that this author states. Be sure that you base your answers on what the passage states, not on ideas that you think are right or that you have learned from other sources. The correct answer is d.

Question 5

5. The author warns against titles that promise more than they deliver because they
   a. are dishonest.
   b. may make a reader angry.
   c. grab a reader's attention.
   d. lead to reader disappointment.

SECTION A

SECTION B

SECTION C

COMPREHENSIVE PRACTICE Test 1

COMPREHENSIVE PRACTICE Test 2

COMPREHENSIVE PRACTICE Test 3

This type of question asks you to be accurate in finding details in the passage. In the fifth paragraph, the author states: "This practice of . . . exaggerating what's in the copy only serves to anger and alienate the reader." This suggests that b is the correct answer.

Be careful about answer choices that are close to what is mentioned in the passage but not precisely the same. Although the fifth paragraph says that titles "should honestly lure the reader into the rest of the paper," it does not single out dishonesty, as answer a does, as the reason for avoiding exaggeration. Also watch out for examples of ideas that are not actually stated in the passage, as in answer d—lead to reader disappointment. Disappointment might be a result of an exaggerated title, but this reaction is never mentioned in the passage. Answer c—grab a reader's attention—is one of the purposes of any title and far too general to be right. It also does not answer the question, which asks for something the author warns against. He would not warn against grabbing the reader's attention. The correct answer is b.

Question 6

6. The writer's intended audience was probably
    a. newspaper reporters.
    b. business executives.
    c. student writers.
    d. magazine editors.

This question asks you to be an observant, thorough reader and to infer ideas from the passage as a whole. The author addresses writers in the opening paragraph: "It's your decision as the writer" suggests that her intended audience is probably not business executives or magazine editors, ruling out answers b and d. The tone and style of the writing also sound as if they are meant for students, not for professional reporters, making answer c more likely than answer a. Finally, when you read passages on comprehension tests, do not overlook any material that tells you about the source of the article or its publication history. Often, these explanations can give you clues about the author's tone and purpose. In this case, the citation at the end of the article reads in part, "Reprinted by permission of Scholastic Books Service, a division of Scholastic, Inc.," and Scholastic publishes mainly to students and teachers. The correct answer is c.

A FINAL WORD

When you take reading comprehension tests—or any test, for that matter—it is crucial to maintain your focus and, especially, to avoid panic attacks that muddle your thinking and slow you to a standstill. Being nervous before a test does not hurt as long as you convert that nervous energy into positive energy and focus once the test is underway.

The best way to avoid the kind of nervousness that destroys concentration is to practice taking the tests. If you feel positive about your skills and know what you are going to find on the day of the real test, you are much more likely to do well. Build up your confidence by doing lots of practice questions, at first without timing yourself. Work out the answers carefully. Later, if you wish, you can make your practice sessions more like the real thing by timing yourself.

On test day, if you find questions very difficult, do not let them rattle you. Skip over them—making sure that you keep track of where you are on your answer sheet. Then come back to them after you feel that you have answered several questions correctly and are working efficiently with reestablished focus.

The best test takers are usually people who have fun taking tests. You may not be one of those lucky individuals, but with preparation, practice, and reasonable goals you can at least take tests with confidence, knowing that your score will truly reflect your ability.

SECTION A

SECTION B

SECTION C

COMPREHENSIVE PRACTICE Test 1

COMPREHENSIVE PRACTICE Test 2

COMPREHENSIVE PRACTICE Test 3

I. Verbal Ability

Word Knowledge and Reading Comprehension

45 minutes per test

DIRECTIONS

This section contains three tests, each with two sections: Word Knowledge and Reading Comprehension. You should be able to answer all the questions in 45 minutes per test. Since it is important to answer all the questions in the allotted time, it is a good idea to use a timer.

Each test question consists of an incomplete sentence or question, followed by four choices. Read each question carefully; then decide which choice is the best answer. After you have completed the test, check your answers against those at the back of this section.

Your score will be the total number of correct answers. Answer a question even if you are not completely sure of the correct answer. Do not spend too much time on any one question. If you cannot answer a question, go on to the next one.

If you finish the Verbal Ability test before the 45 minutes are up, go back and check your work.

WORD KNOWLEDGE: Read each sentence carefully. Then, *on the basis of what is stated in the sentence*, select the answer that best completes the statement. (The correct answers are at the end of Section A.)

1. When Vincent wanted to finish the race, I dissuaded him.
   Dissuaded means
   a. deserted.
   b. discouraged.
   c. disqualified.
   d. prevented.

2. The dispute was settled by a judicial decision.
   Judicial means
   a. majority.
   b. court-related.
   c. reached by arbitration.
   d. wise.

3. The rubber band was stretched to a great length and thinness. It was
   a. elided.
   b. concerted.
   c. elongated.
   d. prolonged.

4. Harry constantly gets sinus infections. With respect to these infections, he is
   a. habituated.
   b. resistant.
   c. susceptible.
   d. reactive.

5. She read the apartment lease carefully to see what it stipulated.
   Stipulated means
   a. specified.
   b. advised.
   c. proposed.
   d. meant.

6. An agrarian community is one that is based on
   a. mining.
   b. religion.
   c. farming.
   d. politics.

7. Directors and actors sometimes quibble about the shade of a spotlight gel. Their argument is
   a. abrasive.
   b. halfhearted.
   c. playful.
   d. petty.

8. The unstable food supply caused the tribes in the region to become nomads.
   Nomads are
   a. wanderers.
   b. farmers.
   c. mystics.
   d. cannibals.

9. Her paper was about an important epoch in history.
   An **epoch** is a
   a. saga.
   b. period in time.
   c. turning point.
   d. renaissance.

10. She always wore a great deal of tawdry jewelry.
    Tawdry means
    a. antique.
    b. gaudy.
    c. ugly.
    d. expensive.

11. The window shade blocked most of the sun's rays. The shade was
    a. alabaster.
    b. motley.
    c. prismatic.
    d. opaque.

12. The secret agent was spying for both sides. The agent was acting with
    a. duplicity.
    b. travesty.
    c. circumspection.
    d. discrimination.

13. A person who is uncouth is
    a. uncomfortable.
    b. unpolished.
    c. uninquisitive.
    d. undappled.

14. The fortune-teller's remarks seemed to have hidden meaning. The remarks were
    a. grotesque.
    b. fulsome.
    c. morbid.
    d. cryptic.

15. The plant had variegated leaves.
    Variegated means
    a. uneven in length.
    b. differing in color.
    c. synthetic.
    d. elastic.

16. At one time, people were not protected by law from being used as chattel.
    Chattel means
    a. scientific subject.
    b. child laborer.
    c. piece of property.
    d. prostitute.

17. The donkey is known to have an adamant nature.
    Adamant means
    a. stupid.
    b. obstinate.
    c. friendly.
    d. patient.

18. The girl looked wistfully at the beautiful things in the store.
    Wistfully means
    a. longingly.
    b. enviously.
    c. hopefully.
    d. slowly.

SECTION A
SECTION B
SECTION C
COMPREHENSIVE PRACTICE Test 1
COMPREHENSIVE PRACTICE Test 2
COMPREHENSIVE PRACTICE Test 3

19. Jim tried to wrest the ball from Alex.
    Wrest means
    a. conceal.
    b. retrieve.
    c. steal.
    d. snatch.

20. She has an extreme dislike of strangers. She is a
    a. xenophobe.
    b. dilettante.
    c. paragon.
    d. peccadillo.

21. The glue was said to adhere to any surface.
    Adhere means to
    a. cooperate.
    b. diffuse.
    c. orient.
    d. stick.

22. The patient became increasingly listless.
    Listless means
    a. sluggish.
    b. anxious.
    c. helpless.
    d. hopeless.

23. When the prisoners begged for mercy, the king was inexorable.
    Inexorable means
    a. relentless.
    b. indifferent.
    c. compassionate.
    d. discomforted.

24. The judge told the witness to reiterate his statement. The witness was expected to
    a. explain it.
    b. withhold it.
    c. reconsider it.
    d. repeat it.

25. There has been a dearth of information about certain prehistoric periods.
    Dearth means
    a. growth.
    b. loss.
    c. scarcity.
    d. absence.

26. Julia's clothes were always the epitome of fashion. Her clothes were
    a. a poor imitation.
    b. the most chic.
    c. the most expensive.
    d. the cheapest.

27. The community's cleanup efforts were laudable. Their efforts were
   a. disorganized.
   b. successful.
   c. praiseworthy.
   d. useless.

28. The evidence given at the trial was relevant to the case. The evidence was
   a. new.
   b. applicable.
   c. helpful.
   d. vital.

29. During the inquiry the witness gave a candid account. The account was
   a. matter-of-fact.
   b. colorful.
   c. helpful.
   d. frank.

30. When the house was sold, its fixtures, curtains, carpeting, and appliances were included in the sale. The house was sold with
   a. appurtenances.
   b. encumbrances.
   c. endowments.
   d. attenuations.

READING COMPREHENSION: There are five reading passages in this section. Read each passage carefully. Then, *on the basis of what you have read in the passage*, select the best answer for each of the questions following the passage.

I

Whatever happened to the fine old art of political insult? Maybe it's because they've been squeezed through too many TV tubes, but don't modern politicians seem a bit bland?

With no polls, PR wizards or slick video ads to rely on, candidates used to go into combat armed with razor wits and luxuriant vocabularies. Maledictions sizzled through the air like rockets. And a sharpened slur could be lethal.

For instance: the eloquent John Randolph, of Virginia, was not fond of his fellow Congressman, Henry Clay, of Kentucky. One day, brimming with bile, Randolph shot off this description of Clay: "This being, so brilliant yet so corrupt, which, like a rotten mackerel by moonlight, shines and stunk."

Slapped with a sentence like that, a man might forever smell faintly of fish. That sort of invective led one foreign observer of our political style to note that Americans were the only people he knew to pass from barbarism to decadence without experiencing civilization.

Disgusted with a campaigner who was trampling all over the facts, a reporter told fellow newsman Heywood Broun, "He's murdering the truth!" "Don't worry," Broun replied. "He'll never get close enough to do it any harm." New York attorney Roscoe Conkling, asked to campaign for Presidential candidate James G. Blaine, replied, "I do not engage in criminal practice."

SECTION A

SECTION B

SECTION C

COMPREHENSIVE PRACTICE Test 1

COMPREHENSIVE PRACTICE Test 2

COMPREHENSIVE PRACTICE Test 3

It was Theodore Roosevelt who inspired one of the neatest political barbs. Teddy had just left on a much-publicized lion-hunting safari in Africa when the following notice appeared on a wall at the New York Stock Exchange: "Wall Street expects every lion to do his duty."

Politicians weren't the only ones with sharp tongues. Hecklers, too, knew the potency of a booby-trapped sentence, as William Jennings Bryan discovered. During a political speech he unleashed his famous oratorical ability, crying, "I wish I had the wings of a bird to fly to every village and hamlet in America to tell the people about this silver question." Cried a voice from the audience, "You'd be shot for a goose before you've flown a mile."

(Reprinted with permission of the author, Richard Wolkomir © 1980. Originally appeared in the June 1980 *Smithsonian Magazine*.)

31. The best title for this selection is
    a. "Political Campaigns of Yesteryear"
    b. "The Fine Art of Political Insult"
    c. "From Barbarism to Decadence"
    d. "Murdering the Truth"

32. The passage contrasts
    a. political styles of yesterday and today.
    b. candidates and reporters.
    c. barbarism and decadence.
    d. politicians and hecklers.

33. It can be inferred from the passage that "brimming with bile" refers to John Randolph's
    a. brilliance.
    b. eloquence.
    c. anger.
    d. impatience.

34. The person correctly paired with his position is
    a. Theodore Roosevelt—financier.
    b. John Randolph—congressman.
    c. Roscoe Conkling—presidential candidate.
    d. William Jennings Bryan—newsman.

35. Henry Clay was described as resembling
    a. bile.
    b. moonlight.
    c. a goose.
    d. a fish.

36. A person well-known as a public speaker was
    a. Roscoe Conkling.
    b. Heywood Broun.
    c. William Jennings Bryan.
    d. Theodore Roosevelt.

Word Knowledge and Reading Comprehension   35

SECTION A
SECTION B
SECTION C
COMPREHENSIVE PRACTICE Test 1
COMPREHENSIVE PRACTICE Test 2
COMPREHENSIVE PRACTICE Test 3

II

Geologists use it to search for hidden minerals. Forest rangers use it to look for the spread of tree diseases. Farm experts use it to study crop growth. And biologists use it to check for lake pollution.

What is it that all these people use for such different purposes?

A satellite! A satellite called Landsat, developed by the United States government to help scientists study the world's natural resources.

Since 1972, a total of five Landsat satellites have been put into orbit. While only two are still working, altogether the five have taken millions of pictures of our planet.

Landsat zips around the globe in an orbit 425 miles in space. The satellite passes over each spot on the earth every sixteen days.

On board each satellite are instruments that look at earth. These instruments "see" the different colors of forests, rocks, waters, crops, and other objects, just as you do.

But the satellite can also see certain "colors" of light (infrared light, for instance) that a person cannot see. By looking at all of these colors, Landsat can tell scientists a lot about the earth. For example, healthy plants are a different color than diseased plants. Clear lakes differ from polluted ones. And so on.

The information that Landsat gathers is beamed to earth and stored on computer tapes for later use by scientists.

Of course, there can be a few problems with using Landsat. Sometimes clouds are in the way and the satellite cannot see the earth. Sometimes Landsat's instruments don't work as they should. And sometimes the colors that Landsat sees just aren't different enough from each other to tell scientists very much.

However, Landsat does gather certain information that scientists cannot get in other ways. And Landsat gives scientists their first look at many hard-to-get-to parts of the planet.

Landsat is an eye in the sky that gives us a helping hand.

(From "Satellites, Scientists, and Secrets of the Earth," by Robert Meredith. Copyright © *Highlights for Children*, July–August 1986.)

37. Which of these titles would be best for this passage?
    a. "Spying on the Earth"
    b. "An Eye on High"
    c. "The Story of the Earth"
    d. "Rockets in Outer Space"

38. We can infer that when the Landsat satellites stop working, they
    a. crash to earth.
    b. are brought back to earth.
    c. are destroyed in space.
    d. remain in orbit.

39. The pictures sent to earth by Landsat are taken by
    a. special instruments.
    b. an astronaut.
    c. trained primates.
    d. trained rats.

40. Information received from Landsat could help farmers to
    a. avert land erosion.
    b. regulate planting time.
    c. locate areas of plant disease.
    d. forecast drought.

41. The term "Landsat" probably means
    a. land surveillance.
    b. land satellite.
    c. land saturation.
    d. land security.

42. According to this article, the use of the Landsat satellite is still problematic because of
    a. radio interference.
    b. its distance from earth.
    c. air pollution.
    d. faulty instruments.

III

Where does all the material come from to build the various structures in space? Earth's resources are being stretched thin for the needs of Earth's own population. And even if enough can be found for delivery to space, the act of delivery would be very expensive.

Fortunately, there is an enormous piece of real estate that we can reach, real estate that we already have reached with old-fashioned, nonreusable spaceships. It is the moon.

Once we have space stations in orbit, it will be only a matter of time before we return to the moon. This time, it will not be for temporary visits, but to stay—at least in relays. Once we have a permanent lunar presence, we will be able to study the moon in detail and use it as a stable, airless base on which to establish a huge astronomical observatory.

More than that, we can establish a mining station there. Detailed studies have been made concerning the gathering of ore from the lunar surface. It could be hurled into space electromagnetically (not difficult, since the moon's escape velocity is not much more than one-fifth that of the Earth's), and there, in space, it could be smelted with the use of solar energy.

Lunar material can serve as a source of structural metals, cement, concrete, glass, and even oxygen. With the sun supplying energy and the moon supplying material, it will be possible for human beings to build space structures without calling upon Earth itself for excessive supplies of energy or matter. One might argue that Earth would have to supply people, but even that is not necessarily so.

Among the structures that will be built in space might be space stations so large that they could hold thousands of people, rather than a dozen; so large that rotation at a

Word Knowledge and Reading Comprehension 37

SECTION A

SECTION B

SECTION C

COMPREHENSIVE PRACTICE Test 1

COMPREHENSIVE PRACTICE Test 2

COMPREHENSIVE PRACTICE Test 3

not-excessive speed would supply a centrifugal effect that would prove an adequate substitute for gravity. This would avoid the deleterious effects of zero gravity. In such stations, human beings might be able to live lifelong, generation after generation.

The space settlements could control the quantity of sunshine they receive and would be free of bad weather. They would keep out deleterious life forms (at least to a greater extent than we can on Earth). Conditions on space settlements might thus prove ideal for farming.

Using the knowledge gained when greenhouses were added to the original space stations, the settlements could make use of adequate cycling procedures and minimal supplies of fertilizer from Earth to produce plants and even small animals in supplies far greater than they themselves would need.

(Reprinted from *Popular Mechanics*, July 1986. Copyright © The Hearst Corporation. All rights reserved.)

43. The reader can infer that the spaceships that have been used so far to fly to the moon were
    a. disposable.
    b. sturdy.
    c. failures.
    d. roomy.

44. According to the article, the energy needed to build structures in space would come from
    a. electromagnetism.
    b. smelted lunar ore.
    c. the sun.
    d. Earth.

45. The article suggests that the people needed to build space structures would come from
    a. lunar mining stations.
    b. farming communities on Earth.
    c. the Earth's homeless population.
    d. space-born descendants of space settlers.

46. According to the article, the effect of the centrifugal force resulting from the rotation of a space structure would substitute for
    a. solar energy.
    b. fresh air.
    c. changing weather.
    d. Earth's gravity.

47. The article implies that space settlements could raise enough crops and animals to
    a. produce a surplus for export.
    b. supplement shipments from Earth.
    c. provide a basis for farming experiments.
    d. feed the hungry on Earth.

48. Future space settlers may be better suited than Earth dwellers for taking long flights into space because the settlers will probably
    a. have a longer lifespan.
    b. undergo mutations that allow them to adapt to space.
    c. be accustomed to conditions in space.
    d. mature and reproduce more rapidly.

IV

The term "addiction" was once reserved for dependence on drugs. Today it is applied to a range of compulsive behaviors as disparate as working too hard and eating too much chocolate. The fact is that there are essential biological, psychological, and social common denominators between drug use and other habitual behaviors. Whether your pleasure is meditation or mescaline, cocaine or cults, you are addicted if you cannot control when you start or stop the activity.

Although it is commonly accepted that loss of control is a primary feature in all addictive disturbances, there is no generally accepted definition of addiction. We define it as self-induced changes in neurotransmission (a type of brain activity) that result in problem behaviors. This definition encompasses a multidisciplinary understanding of compulsive problem behaviors that involves personal responsibility (they are self-induced), biochemical effects (changes in neurotransmission), and social reactions.

Neurotransmission is the mechanism by which signals or impulses are sent from one nerve cell to another. The more rapid the transmission in certain pathways of the brain, the more intense the feeling. Individuals repeat a behavior (activity or substance intake) to bring about neurotransmission consistent with how they want to feel. The desired feeling differs among addicted individuals and determines the activity or substance they choose to abuse.

How rapidly neurons fire is determined by the concentration of molecules known as neurotransmitters present in the synapse (junction) between neurons: The more neurotransmitters in the junction, the faster the rate of firing. Ordinarily, neurotransmitters are pumped back into the pre-synaptic neuron and stored there.

Certain drugs, however, block this pump and keep the neurotransmitter molecules in the synapse, where their presence brings about more rapid neurotransmission. This creates the elevated mood sought by cocaine users, for example.

Why do people become addicts? Most researchers in the field—even those who disagree about other matters of causation and treatment—agree that low self-regard is a crucial factor in addiction. Manifest or masked, it is basic to most dysfunctional lifestyles.

One way of coping with feelings of worthlessness is to immerse oneself in mood-altering behavior. Depression, for example, can be lessened through exciting activities. Skydivers are unlikely to experience sadness during the "rush" of being airborne. Such potent emotional shifts are related to chemical alterations in the brain, which the individual learns to recreate, through either commodities (drugs or food) or activity. Workaholics, for example, find temporary relief from loneliness or low self-regard in their jobs; overeaters find it in chocolate éclairs.

Although these activities provide a brief reprieve from conflict, overindulgence can lead to progressive physical, social, or economic deterioration. Harvard psychologist Howard

Shaffer calls addiction "a two-edged sword; it serves as it destroys." Whether the gratifying behavior is work, gambling, or chanting, some people lose control and continue despite the consequences. Compulsive runners, for example, may continue jogging despite damage to their knees, ankles, and other parts of their skeletal systems.

(Reprinted with permission from *Psychology Today Magazine*, Copyright © 1983 Sussex Publishers, Inc.)

49. According to this passage, cocaine has the effect of
    a. depressing the nervous system.
    b. producing feelings of guilt and anger.
    c. causing repetitive speech and behaviors.
    d. increasing the rate of brain activity.

50. According to this passage, the most important factor in an individual's potential for addiction seems to be
    a. self-esteem.
    b. age.
    c. the size of the neurons in the brain.
    d. childhood experiences.

51. Considering the nature of the addictive activities mentioned in this passage, we might draw the conclusion that
    a. all addictive activities are socially unacceptable.
    b. most addictive activities ultimately result in the addict's death.
    c. some addictive activities can bring the addict lasting inner peace.
    d. even initially healthy pursuits can become addictive activities.

52. From this passage, we can infer that drug addicts
    a. have brains that function more rapidly than average.
    b. have much in common with persons who have other addictions.
    c. can give up their addiction by exercising self-control.
    d. are compulsive overeaters.

53. One activity the author does not mention as producing addictively "desirable" chemical activity in the brain is
    a. overeating.
    b. jogging.
    c. smoking.
    d. skydiving.

54. Neurotransmitters are composed of
    a. synapses.
    b. neurons.
    c. drugs.
    d. molecules.

V

Ask an architect to define a skyscraper, and he will say it's any building with a height/width ratio greater than 7 to 1. But ask a structural engineer, and he'll tell you a skyscraper is any

SECTION A

SECTION B

SECTION C

COMPREHENSIVE PRACTICE Test 1

COMPREHENSIVE PRACTICE Test 2

COMPREHENSIVE PRACTICE Test 3

building whose major load is due to the wind. Architects work at drawing boards on dreams. But engineers have to deal with the real world, and their definition is perhaps more useful.

The forces exerted even by a gentle breeze, acting on a lever that can be thousands of feet long, do apply tremendous loads to a skyscraper. In a hurricane, the stress factor is truly awe-inspiring.

In the design of a tall building, breaking is out of the question, but bending is permissible. The upper floors of skyscrapers can sway several feet in a high wind.

To find out how different building structures are made to deal with the physical problems, you have to go under the structure's skin. All tall buildings have one thing in common: They can be considered as a beam cantilevered upward from its foundation. The greatest strength and stiffness are achieved by placing all of the support in the building's perimeter. And the lowest cost is reached by using all the supporting structure to resist bending and carrying weight.

The classic design is a frame-curtain-wall construction. New York's Empire State Building is the greatest example. Its heavy stone walls provide most of the building's stiffness. But the Empire State Building was built more heavily and more expensively than more recent competitors and future tall buildings. For a lighter, roomier, and less expensive construction, engineers have followed by building with structural supports as outboard as possible for maximum rigidity. Load-bearing walls are placed against a framed tube in this construction.

The Sears Tower in Chicago—still the world's tallest building—uses a bundled-tube construction technique, which allows lighter-weight walls and more window space. In the future, the tallest building will use a trussed tube design, which bears even greater load per square foot of lighter construction materials.

A 135-story building that had been planned for New York's Columbus Circle was expected to make use of the trussed tube method, opening a new era of tall buildings.

(Reprinted from *Popular Mechanics,* July 1986. Copyright © The Hearst Corporation. All rights reserved.)

55. Which of these titles would be best for this article?
    a. "Why Skyscrapers Sway in the Wind"
    b. "The Various Structures of Skyscrapers"
    c. "Famous Skyscrapers of the United States"
    d. "Skyscrapers of the Future"

56. According to this article, the most important technical consideration in building a skyscraper is
    a. the 7-to-1 ratio.
    b. the number of windows.
    c. the stress factor.
    d. the elevation of the site.

57. It can be inferred that the factor that made skyscrapers possible was the development of
    a. flexible structures.
    b. steel beams.
    c. unbreakable glass.
    d. reinforced concrete.

58. The article says that structural supports have been placed as outboard as possible for maximum rigidity.
    Rigidity means
    a. stiffness.
    b. strength.
    c. economy.
    d. space.

59. Considering the points discussed in this article, a person who wanted to become an architect or an engineer would be well-advised to study
    a. esthetics.
    b. ecology.
    c. physics.
    d. chemistry.

60. The article implies that in the future, skyscrapers will probably have which of these characteristics?
    a. They will be built of artificial materials.
    b. They will bear a greater load than was possible with past construction techniques.
    c. They will be made with less glass.
    d. They will be less attractive due to their strictly functional designs.

SECTION A

SECTION B

SECTION C

COMPREHENSIVE PRACTICE Test 1

COMPREHENSIVE PRACTICE Test 2

COMPREHENSIVE PRACTICE Test 3

II. Verbal Ability

Word Knowledge and Reading Comprehension

45 minutes per test

WORD KNOWLEDGE: Read each sentence carefully. Then, *on the basis of what is stated in the sentence,* select answer that best completes the statement. (The correct answers are at the end of Section A.)

1. The nurse was able to adapt easily from one kind of assignment to another. The nurse was very
   a. versatile.
   b. harried.
   c. misguided.
   d. complex.

2. The clinic checkbook and the bank statement differ; there is a
   a. misdemeanor.
   b. contortion.
   c. credential.
   d. discrepancy.

3. The athlete was famished after her long workout.
   Famished means
   a. exhausted.
   b. strained.
   c. hungry.
   d. well-known.

4. Fred forgot to check the schedule. He had a momentary
   a. lapse.
   b. jaunt.
   c. legend.
   d. record.

5. The news report from the war-torn country was authentic.
   Authentic means
   a. distorted.
   b. genuine.
   c. thorough.
   d. current.

SECTION A

SECTION B

SECTION C

COMPREHENSIVE PRACTICE Test 1

COMPREHENSIVE PRACTICE Test 2

COMPREHENSIVE PRACTICE Test 3

6. The hospital employee failed to perform the required duties. The employee was
   a. devious.
   b. delinquent.
   c. decisive.
   d. dejected.

7. I needed a horse that was easy to handle. It had to be
   a. docile.
   b. domestic.
   c. demure.
   d. dormant.

8. The small suitcase I carried on board the plane is called a
   a. valet.
   b. livery.
   c. canvas.
   d. valise.

9. The sailor abetted the mutiny, although he was careful not to take part in it.
   Abetted means
   a. avoided.
   b. encouraged.
   c. watched.
   d. initiated.

10. Marta was not born here, but she has become a citizen of this country. She is a
    a. primary candidate.
    b. surplus alien.
    c. naturalized citizen.
    d. mobilized combatant.

11. The candidate was embarrassed because he had failed the surgical examination.
    The candidate was
    a. dispelled.
    b. chagrined.
    c. foreboding.
    d. unerring.

12. Because this court case will be used as an example for future decisions, it sets a
    a. pretext.
    b. priority.
    c. precept.
    d. precedent.

13. The climate in the spring and fall is quite temperate.
    Temperate means
    a. changeable.
    b. humid.
    c. moderate.
    d. predictable.

14. The grandfather lamented the loss of the friends he knew in the "good old days."
    Lamented means
    a. described.
    b. mourned.
    c. recalled.
    d. disregarded.

15. The students were subjected to a long, fervent speech against marijuana. The speech was actually a
    a. truism.
    b. wrangle.
    c. tirade.
    d. premonition.

16. The music warned us that something evil was going to happen. The music was
    a. pessimistic.
    b. vibrant.
    c. ominous.
    d. odious.

17. Although the patient was in pain, she seemed indifferent to it. Her behavior is best described as
    a. pathetic.
    b. stoic.
    c. languid.
    d. nondescript.

18. They were unable to catch the butterfly in the net. It kept
    a. enfolding them.
    b. eluding them.
    c. engaging them.
    d. endowing them.

19. To indicate that it catered to guests who stay for a short time, the hotel displayed a sign saying,
    a. "Transients."
    b. "Incumbents."
    c. "Nocturnals."
    d. "Expedients."

20. In handling the medical supplies, the aide was generally careless, paying little attention to cleanliness and order. The aide was
    a. slovenly.
    b. fastidious.
    c. profane.
    d. distraught.

21. The belligerent pupil refused to obey the teacher's request.
    Belligerent means
    a. arrogant.
    b. disrespectful.
    c. righteous.
    d. quarrelsome.

22. The political conditions in the undeveloped country were very volatile. **Volatile** means
    a. intolerable.
    b. biased.
    c. discouraging.
    d. explosive.

23. To say that William Shakespeare typed his plays is an
    a. affinity.
    b. antithesis.
    c. anachronism.
    d. atrophy.

24. The art gallery was showing the body of the artist's work. The exhibit was a
    a. restoration.
    b. resurrection.
    c. retribution.
    d. retrospective.

25. The patient showed little or no emotion when informed of the results of the laboratory tests. The patient was
    a. stolid.
    b. submissive.
    c. indispensable.
    d. deliberate.

26. Dr. Stone showed great animosity toward his colleagues. He treated them with
    a. gratitude.
    b. respect.
    c. discernment.
    d. hatred.

27. The music played at the funeral was a
    a. benediction.
    b. crypt.
    c. dirge.
    d. wake.

28. The conduct of all those present at the nursing staff meeting was staid. The people were
    a. sedate.
    b. grim.
    c. determined.
    d. tense.

29. The patient sitting alone was so reluctant to join in the conversation that he could be described as
    a. terse.
    b. taciturn.
    c. insidious.
    d. agitated.

SECTION A

SECTION B

SECTION C

COMPREHENSIVE PRACTICE Test 1

COMPREHENSIVE PRACTICE Test 2

COMPREHENSIVE PRACTICE Test 3

30. To receive a doctorate, most students are required to submit a long written essay, or
    a. theorem.
    b. proposition.
    c. disclosure.
    d. dissertation.

READING: There are five reading passages in this section. Read each passage carefully. Then, *on the basis of what you have read in the passage,* select the best answer for each of the questions following the passage.

I

In demographic terms, there are deaf people and deaf people. Of the 2 million Americans who can't hear speech, about a quarter lost that ability before the age of 19, and roughly one in eight either was born without it or lost it before the age of 3. Possibly half the deaf are elderly, and many more are approaching old age. But deafness has social as well as physical consequences; when it strikes early and hard, it has educational ones as well.

Americans who lose their hearing early in life do form a distinctive social and cultural group, a society strongly cohesive. This is especially true for sign-language users, but even among those who communicate largely in oral language, relying more or less on hearing aids, or lipreading, four out of five marry a deaf spouse rather than a hearing one. And most prevocationally deaf spend nearly all their leisure time and find their basic personal identity in the company of others like themselves.

Overwhelmingly, they find employment in industries engaged in manufacture of nondurable goods and in trades such as printing and sewing, where they can get by with stereotyped, and thus reasonably predictable, oral communication. It's no surprise, therefore, that the prevocationally deaf earn much less than the hearing. Deaf people average a bit more than 70 percent of the earnings of the nondeaf.

It might seem, at first innocent glance, that a person is deaf who cannot hear. If one can hear imperfectly, but well enough for many purposes, then he or she is probably hard-of-hearing. And probably anyone with hearing defective to any degree is hearing-impaired. But logic rarely helps when dealing with belief, and the field of hearing impairment has been rent for centuries by a conflict as fierce as any that ever sundered a party cell or a religious denomination. . . .

The plain truth is that "deaf" and "hearing-impaired," when used by people in the field, usually do not describe physiological conditions but signal loyalties in a continuing war over communication and, ultimately, over the place of the hearing-handicapped in society. Those who favor manual communication tend to describe people with serious hearing losses as "deaf"; those who oppose it tend to call them "hearing-impaired."

(From "Dialogue of the Deaf" by Beryl Lieff Benderly. Reprinted from *Psychology Today* and with permission of the author. Copyright © October 1980.)

SECTION A

SECTION B

SECTION C

COMPREHENSIVE PRACTICE Test 1

COMPREHENSIVE PRACTICE Test 2

COMPREHENSIVE PRACTICE Test 3

31. The main idea of this passage is that
    a. demographers do not understand the world of the deaf.
    b. sign language is the best means of communication for the deaf.
    c. the field of hearing impairment is marked by differing definitions and philosophies.
    d. a hearing impairment is a handicap that can ruin people's lives.

32. According to this passage, how many Americans lost their hearing before they were 19 years old?
    a. two million
    b. one million
    c. a half million
    d. a quarter million

33. According to the passage, people who have been deaf since an early age
    a. often cannot communicate at all.
    b. earn less money than nondeaf people.
    c. are often highly successful in business.
    d. usually develop other physical problems.

34. We can infer from this passage that the *prevocationally* deaf are those who
    a. were fired from their jobs when they lost their hearing.
    b. lost their hearing before they were regularly employed.
    c. can work only with other deaf people.
    d. are unable to work because of their deafness.

35. In the phrase "the field of hearing impairment has been rent for centuries," **rent** means
    a. occupied.
    b. split.
    c. involved.
    d. troubled.

36. The use of the terms "deaf" and "hearing-impaired" by people in the field reflects a conflict over whether deaf people should
    a. be paid higher wages.
    b. use sign language.
    c. form a political action group.
    d. learn lipreading.

II

Originally the term "textiles" referred only to fabrics produced by weaving. Today, it includes not only woven products, but those made by knitting, twisting, or any other means. It also includes fabrics produced from man-made fibers and materials. It also includes threads and yarns from which fabrics are made, and even artificial leather, oilcloth, string, and rope.

Until very recently in man's history, textiles were made only from fibers that were produced by plants and animals. These fibers include cotton, flax, wool, and silk. Then, in 1885, a French scientist, Hilaire Chardonnet, discovered how to make artificial silk fibers from the cellulose materials of cotton. Later, cellulose from wood pulp was also used. In the United States, artificial silk was first manufactured in 1910, but it took about ten to fifteen years before it became important commercially. In 1924, it was given the commercial name of rayon. Rayon, as you probably know, still is a very important product in the textile industry of the United States and several other nations, especially Japan. As a shiny, silk-like material, it cut greatly into the world market for the more expensive real silk.

In the 1920s and 1930s, research workers of the chemical firm of Du Pont de Nemours and Company experimented in making artificial, or synthetic, fibers from several different kinds of raw materials. By 1935, Dr. W. H. Carothers, of the Du Pont firm, successfully produced synthetic fibers from coal, air, and water. The name nylon was given to these fibers. Nylon was first marketed in 1938 and was used particularly for nylon stockings. Today, nylon is used for many things, from stockings, underwear, and dresses to fishing line, carpets, and cord for auto tires.

Since 1938, many new synthetic fibers, such as dacron, orlon, and acrilan, have appeared. They are made chiefly from coal, natural gas, petroleum, and air and water. The synthetic fibers now offer very serious competition to natural fibers. However, in spite of the competition of synthetics, far more cotton textiles are produced than any other type.

(From *Your Country and the World,* New Edition of the Tiegs-Adams Series. Copyright © 1966, by Ginn and Company [Xerox Corporation]. Used with permission.)

37. In its earliest meaning, a textile was defined only as a fabric that was
    a. constructed of separate threads and yarns.
    b. created by a weaving process.
    c. made from plant or animal fibers.
    d. produced from man-made materials.

38. Synthetic fibers include
    a. wool and silk.
    b. rayon and nylon.
    c. cotton and flax.
    d. all of these.

39. An artificial textile that is made from parts of plants is
    a. rayon.
    b. nylon.
    c. dacron.
    d. flax.

40. The first successful synthetic fiber was made from
    a. coal, air, and water.
    b. natural gas, air, and water.
    c. wood pulp.
    d. cotton cellulose.

41. The person who first developed nylon was
    a. Chardonnet.
    b. a Japanese scientist.
    c. Carothers.
    d. Du Pont de Nemours.

Word Knowledge and Reading Comprehension   49

SECTION A
SECTION B
SECTION C
COMPREHENSIVE PRACTICE Test 1
COMPREHENSIVE PRACTICE Test 2
COMPREHENSIVE PRACTICE Test 3

42. According to the text, the majority of textiles produced today are made of
   a. wool.
   b. nylon.
   c. rayon.
   d. cotton.

III

Fevers above 103 in an adult may upset mental processes temporarily, causing a lack of judgment, confusion, or even delirium. Young children can suffer convulsions from a very rapid rise in body temperature, but once a high fever develops, convulsion is unlikely. According to the best available evidence, these febrile convulsions, though frightening, are not dangerous and do not cause brain damage.

The higher your fever, the worse you're likely to feel. But it doesn't necessarily follow that you're more seriously ill when your fever is high than when it's only a degree or two above normal. Babies and young children have incompletely developed heat-regulating systems, so they tend to run high temperatures even from minor infections.

A child with a strep throat that requires medical treatment may have a temperature of only 100, whereas a flulike illness that needs only symptomatic care may send the temperature soaring to 104. Premature infants and elderly persons, on the other hand, rarely run high fevers. They can have serious infections and no fever at all.

How can you know, then, when to take a fever seriously? In children, any of the following circumstances should prompt a call to the doctor:

   —If a temperature above 101 orally or 102 rectally persists for more than a day.
   —If a fever of 104 or higher lasts for four hours and doesn't go down in response to fever-reducing drugs.
   —If any fever, even a low one, persists for four or more days.
   —If the child is less than four months old.
   —If other worrisome symptoms are present, such as rash, sore throat, earache, bad cough, breathing difficulties, extreme lethargy, vomiting, diarrhea, or stiff neck.

An adult should also check out a persistent temperature or one associated with possibly serious symptoms such as the above.

In reporting a fever to the doctor, note the time of day, how it was measured, and any trends. Body temperature normally fluctuates during the day—usually lowest first thing in the morning, highest in the late afternoon or evening. A child sent to school with a normal temperature in the morning may come home feverish at 3 o'clock. If a child has been sick with a fever, it's usually wise to keep him or her home for one extra day after the temperature returns to normal.

(© 1979 by The New York Times Company. Reprinted by permission.)

43. This passage is primarily concerned with the
   a. effects of high fever on children and adults.
   b. conditions under which fever should be taken seriously.
   c. differences in temperature range with age.
   d. heat-regulating systems of the body.

44. A high fever would be considered most unusual in an
    a. infant of six months.
    b. adolescent.
    c. adult of forty.
    d. elderly person.

45. According to the passage, the higher the fever is,
    a. the older the patient is likely to be.
    b. the more uncomfortable the patient will be.
    c. the more serious the illness is.
    d. the more frequently the doctor should be seen.

46. Of the following conditions mentioned in the passage, the one most likely to be accompanied by a low fever is
    a. delirium in an adult.
    b. febrile convulsions.
    c. strep throat.
    d. the flu.

47. According to the advice given in the passage, an adult should consult a doctor when a fever
    a. gets as high as 104 degrees.
    b. fluctuates between 101 and 102 degrees.
    c. is over 100 degrees for 24 hours.
    d. persists for several days.

48. The passage suggests that the effect of fever-induced convulsions in children is not definitely known. This is indicated by which of these phrases?
    a. "may upset mental processes temporarily"
    b. "it doesn't necessarily follow"
    c. "According to the best available evidence"
    d. "these febrile convulsions, though frightening, are not dangerous"

IV

While toys have existed since ancient times, only in recent years have we come to understand their more extensive role and the meaning of play to a child's growth and development.

In more primitive, simple societies, children learned through play to familiarize themselves with their environment and to develop skills which would help them find food and provide shelter in order to survive. In an increasingly complex society, children today must learn more for survival. They must develop physically, mentally, emotionally, and socially in order to cope.

This learning process begins for children through their play, and toys are the educational tools to aid in this development. Though no toy can teach a child anything all by itself, with proper interaction between a child, his toys, and other people—and particularly with his parents—toys can teach many things.

Toys can help children in the development of specific skills such as walking, talking, reading, and generally, to develop confidence in the process of learning.

It is considerably more difficult for children today to mature from child to adult. Life patterns are more complex and a child is not always sure of his adult role. Toys are important

Word Knowledge and Reading Comprehension

51

SECTION A

SECTION B

SECTION C

COMPREHENSIVE PRACTICE Test 1

COMPREHENSIVE PRACTICE Test 2

COMPREHENSIVE PRACTICE Test 3

in helping them prepare for adulthood by increasing their confidence, flexibility, and self-expression. They help introduce children to modern technology and contemporary living by emulating current social trends, attitudes, and interests.

Children gain a sense of values from their toys. As we said, toys by themselves cannot shape a child, but they can help to reinforce the lessons we teach them.

Toys help children get along better with others and to be more responsive to the needs of other people. Scientists refer to this as the development of interpersonal relationships.

Perhaps most important of all, toys teach children to love. They have traditionally provided companionship and security and served as objects of love for children. A favorite doll, a teddy bear, or another special toy has helped many children cope with difficult moments in their young lives. Children have to learn to love and they learn partly from loving their toys.

(Passage from *Toys Are Teaching Tools*, published by Toy Industry Association, Inc., New York. Reprinted with permission.)

49. A good title for this passage would be
   a. "The Benefit of Toys"
   b. "The History of Toys"
   c. "The Study of Children's Toys"
   d. "Children's Social Development"

50. It can be inferred from the passage that boys in primitive societies would most likely play with toy
   a. weapons.
   b. animals.
   c. musical instruments.
   d. money.

51. According to the passage, toys can serve as a means for a child to
   a. play independently.
   b. acquire intelligence.
   c. develop a role model.
   d. become grown up.

52. The author suggests that a child should be expected to
   a. make use of each toy he owns.
   b. develop an attachment to a toy.
   c. require complex toys in a complex society.
   d. mature quickly because of play with toys.

53. One toy mentioned in the passage is a
   a. bow and arrow.
   b. teddy bear.
   c. top.
   d. talking doll.

54. This passage would most likely have appeared in a
   a. weekly news magazine.
   b. toy catalogue.
   c. trade journal.
   d. child development text.

V

Some psychologists and sociologists argue that women, especially, are taught to fear success in our society. Beginning in junior high, experts observe, girls are advised not to do better than boys in athletic and intellectual encounters.

In the early '60s, psychologist Matina Homer studied the way male and female college students felt about success. She gave male and female undergraduates at the University of Michigan a story and asked them to complete it. The men's version featured a man's name; the women's version, a woman's name.

The story began, "At first term finals, Anne/John finds herself/himself at the top of the medical school class." Homer asked students to finish the story.

The men's stories depicted John as successful and happy. Ninety percent of the men showed strong positive feelings, like confidence in themselves and high hopes for their futures.

Women's responses to the story were very different. They typically described Anne deliberately lowering her grades to avoid competing with a husband or boyfriend, or quitting school entirely. Many chalked up the success to luck, or described Anne as a lonely reject.

Homer concluded that a majority of these young women were afraid to succeed. Later studies showed that fear of success increased as women went further in their educations.

A 1976 study by psychologists at the University of Southern California (USC) reached slightly different conclusions. Researchers found that women's attitudes toward success depended on the expectations of others.

The experiment involved young women who had scored high on a fear-of-success test. They were put into a situation in which they were either punished or rewarded for doing well. The researchers told subjects the study was about how people form impressions. A psychologist, the women were told, would form an impression of them based on an intelligence test. After taking what they were told was a practice test, half the women were told the psychologist approved of high intelligence. Half were told the psychologist disapproved of high intelligence.

The women who were told that their braininess would be appreciated scored much higher on a second intelligence test. The women who were told their intelligence would not be appreciated did the same or worse on the tests. The experiment seems to confirm that other people's expectations influence fear of success.

Experts like Homer and Dr. Renee Jackson-White of USC think that as stereotyped notions of masculinity and femininity change, women's attitudes toward success also will change.

(Reprinted from *Career World*, October 1979. Copyright © 1979 by Curriculum Innovations, Inc.)

55. In Homer's study, positive expectations for future success were shown by
    a. most of the male and female college students.
    b. few of the male and female students.
    c. the majority of the male subjects, but few of the female subjects.
    d. those female students who were told that their intelligence was appreciated.

56. Subjects in a study conducted at the University of Southern California
    a. were punished or rewarded for doing well.
    b. studied how people form impressions.
    c. were encouraged to raise their intelligence test scores.
    d. were given two fear-of-failure tests.

57. Homer assumed that students' stories would
    a. reflect their own feelings.
    b. have no relationship to their prior experiences.
    c. be similar for both sexes.
    d. predict future achievement.

58. In the University of Southern California study, telling women that the psychologist approved of high intelligence was considered
    a. a threat.
    b. a stereotype.
    c. a reward.
    d. an indicator of IQ.

59. In Homer's research, male and female college students were asked to complete stories that differed in the main character's
    a. sex.
    b. career expectations.
    c. personality.
    d. academic success.

60. Homer interpreted the female students' responses to incomplete stories as reflecting
    a. the influence of boyfriends or husbands.
    b. the students' own lack of success in school.
    c. stereotyped notions of femininity.
    d. a desire to satisfy the researcher's expectations.

SECTION A

SECTION B

SECTION C

COMPREHENSIVE PRACTICE Test 1

COMPREHENSIVE PRACTICE Test 2

COMPREHENSIVE PRACTICE Test 3

III. Verbal Ability

Word Knowledge and Reading Comprehension

45 minutes per test

WORD KNOWLEDGE: Read each sentence carefully. Then, *on the basis of what is stated in the sentence*, select the answer that best completes the statement. (The correct answers are at the end of Section A.)

1. The supervisor said, "Please make sure your watches all have the same time." The watches should be
   a. synthesized.
   b. synchronized.
   c. syndicated.
   d. systematic.

2. Sunday morning brunch at nursing school followed an established procedure. It was really a
   a. ritual.
   b. forum.
   c. revel.
   d. farce.

3. John's thoughts were dominated by his desire to run the marathon. Running the marathon became an
   a. ultimatum.
   b. addiction.
   c. obsession.
   d. enticement.

4. When you do a friend a favor in return for a similar favor done for you, you
   a. replenish.
   b. retaliate.
   c. reminisce.
   d. reciprocate.

5. The nurse's aide who received the award made an impromptu speech. **Impromptu** means
   a. well prepared.
   b. spontaneous.
   c. appropriate.
   d. terse.

54

6. Instead of writing "horseback rider" on her application, Ann wrote that she was
   a. a pedestrian.
   b. an equestrian.
   c. a hackney.
   d. an envoy.

7. The head nurse was very honest in her comments about the staff. She was
   a. conducive.
   b. sarcastic.
   c. candid.
   d. condescending.

8. The laboratory tests corroborated the diagnosis made by the doctor. The doctor's diagnosis was
   a. supplemented.
   b. supported.
   c. contradicted.
   d. questioned.

9. An unproven theory that temporarily provides a basis for further investigation is a
   a. postulate.
   b. theorem.
   c. maxim.
   d. hypothesis.

10. The nurse stayed awake to watch her patient's progress. She was keeping a
    a. vigil.
    b. reign.
    c. regimen.
    d. reverie.

11. Parliament demanded that the king give up his throne; so he
    a. abstained.
    b. abdicated.
    c. revoked.
    d. detracted.

12. The demented patient was extremely difficult to handle.
    Demented means
    a. skeptical.
    b. obstinate.
    c. insane.
    d. bewildered.

13. A person who rejects the beliefs of an established religious group is
    a. a disciple.
    b. an impostor.
    c. a heretic.
    d. an idolater.

SECTION A

SECTION B

SECTION C

COMPREHENSIVE PRACTICE Test 1

COMPREHENSIVE PRACTICE Test 2

COMPREHENSIVE PRACTICE Test 3

14. The surgeon was profuse in his praise of those who helped him with the operation.
    Profuse means
    a. lavish.
    b. sparing.
    c. grateful.
    d. superficial.

15. The advice given to the young nurse by her supervisor was invaluable. The advice was
    a. needless.
    b. priceless.
    c. senseless.
    d. worthless.

16. The filament was white with heat; it was
    a. incited.
    b. accentuated.
    c. excited.
    d. incandescent.

17. The police asked the witness to give a pictorial account of the accident. They wanted him to be
    a. abstract.
    b. concise.
    c. graphic.
    d. composed.

18. Your community health paper must include a list of the books you used. This list will be called the
    a. biography.
    b. appendix.
    c. preface.
    d. bibliography.

19. There were many impediments to the student getting the nursing diploma
    Impediments are
    a. requirements.
    b. advantages.
    c. obstacles.
    d. stages.

20. The arrival of the paramedic was most opportune.
    Opportune means
    a. unexpected.
    b. fortunate.
    c. timely.
    d. surprising.

21. A person formally charged by a grand jury with the commission of a crime has been
    a. indicted.
    b. convicted.
    c. arrested.
    d. impeached.

22. The students of pediatrics had taken copious notes during the lecture. The notes were
    a. copied.
    b. in shorthand.
    c. concise.
    d. abundant.

23. The leader was an unwitting ally of those who wished to overthrow him. The leader's aid to his enemies was
    a. unrestrained.
    b. unintentional.
    c. unremitting.
    d. uninformed.

24. Because the large dog frightened strangers and kept them from entering the gate, he was considered a(n)
    a. deterrent.
    b. denouncer.
    c. marauder.
    d. encumbrance.

25. The audience did its best to disconcert the musician. They tried to
    a. show he was out of tune.
    b. indicate their pleasure.
    c. encourage him to play another piece.
    d. upset his composure.

26. The new nurses emulated the actions of the supervisor.
    Emulated means
    a. criticized.
    b. imitated.
    c. admired.
    d. described.

27. The effects of an unbalanced diet can be most harmful. The effects can be
    a. opprobrious.
    b. impervious.
    c. meritorious.
    d. deleterious.

28. A narrow strip of land bordered on both sides by water and connecting two larger bodies of land is called a(an)
    a. isthmus.
    b. island.
    c. peninsula.
    d. delta.

29. The hospital workers wanted to abrogate the agreement that had been reached with their employer. They wanted the contract
    a. amended.
    b. canceled.
    c. extended.
    d. fulfilled.

SECTION A

SECTION B

SECTION C

COMPREHENSIVE PRACTICE Test 1

COMPREHENSIVE PRACTICE Test 2

COMPREHENSIVE PRACTICE Test 3

30. A standard by which the value of something can be measured is
    a. a consensus.
    b. an appraisal.
    c. an evaluation.
    d. a criterion.

READING: There are five reading passages in this section. Read each passage carefully. Then, *on the basis of what you have read in the passage,* select the best answer for each of the questions following the passage.

I

Lacey Taylor's parents thought they were helping to protect her against winter colds with massive doses of vitamin A. Instead it almost killed her.

The 3-year-old was hospitalized suffering from itching, dehydration, and a severe tremor. Tests at Sparrow Hospital disclosed the child had a blood calcium level so high that it could have stopped her heart, and doctors worked on her for six days, thinking she had Reye's Syndrome.

Finally they discovered that her puzzling condition, normally associated with excess vitamin D, was linked to an overdose of vitamin A from over-the-counter pills. The child, they determined, had been given doses of 200,000 units of vitamin A, 100 times the daily requirement of 2,000 units.

Lacey has both liver and kidney damage but will recover from both, her doctors say.

Dr. Donald F. Knickerbocker described the incident as a "totally innocent misuse of what was thought to be a proper use of over-the-counter materials."

"It has been an amazing case which we will undoubtedly be reporting in the medical literature," said Dr. William Weil.

"The overdose was potentially fatal because it altered her heart rate, her heart rhythm," Dr. Weil said. "Conceivably her heart could have stopped at that level of calcium and that was a major danger."

"The body stores vitamin A," Dr. Weil said. "It is unlike vitamin C, which is excreted if not used by the body. You don't know how much excess vitamin any one person can tolerate because sensitivity varies. The real message in this case is that although vitamins are important for one's health, an excess can be very damaging—particularly of vitamins A and D."

31. The doctors in the hospital initially believed that Lacey had
    a. Reye's Syndrome.
    b. an overdose of vitamin A.
    c. too much vitamin A and D in combination.
    d. an excess of vitamin D.

32. The symptoms that Lacey had are typically found with
    a. Down's Syndrome.
    b. an excess of vitamin A.
    c. an excess of vitamin C.
    d. an excess of vitamin D.

33. The recommended daily requirement of vitamin A for a 3-year-old is
    a. 100 units.
    b. 2,000 units.
    c. 20,000 units.
    d. 200,000 units.

34. The change in Lacey's heart rate and rhythm was a direct result of
    a. the severity of dehydration.
    b. liver and kidney damage.
    c. the high level of blood calcium.
    d. excess vitamin D.

35. It can be inferred from the passage that, once Lacey regains her health, she will
    a. have no remaining symptoms.
    b. suffer from heart irregularity.
    c. retain a high blood calcium level.
    d. have some liver and kidney damage.

36. Evidence that this incident is of particular interest to the medical profession is suggested by the fact that
    a. the patient required a long hospitalization.
    b. two doctors were called in to treat the patient.
    c. many tests were necessary to make a diagnosis.
    d. the case will be described in medical publications.

II

When people talk about chauvinism nowadays, more often than not they mean male chauvinism: the belief that men are superior to women, and the behavior resulting from this assumption. Male chauvinists do not want to face the obvious fact that girls can do almost anything boys can do—and quite a few things that they can't. Of course, since most of the power in society has long been held by men, there has been a tendency for this silly and fraudulent theory to become a self-fulfilling prophecy.

"Chauvinism" is the belief that one's own nation, or one's own sex, or one's own anything, is naturally superior to all others, especially when such patriotism is carried to a ridiculous extreme. It was a Frenchman who gave his name to this aberration: one Nicolas Chauvin, a trooper who served in Napoleon's army. Wounded no less than seventeen times, Chauvin was eventually put out to pasture with a miserable two hundred francs a year as veteran's pension and a decorative saber as a souvenir. Another man might have been disillusioned by such high-handed treatment. Not so with Chauvin, who continued to champion Napoleon long after his fall from power and popularity. So high-pitched were his praises for the former emperor that his mad loyalty to this lost cause inspired a whole series of comic plays with Chauvin as the main figure of fun.

Do not jump to the conclusion that because Chauvin was French, the French are any more chauvinistic than anyone else. The British have their own brand of chauvinism, known as "jingoism." The original Jingoists were a minority of English politicians who wanted to fight Russia when she was invading Turkey in 1878. Their marching song was a music-hall ditty of the time which went, "We don't want to fight, yet by jingo! if we do, we've got the ships, we've got the men, and got the money too."

As for home-grown American flag-waving, there is a word for that too: Inflated or boastful talk about the United States is known, by reference to the nation's emblem, an eagle, as "spread-eagleism."

(Copyright © 1979 by Donald Smith. Reprinted by permission of Scholastic, Inc.)

37. The passage points out that chauvinism is
   a. un-American.
   b. uniquely French.
   c. confined to the military.
   d. universal.

38. Nicolas Chauvin became an object of
   a. admiration.
   b. mockery.
   c. courage.
   d. envy.

39. The passage implies that Chauvin was
   a. unrealistic.
   b. unpopular.
   c. successful.
   d. miserable.

40. Chauvinism, jingoism, and spread-eagleism are all forms of
   a. national flag-waving.
   b. minority resistance.
   c. military power and popularity.
   d. music hall playacting.

41. The passage implies that Chauvin's loyalty to Napoleon was
   a. well-founded.
   b. hopeless.
   c. popular.
   d. short-lived.

42. Male chauvinism has become a self-fulfilling prophecy because
   a. males are born stronger than females.
   b. girls can do almost anything boys can do.
   c. men have held most of the power in society.
   d. the theory is silly and fraudulent.

SECTION A

SECTION B

SECTION C

COMPREHENSIVE PRACTICE Test 1

COMPREHENSIVE PRACTICE Test 2

COMPREHENSIVE PRACTICE Test 3

III

Transactions within groups satisfy a person's need for establishing and maintaining his interdependency within the social, cultural, and economic environments. As we have advanced in our technological development, so too have our interdependent needs expanded within these environs. History reveals, with each era, shifts in the priorities of needs that affect interpersonal relationships—to man, with one or several others, and with our environment. The twentieth century is an era of complex interdependent relationships. This complexity is manifested through the types of group relationships that individuals form.

Group relationships are divided into three major categories—primary, secondary, and tertiary. The rationale for this categorization is based on the individual's need to set priorities in his search for fulfillment.

A *primary* group can be defined as a unit composed of close-knit, mutually interdependent and reciprocal memberships. In other words, the primary group is any small group to which an individual belongs because of a vested interest, specialized activity, or fulfillment of need gratification. Familial, peer, or religious groups are examples of primary groups. It is in conjunction with the primary group that the individual establishes the norms and mores for his particular position in life. It is through his continuous involvement with this type of group relationship that the individual finds validation for his ideas, thoughts, actions, and feelings. This type of group relationship provides the members with group security and a means of identity, establishes role expectations and functionings, and contributes a sense of belonging and acceptance.

Secondary groups are those formed for the purpose of enrichment and refinement of the individual's total living experience. The kinds of interdependent relationships formed within this category manifest a moderate degree of intimacy. The individual retains freedom to move in and out of secondary groups as his priorities change. This freedom of movement is unique to secondary groups and is another characteristic that distinguishes it from the primary group. A work group, a social club, an art class, or a professional organization exemplifies this secondary group category. Secondary group memberships are formed because they serve as a necessary and significant vehicle for the individual to meet his social, cultural, and financial needs.

Tertiary groups are those in which there exists between members a limited degree of intimacy and involvement. Membership is based on the necessity for gratifying immediate needs. The relationships formed within the group are not designed to be continuous. They are based on priorities which, most likely but not exclusively, have been established by the individual within his primary or secondary groups. Participating in a fundraising campaign, becoming a member of a committee, joining a vacation tour group, or taking part in a community action group is identified as a tertiary type of interpersonal group relationship.

(Kreigh & Perko, *Psychiatric and Mental Health Nursing: Commitment to Care and Concern,* 1979, pgs. 58–59. Reprinted with permission of Pearson Education, Inc., Upper Saddle River, New Jersey.)

43. The major subject of this passage is
    a. the rules governing social behavior in three types of groups.
    b. the differences between group relationships of the present and those of earlier times.
    c. the distinctive characteristics of different types of groups.
    d. the changes made by technological advances on the nature of group participation.

44. The three kinds of groups discussed in this passage differ from each other primarily by
    a. the emotional closeness of the members of the group.
    b. the success with which the members' needs are met by the group.
    c. the variety of activities carried out by the group.
    d. the status that the community gives to the group.

45. Which of these statements describes a characteristic of any interdependent relationship?
    a. Participants in the relationship have equal status.
    b. Participants in the relationship satisfy each other's needs.
    c. The relationship is essential to the participants' well-being.
    d. The relationship is based on priorities established in adulthood.

46. The term "validation," as it is used in the third paragraph, can best be defined as
    a. a sense of individuality.
    b. an acceptable explanation.
    c. consistent satisfaction.
    d. sound support.

47. One might infer from this passage that
    a. primary groups have the greatest influence on an individual's personality development.
    b. people are attracted to a particular category of group according to their personalities.
    c. group relationships fulfill only needs that cannot be fulfilled by one-to-one relationships.
    d. tertiary groups are characterized by a similarity in the members' educational backgrounds.

48. This passage implies that the purpose of studying groups is to help a person
    a. participate more effectively in groups.
    b. understand human behavior.
    c. select those groups that are most suited to his needs.
    d. understand the quest for self-identity.

IV

One of the major triumphs of the print and electronic media during the 1960s and 1970s was the turnaround in people's attitude toward endangered species. Before 1960, the very mention of "endangered" or "threatened" species drew a blank stare or a mumbled remark about how well we have been doing without the dinosaur and the dodo. Twenty years of drumming by the media and conservation organizations has worked miracles. Not many politicians today would dare proclaim that when you have seen one redwood you have seen them all. Some, but not many.

After public awareness came conscience, and from conscience grew conscientiousness. Although plant and animal species are vanishing every day, we are saving others from extinction. But saving them is only the first step. After we do that, we have to find someplace to put them.

To date, habitat has not been too much of a problem. When the rare Hawaiian goose, or nene, was on the brink of extinction, the few dozen birds left were captured and packed off

Word Knowledge and Reading Comprehension

63

SECTION A

SECTION B

SECTION C

COMPREHENSIVE PRACTICE Test 1

COMPREHENSIVE PRACTICE Test 2

COMPREHENSIVE PRACTICE Test 3

to Slimbridge, on the Severn Estuary, in southern England, where Sir Peter Scott has his Wildfowl Trust. The birds were bred back up to strength and distributed to satellite breeding stations around the world. The redeemed goose is so plentiful now that some areas of the Hawaiian Islands—its original habitat—are being restocked.

It is hardly news that there were once vast herds of bison in North America. But their habitat was usurped for farmland, their water supplies were denied them, their migratory routes were interrupted, and they were slaughtered in incredible numbers in one of the worst bloodbaths in the long, sordid history of man and animal on this planet. Conservation efforts saved them. The bison herd in North America now numbers about 35,000. The buffalo is safe, so safe that we are turning some into buffalo burgers.

The slightly less impressive European bison, or wisent, was similarly saved at the last minute, and that herd has been bred back up too. The point here is that there is available space for both the buffalo and the wisent. They are not likely to become a problem in the foreseeable future.

But this hopeful picture is not worldwide. After the species crisis comes the space crisis, at least for most species. In a word, all will have been for naught unless we recognize the real natural history imperative of the 1980s—habitat.

(From "Saving Animals—For What?" by Roger Caras. *The Dial*, December 1980.)

49. The author attributes public concern for some endangered species to the efforts of
   a. electronic and print media.
   b. politicians.
   c. wildlife trusts.
   d. satellite breeding stations.

50. According to the passage, the nene and the North American bison have in common the fact that they
   a. are again faced with extinction.
   b. have been distributed around the world.
   c. were denied their water supplies.
   d. are back in their native habitat.

51. To save animals from extinction, capturing them is the first step. The second is
   a. making politicians act.
   b. rousing public awareness.
   c. setting up breeding stations.
   d. finding them a habitat.

52. Evidence that buffalo have been bred to a desired population is the fact that
   a. there is no space for any more buffalo.
   b. farmland has been converted to buffalo habitat.
   c. some buffalo are being used for food.
   d. the migratory routes of buffalo have been reestablished.

53. Compared to the American bison, the European bison is probably
   a. in less danger of extinction.
   b. of smaller size.
   c. less likely to find a habitat.
   d. of little interest to conservationists.

54. The attitude of the author is one of
    a. general unconcern.
    b. broad pessimism.
    c. limited optimism.
    d. heartfelt gratitude.

V

Mr. Hebert has been interested in the possibilities of using problem-solving approaches in his classes in order to make learning more interesting and to teach students to learn more "on their own." He tries this out in his literature class by having the students read a story for homework, and then presenting them with a problem in analysis the next day in class. He does this first with the whole class, rather than breaking them down into discussion groups, because he feels that they are going to need some help with the process. After giving them the problem, he lets them think about it, and then begins to solicit questions from them. They are seated at an oval table, and there are only about twenty-two students, so it is not a bad setting although the group is a bit large for this kind of thing.

There are very few opinions or ideas offered, and Mr. Hebert begins to feel a little uncomfortable. So do the students, so one of them gives a response to the problem. It is a really ridiculous one, however, and Mr. Hebert has an uncontrollable impulse to tell the student so. This does not exactly help the situation, because then there is even less tendency to try solutions. Mr. Hebert recognizes his error, and decides to talk with them a little about problem solving and about the need to risk ideas. He also decides that he will have to be more careful about accepting their ideas and not turning them off by his reactions to them. He then discusses this new process with them, and assigns them to small groups, each with a good student as a leader, and each with one or two questions to discuss about the reading. As he circulates he finds that they are still hesitant about taking part, and begins to realize how frightened these students are of making a mistake—even in front of each other, much less in front of him. He decides that he is going to have to have a period of training, where he desensitizes them of their fear of errors and builds participation and problem-solving strategies.

Mr. Hebert revises his approach, then, and returns to something very much like his old way of doing things. However, he also begins to inject into his classes occasional simple problems, giving plenty of guidance, and as the year goes on he gives more and more problems, with less and less guidance, so that the students gradually learn how to learn through this method.

(From M. Daniel Smith, *Educational Psychology and It's Classroom Applications*. Copyright © 1975 by Allyn and Bacon, Inc., Boston. Reprinted with permission.)

55. The main purpose of Mr. Hebert's using the new approach in his classroom was to
    a. teach literature to his class.
    b. stimulate class discussion.
    c. help students overcome fear.
    d. help students learn on their own.

56. At first Mr. Hebert tried his approach with the class as a whole because he believed that
    a. the class was small enough for the approach used.
    b. working with students individually would be too threatening.
    c. all students would need some guidance from him.
    d. students would be more hesitant in small groups.

57. The students' reactions to Mr. Hebert's approach were due mainly to their
    a. lack of knowledge of the subject matter.
    b. inability to ask questions.
    c. fear of making errors.
    d. misunderstanding of what they were expected to do.

58. When Mr. Hebert assigned the students to small groups, he made sure that each group included
    a. a good student leader.
    b. students who felt comfortable with each other.
    c. some people who were not afraid to risk ideas.
    d. someone who already had learned problem-solving skills.

59. This passage implies all of the following conclusions *except* that
    a. students are reluctant to talk in class.
    b. no student is exactly like another student.
    c. a teacher can learn from his mistakes in the classroom.
    d. students must be taught to risk ideas in classroom discussions.

60. In the end Mr. Hebert decided to
    a. continue his new problem-solving approach with the class as a whole.
    b. use the new problem-solving approach only when the students were in small groups.
    c. return to his old method of teaching without a problem-solving approach.
    d. use his original teaching method, adding some problem-solving activities.

SECTION A

SECTION B

SECTION C

COMPREHENSIVE PRACTICE Test 1

COMPREHENSIVE PRACTICE Test 2

COMPREHENSIVE PRACTICE Test 3

Answers

I. VERBAL ABILITY: WORD KNOWLEDGE AND READING COMPREHENSION

1.	b	21.	d	41.	b
2.	b	22.	a	42.	d
3.	c	23.	a	43.	a
4.	c	24.	d	44.	c
5.	a	25.	c	45.	d
6.	c	26.	b	46.	d
7.	d	27.	c	47.	a
8.	a	28.	b	48.	c
9.	b	29.	d	49.	d
10.	b	30.	a	50.	a
11.	d	31.	b	51.	d
12.	a	32.	a	52.	b
13.	b	33.	c	53.	c
14.	d	34.	b	54.	d
15.	b	35.	d	55.	b
16.	c	36.	c	56.	c
17.	b	37.	b	57.	a
18.	a	38.	d	58.	a
19.	d	39.	a	59.	c
20.	a	40.	c	60.	b

II. VERBAL ABILITY: WORD KNOWLEDGE AND READING COMPREHENSION

1.	a	6.	b	11.	b
2.	d	7.	a	12.	d
3.	c	8.	d	13.	c
4.	a	9.	b	14.	b
5.	b	10.	c	15.	c

16.	c	31.	c	46.	c
17.	b	32.	c	47.	d
18.	b	33.	b	48.	c
19.	a	34.	b	49.	b
20.	a	35.	b	50.	a
21.	d	36.	b	51.	d
22.	d	37.	b	52.	b
23.	c	38.	b	53.	b
24.	d	39.	a	54.	c
25.	a	40.	d	55.	c
26.	d	41.	c	56.	a
27.	c	42.	d	57.	a
28.	a	43.	b	58.	c
29.	b	44.	d	59.	a
30.	d	45.	b	60.	c

III. VERBAL ABILITY: WORD KNOWLEDGE AND READING COMPREHENSION

1.	b	17.	c	33.	b
2.	a	18.	d	34.	c
3.	c	19.	c	35.	a
4.	d	20.	c	36.	d
5.	b	21.	a	37.	d
6.	b	22.	d	38.	b
7.	c	23.	b	39.	a
8.	b	24.	a	40.	a
9.	d	25.	d	41.	b
10.	a	26.	b	42.	c
11.	b	27.	d	43.	c
12.	c	28.	a	44.	a
13.	c	29.	b	45.	b
14.	a	30.	d	46.	d
15.	b	31.	a	47.	a
16.	d	32.	d	48.	b

SECTION A

SECTION B

SECTION C

COMPREHENSIVE PRACTICE Test 1

COMPREHENSIVE PRACTICE Test 2

COMPREHENSIVE PRACTICE Test 3

49.	a	53.	b	57.	c
50.	d	54.	c	58.	a
51.	c	55.	d	59.	b
52.	c	56.	c	60.	d

BIBLIOGRAPHY

Vocabulary Study

Levine, Harold. *Vocabulary for the College-Bound Student*. New York: Amsco, 1994.
Miller, Ward S. *Word Wealth*. New York: Holt, Rinehart and Winston, 1978.

Reading Study

Coman, Marcia J., and Heavers, Kathy L. *Improving Reading Comprehension and Speed, Skimming and Scanning, Reading for Pleasure*. New York: NTC, 1997.
Kump, Peter. *Breakthrough: Rapid Reading*. Upper Saddle River, NJ: Prentice Hall, 1979.
McWhorter, Kathleen T. *Effective and Flexible Reading*. New York: Longman, 1998.

Mathematics Review

This section is intended to give you a basic overview of the math required for this exam. The topics included are basic vocabulary; integers; fractions; decimals; percentages; converting between decimals, fractions, and percentages; converting between measurements; ratio and proportion; basic algebra; and basic geometry.

BASIC VOCABULARY

Here are a few basic terms with which you should be familiar. Take some time to learn their definitions:

addends	two or more numbers you add together
sum	the answer to an addition problem
minuend	the number you subtract from in a subtraction problem
subtrahend	the number you subtract in a subtraction problem
difference	the answer to a subtraction problem
factor	a number that is multiplied by another number
product	the answer to a multiplication problem
divisor	the number that divides into another number
dividend	the number that is divided by the divisor
quotient	the answer to a division problem
rational numbers	numbers that can be expressed as fractions
whole number	any positive, nonfraction or nondecimal number, such as 1, 2, 3, and so on

Place Value

Our counting system is based on *place value*. Each of the digits making up a number has a value based on units of ten. In the following example, note the place value of each digit from right to left. The rightmost digit represents ones; the digit to the immediate left represents tens; and so on.

EX: 1,234,567

7 = ones (or units) place	→ 7·1 = 7
6 = tens place	→ 6·10 = 60
5 = hundreds place	→ 5·100 = 500
4 = thousands place	→ 4·1,000 = 4,000
3 = ten-thousands place	→ 3·10,000 = 30,000
2 = hundred-thousands place	→ 2·100,000 = 200,000
1 = millions place	→ 1·1,000,000 = 1,000,000

This number is read, "One million, two hundred thirty-four thousand, five hundred sixty-seven."

When you add or subtract, be sure to line up the digits according to their place value:

EX:
```
 23,345          3,875
+   368         - 905
 23,713          2,970
```

Rounding

Sometimes the answer to a problem must be rounded off to a whole number or to some other specified place value. Whether you are rounding whole numbers or rational numbers, the rules are the same.

1. Underline the place value to which you are rounding.

2. Examine the number immediately to the right of the underlined number.

3. If the number to the right is 5 or greater, round the underlined number up by one.

4. If the number to the right is less than 5, leave the underlined number unchanged.

EX:

Round to the nearest one:

84.71 = 84.71 = 85

123.38 = 123.38 = 123

Round to the nearest hundred:

8,245 = 8,245 = 8,200

3,729 = 3,729 = 3,700

Round to the nearest tenth:

458.296 = 458.296 = 458.3

35.62 = 35.62 = 35.6

SECTION A

SECTION B

SECTION C

COMPREHENSIVE PRACTICE Test 1

COMPREHENSIVE PRACTICE Test 2

COMPREHENSIVE PRACTICE Test 3

Prime Numbers

Prime numbers are whole numbers that have exactly two whole number factors: 1 and the number itself. The first 10 prime numbers are 2, 3, 5, 7, 11, 13, 17, 19, 23, and 29. The only even prime number is 2. (All other even numbers have 2 as a factor and therefore have more than two factors.) The opposite of a prime number is a *composite number*, which is a whole number (other than 0) with more than two factors. Note: 0 and 1 are neither prime nor composite numbers.

Divisibility Rules

The following rules help you determine whether a given number is evenly divisible by another:

- If the last digit of the number is 0, 2, 4, 6, or 8, then it is divisible by 2.
- If the sum of the digits of the number is a multiple of 3, then it is divisible by 3.
- If the last digit of the number is 5 or 0, then it is divisible by 5.
- If the number is divisible by 2 and 3, then it is divisible by 6.
- If the sum of the digits of the number is a multiple of 9, then it is divisible by 9.
- If the last digit of the number is 0, then it is divisible by 10.
  - If the number is a multiple of 3 *and* 4, then it is divisible by 12.

Average

The *average* of a group of numbers is the sum of the numbers, divided by the number of numbers added.

EX: The average of 5, 9, and 10 is calculated as follows:

$$\frac{5 + 9 + 10}{3} = \frac{24}{3} = 8$$

Exponents

An *exponent* (or *power*) tells you how many times to multiply the base by itself.

EX: In the number 5^2, 2 is the exponent and 5 is the base. Therefore, $5^2 = 5 \times 5 = 25$.

EX: In x^4, 4 is the exponent, and x is the base. Therefore, $x^4 = x \cdot x \cdot x \cdot x$.

EX: In 6^{-3}, -3 is the exponent, and 6 is the base. Therefore, $6^{-3} = \frac{1}{6^3} = \frac{1}{6 \times 6 \times 6} = \frac{1}{216}$.

$$x^{-n} = \frac{1}{x^n}$$

When the exponent is 2, the expression is called a *square*, or *perfect square*. You can read 4^2 as "four squared," and 16 is said to be the square of 4. When the exponent is 3, the expression is called a *cube*, or *perfect cube*. Read 4^3 as "four cubed;" 64 is the cube of 4. The following list contains common squares and cubes with which you should be familiar.

$$1^2 = 1 \qquad\qquad 1^3 = 1$$
$$2^2 = 4 \qquad\qquad 2^3 = 8$$
$$3^2 = 9 \qquad\qquad 3^3 = 27$$
$$4^2 = 16 \qquad\qquad 4^3 = 64$$
$$5^2 = 25 \qquad\qquad 5^3 = 125$$
$$6^2 = 36 \qquad\qquad 6^3 = 216$$
$$7^2 = 49 \qquad\qquad 7^3 = 343$$
$$8^2 = 64 \qquad\qquad 8^3 = 512$$
$$9^2 = 81 \qquad\qquad 9^3 = 729$$
$$10^2 = 100 \qquad\qquad 10^3 = 1{,}000$$
$$10^{-1} = .1 \qquad\qquad 10^{-2} = .01$$

Square Roots and Cube Roots

The square of 4 is 16. Conversely, 4 is called the *square root* ($\sqrt{}$) of 16. A *square root* is the number that is multiplied by itself to obtain another number.

EX: $\sqrt{16} = 4$, because $4 \times 4 = 16$.

The symbol used ($\sqrt{}$) is called the *radical*, and the number underneath the symbol ($\sqrt{16}$) is called the *radicand*.

EX: In the equation $\sqrt[3]{36} = 6$, $\sqrt{}$ is the radical, 36 is the radicand, and 6 is the square root.

Similarly, a *cube root* is the number that is multiplied by itself three times to obtain another number.

EX: Four is called the cube root ($\sqrt[3]{}$) of 64 because 64 is the cube of 4. $\sqrt[3]{8} = 2$, because $2 \times 2 \times 2 = 8$.

The terminology for cube roots is the same as for squares.

EX: In the equation $\sqrt[3]{64} = 4$, $\sqrt[3]{}$ is the radical, 64 is the radicand, and 4 is the cube root.

Radicals work in a similar fashion for fourth roots, fifth roots, and so on.

Here are two rules that apply to multiplying and dividing *radical expressions* (expressions containing square roots, cube roots, other kinds of roots).

1. $\sqrt{AB} = \sqrt{A} \times \sqrt{B}$ 2. $\sqrt{\dfrac{A}{B}} = \dfrac{\sqrt{A}}{\sqrt{B}}$

EX: $\sqrt{81} = \sqrt{9 \times 9} = \sqrt{9} \times \sqrt{9} = 3 \times 3 = 9$ EX: $\sqrt{\dfrac{9}{25}} = \dfrac{\sqrt{9}}{\sqrt{25}} = \dfrac{3}{5}$

SECTION A

SECTION B

SECTION C

COMPREHENSIVE PRACTICE Test 1

COMPREHENSIVE PRACTICE Test 2

COMPREHENSIVE PRACTICE Test 3

EX: $\sqrt{12} = \sqrt{4 \times 3} = \sqrt{4} \times \sqrt{3} = 2 \times \sqrt{3} = 2\sqrt{3}$

EX: $\sqrt{\dfrac{27}{16}} = \dfrac{\sqrt{27}}{\sqrt{16}} = \dfrac{\sqrt{9 \times 3}}{\sqrt{16}} = \dfrac{3\sqrt{3}}{4}$

Both rules also work in reverse.

1. $\sqrt{A} \times \sqrt{B} = \sqrt{AB}$ $\qquad\qquad\qquad \dfrac{\sqrt{A}}{\sqrt{B}} = \sqrt{\dfrac{A}{B}}$

EX: $\sqrt{3} \times \sqrt{5} = \sqrt{15}$ $\qquad\qquad$ EX: $\dfrac{\sqrt{48}}{\sqrt{12}} = \sqrt{\dfrac{48}{12}} = \sqrt{4} = 2$

EX: $\sqrt[3]{2} \times \sqrt[3]{4} = \sqrt[3]{8} = 2$

You may add or subtract radical expressions only if:

- the radicands are the same, and

- they are the same type of radical (square root, cube root, fourth root, and the like).

EX: These may all be combined: $\qquad\qquad$ None of these may be combined:

$2\sqrt{5} + 4\sqrt{5} = 6\sqrt{5}$ $\qquad\qquad\qquad$ $5\sqrt{3} + 8\sqrt{11}$

$9\sqrt{7} - 2\sqrt{7} = 7\sqrt{7}$ $\qquad\qquad\qquad$ $4\sqrt{7} - 12\sqrt{15}$

$2\sqrt[4]{8} + 3\sqrt[4]{8} = 5\sqrt[4]{8}$ $\qquad\qquad\qquad$ $\sqrt{5} + \sqrt[3]{7}$

You may need to simplify radical expressions before you can combine them.

EX: $\sqrt{60} + 3\sqrt{15} =$ $\qquad\qquad\qquad$ EX: $7\sqrt{3} + 5\sqrt{12} =$

$\sqrt{4 \times 15} + 3\sqrt{15} =$ $\qquad\qquad\qquad$ $7\sqrt{3} + 5(\sqrt{4} \times \sqrt{3}) =$

$2\sqrt{15} + 3\sqrt{15} = 5\sqrt{15}$ $\qquad\qquad\qquad$ $7\sqrt{3} + 5(2\sqrt{3}) =$

$\qquad\qquad\qquad\qquad\qquad\qquad\qquad\qquad$ $7\sqrt{3} + 10\sqrt{3} = 17\sqrt{3}$

INTEGERS

An *integer* is any positive whole number, negative whole number, or zero. Integers may not contain fractions or decimals.

EX: $-212, -6, 0, 234, 287$

The set of integers is just one set of all the kinds of numbers we use. The following table relates the major number sets we use. Beneath the heading for each set of numbers are all of the numbers in the set. As you can see in the table, the set of integers includes all whole numbers and counting numbers. In the same way, the set of real numbers contains all of the numbers in the sets beneath it.

real numbers	all numbers on the number line
rational numbers	numbers that can be expressed as fractions

integers	$\ldots -3, -2, -1, 0, 1, 2, 3 \ldots$
whole numbers	$0, 1, 2, 3, 4, \ldots$
counting (natural) numbers	$1, 2, 3, 4, \ldots$

Adding Integers

When the signs of integers are the same, adding two (or more) integers works just as you might remember:

positive + positive = positive

negative + negative = negative

| EX: $+12 + +17 = 29$ | The positive (plus) sign is usually omitted: $12 + 17 = 29$. |
| EX: $-12 + -17 = -29$ | The negative (minus) sign may or may not be raised, but it means the same thing: a negative number. |

When the signs are different, adding integers is a tad trickier, but not too much:

1. Ignore the signs until the end of your work.

2. Subtract the smaller number from the larger number.

3. Give your answer the same sign as the larger number.

EX: $-7 + 24 \ \rightarrow \ 24 - 7 \ \rightarrow \ 17$. Now put in the correct sign. With the signs removed, 24 is the larger number. Therefore, $-7 + 24 = 17$.

EX: $-25 + 4 \ \rightarrow \ 25 - 4 \ \rightarrow \ 21$. Now put the correct sign in. With the signs removed, 25 is the larger number. Therefore, $4 + -25 = -21$.

Subtracting Integers

One of the easiest ways to subtract integers is to turn subtraction into addition.

- Subtracting a positive is the same as adding a negative:

  EX: $+15 - +5 = +15 + -5 = 10$

  EX: $-20 - +5 = -20 + -5 = -25$

- Subtracting a negative is the same as adding a positive:

  EX: $+15 - -5 = +15 + +5 = 20$

  EX: $-20 - -5 = -20 + +5 = -15$

Multiplying Integers

An *even* number of negative numbers gives you a *positive* product.

EX: $2 \times -5 \times -3 \times 4 = 120$

An *odd* number of negative numbers gives you a *negative* product.

EX: $-2 \times -5 \times -3 \times 4 = -120$

Dividing Integers

positive ÷ positive = positive

EX: $20 \div 5 = 4$

negative ÷ negative = positive

EX: $-220 \div -5 = 4$

positive ÷ negative = negative

EX: $20 \div -5 = -4$

FRACTIONS

A *fraction* is any number that can be written in the form $\dfrac{A}{B}$, where A and B are integers, and B is not zero. (Fractions may not have a denominator of 0, because it is not possible to divide by 0.)

EX: $\dfrac{3}{4}, \dfrac{17}{50}, \dfrac{12}{15}$

In the standard fraction form ($\dfrac{A}{B}$), A is called the *numerator*, and B is called the *denominator*. Think of a fraction as part of something or as a piece of something.
Just be careful: A fraction can represent less than the whole thing, the whole thing, or more than the whole thing. A fraction is just another way of writing a division problem:

EX: $\dfrac{4}{5} = 4 \div 5 = 5\overline{)4}$

You may turn any whole number into a fraction by giving the whole number a denominator of 1.

EX: $5 = \dfrac{5}{1}$ because $5 \div 1 = 5$.

EX: $12 = \dfrac{12}{1}$ because $12 \div 1 = 12$.

SECTION A

SECTION B

SECTION C

COMPREHENSIVE PRACTICE Test 1

COMPREHENSIVE PRACTICE Test 2

COMPREHENSIVE PRACTICE Test 3

proper fraction   a fraction in which A is less than B

EX: $\dfrac{4}{5}$, $\dfrac{25}{100}$

improper fraction   a fraction in which A is greater than or equal to B

EX: $\dfrac{9}{5}$, $\dfrac{12}{12}$

When $A = B$, the fraction is equal to 1 whole (because $12 \div 12 = 1$). When adding or subtracting fractions, it is often useful to rewrite any whole number (e.g., 1, 12, 106, …) as a fraction ($\dfrac{1}{1}$, $\dfrac{12}{1}$, $\dfrac{106}{1}$, …).

mixed number   the sum of a whole number and a fraction, or just another way of writing an improper fraction

EX: $1\dfrac{4}{5}$ really means $1 + \dfrac{4}{5}$.

unit fraction   a fraction $\dfrac{A}{B}$, where $A = 1$

EX: $\dfrac{1}{5}$

complex fraction   a fraction $\dfrac{A}{B}$, where A and/or B are fractions

EX: $\dfrac{\frac{1}{4}}{\frac{4}{5}}$

equivalent fractions   equal fractions

EX: $\dfrac{1}{5} = \dfrac{10}{50} = \dfrac{100}{500}$. Each can be reduced to $\dfrac{1}{5}$.

In addition to types of fractions, here are other important terms to know.

greatest common factor   the largest number that divides evenly into two or more numbers

least common multiple   the smallest number that two or more numbers divide into evenly

relatively prime   term used to describe two or more numbers whose greatest common factor is 1

lowest terms   in a fraction $\dfrac{A}{B}$, where A and B are relatively prime

$$EX: \frac{4}{6} = \frac{2}{3}$$

least common denominator   the smallest denominator that two or more fractions have in common

reciprocal   the resulting fraction when you switch the numerator and denominator. The reciprocal of $\frac{A}{B}$ is $\frac{B}{A}$.

Note: The fraction $\frac{0}{B}$ has no reciprocal.

Converting Fractions

Converting Improper Fractions to Mixed Numbers

Let's take an example.

$$EX: \frac{9}{5} = 1\frac{4}{5}$$

1. Divide the denominator into the numerator: $9 \div 5$.

2. The result is the whole number part of the mixed number: 1.

3. The remainder becomes the numerator part of the mixed number: 4.

4. The original denominator becomes the denominator part of the mixed number: 5.

Converting a Mixed Number into an Improper Fraction

Again, let's use an example.

$$EX: 1\frac{4}{5} = \frac{9}{5}$$

1. Multiply the denominator by the whole number, and add the result to the numerator: $(5 \times 1) + 4$.

2. The answer becomes the numerator of the improper fraction: 9.

3. The denominator of the original mixed number becomes the denominator of the improper fraction: 5.

Reducing Fractions

Reducing fractions to their lowest terms is always a good idea. To reduce a fraction, divide its numerator and denominator by the *largest* number that divides evenly into both.

EX: To reduce $\frac{5}{10}$, divide both the numerator and the denominator by 5.

SECTION A

SECTION B

SECTION C

COMPREHENSIVE PRACTICE Test 1

COMPREHENSIVE PRACTICE Test 2

COMPREHENSIVE PRACTICE Test 3

$$\frac{5}{10} = \frac{5 \div 5}{10 \div 5} = \frac{1}{2}$$

EX: To reduce $\frac{18}{30}$, divide both the numerator and the denominator by 6.

$$\frac{18}{30} = \frac{18 \div 6}{30 \div 6} = \frac{3}{5}$$

Multiplying Fractions

Multiply the numerators, and multiply the denominators.

EX: $\frac{4}{5} \times \frac{2}{3} = \frac{8}{15}$

If you are multiplying mixed numbers, convert them to improper fractions and then multiply.

EX: $1\frac{2}{3} \times 3\frac{1}{2}$ can be converted to $\frac{5}{3} \times \frac{7}{2}$. After multiplying the fractions, the result is $\frac{35}{6}$. This can then be converted to a mixed fraction: $5\frac{5}{6}$.

Remember, you may need to reduce your final answer.

Dividing Fractions

Invert the second fraction, and then multiply the two fractions.

EX: $\frac{1}{5} \div \frac{2}{3} = \frac{1}{5} \times \frac{3}{2} = \frac{3}{10}$

EX: $15 \div \frac{2}{3} = \frac{15}{1} \times \frac{3}{2} = \frac{45}{2} = 22\frac{1}{2}$

Adding and Subtracting Fractions

To add or subtract fractions, all of the fractions in the problem must have the *same* (or *common*) *denominator*. Given common denominators, simply add or subtract the numerators. *Do not* add or subtract the denominators. (Also reduce the answer, if necessary.)

EX: $\frac{4}{15} + \frac{8}{15} = \frac{12}{15} = \frac{4}{5}$

Given *different denominators*, convert the fractions into equivalent fractions with common denominators. In other words, all of the fractions in the problem must have the same denominator. To make this conversion:

- First determine the *lowest common denominator* (*LCD*), which is the smallest number that divides evenly into all denominators in the problem.

EX: To add the fractions $\frac{1}{4} + \frac{5}{6}$, determine the smallest number that 4 and 6 go into (i.e., the LCD). Both denominators (4 and 6) go into 12 (and no lower number), so 12 is the LCD.

- Now convert the original fractions into equivalent fractions with the common denominator. To accomplish this, multiply the numerator and denominator of each fraction by a whole number fraction that makes the denominator equal to the LCD. For the first fraction:

EX: $\frac{1}{4} \cdot \frac{3}{3} = \frac{3}{12}$. The first fraction now has the LCD.

Do the same with any other fraction in the problem. Choose a number that gives each fraction the LCD.

EX: $\frac{5}{6} \cdot \frac{2}{2} = \frac{10}{12}$. The second fraction now has the LCD. The two fractions are equivalent.

Now the fractions can be added.

EX: $\frac{3}{12} + \frac{10}{12} = \frac{13}{12} = 1\frac{1}{12}$

The same procedure applies to subtraction.

EX: $\frac{5}{8} - \frac{1}{5} = \frac{25}{40} - \frac{8}{40} = \frac{17}{40}$

DECIMALS

Like fractions, decimals allow you to represent part of a whole, the entire whole, or more than the whole. To represent these different amounts, decimals use place values to the right of the decimal point. In as much as fractions use different denominators to do the same thing, it seems that decimals are really a type of fraction! Use the following example to review some of the place values used in decimals. The place values in the following example may be continued indefinitely.

EX: 78.123456   1 = tenths place

2 = hundredths place

3 = thousandths place

4 = ten-thousandths place

5 = hundred-thousandths place

6 = millionths place

…

EX:

0.78 is read, "Seventy-eight hundredths."

2.305 is read, "Two and three hundred five-thousandths."

To make the connection between decimals and fractions a little clearer, here are some decimals converted to fractions with denominators of 10, 100, 1,000, and so on.

EX:

$$0.1 = \frac{1}{10}$$

$$0.23 = \frac{23}{100}$$

$$2.75 = 2\frac{75}{100}$$

$$0.005 = \frac{5}{1,000}$$

Converting Between Fractions and Decimals

Fraction to Decimal

To convert a fraction into a decimal, divide the denominator into the numerator.

EX: $\frac{2}{5}$ = 2 divided by 5 = 0.4

EX: $2\frac{3}{4}$ = 2 + (3 divided by 4) = 2.75

Decimal to Fraction

To convert a decimal into a fraction, you must know the place value of the decimal. The place value tells you the denominator of the fraction.

EX: The decimal 0.86 is read as, "Eighty-six hundredths." This means your denominator is 100. Therefore, $0.86 = \frac{86}{100} = \frac{43}{50}$.

The decimal $0.235 = \frac{235}{1,000} = \frac{47}{200}$. (The first fraction was reduced by dividing 5 into the numerator and the denominator.)

Adding and Subtracting Decimals

The only difference between adding or subtracting decimals and whole numbers is the decimal point. To add or subtract decimals, line up the decimals on their decimal points (and, more importantly, on the place values). Lining up the decimal point ensures that you add tenths to tenths, hundredths to hundredths, and so on. You just have to *be careful!*

EX: Given the problem 2.34 + 8.56, set it up as follows:

$$
\begin{array}{r}
2.34 \\
+\ 8.56 \\
\hline
10.90
\end{array}
$$

Or, 23.8 − 7.09 is the same as:

$$
\begin{array}{r}
23.80 \\
-\ \ 7.09 \\
\hline
16.71
\end{array}
$$

(It is OK to add a zero after the decimal point.)

Multiplying Decimals

You do not have to line up the decimal points when you are multiplying decimals. In fact, you do not have to worry about the decimal points until the very end of the problem. To multiply decimals:

1. Multiply the numbers as you would normally.

2. Count the number of decimal places in each number you are multiplying, and add them.

3. Starting from the right end in your product, count from right to left the same number of places as your answer in step 2.

Do not panic! This sounds complicated, but it is really not. Here is an example:

EX: *Step 1: Multiply as you normally would.*

$$
\begin{array}{r}
23.74 \\
\times\ 16.5 \\
\hline
391710
\end{array}
$$

Your answer has no decimal yet, and that is OK!

Step 2: Count the number of decimal places in each number you are multiplying, and add them up.

23.74	2 decimal places
16.5	1 decimal place
3	total decimal places

Step 3: Starting from the right end in your product, count to the left the same number of places as your answer in step 2. The answer is 391.710.

Try another example.

EX: $\begin{array}{r} 42.3 \\ \times\ 1.6 \\ \hline 67.68 \end{array}$ Given a total of 2 decimal places up here …

place a total of 2 decimal places down here.

SECTION A

SECTION B

SECTION C

COMPREHENSIVE PRACTICE Test 1

COMPREHENSIVE PRACTICE Test 2

COMPREHENSIVE PRACTICE Test 3

Multiplying Decimals by Powers of 10

There is a very useful shortcut worth knowing when it comes to *multiplying* decimals by powers of 10 (10, 100, 1,000, and so on): Move the decimal point to the *right* the same number of places as there are zeros in the power of 10.

EX: Given 45.67 × 100, the decimal point moves two places to the right: : 45.67 becomes 4,567.

Given 123.456 × 1,000, the decimal moves three places to the right: 123,456.

Similarly, if you are multiplying by tenths, hundredths, or thousandths, you would move the decimal to the left one, two, or three places.

45.67 × .1 =4.567   the decimal moves one place to the left

334.5 × .01=3.345   the decimal moves two places to the left

Dividing Decimals

You need to learn only a few steps to make dividing decimals as simple as dividing whole numbers:

1. Multiply the divisor by the appropriate power of 10 to make it a whole number.

2. Multiply the dividend by the same power of 10.

3. Bring the decimal point up to the top of the box, and place it directly over the decimal in the dividend.

EX: Given $0.25\overline{)0.625}$, multiply the divisor by the appropriate power of 10, in this case 100, to make it a whole number: 25.

$25\overline{)0.625}$

Multiply the dividend by 100 to turn 0.625 into 62.5.

$25\overline{)62.5}$

Now divide normally. Remember to bring the decimal point up to the top of the box: place it directly over the decimal in the dividend.

$$25\overline{)62.5} \quad \begin{array}{c} 2.5 \\ \end{array}$$

Here is another example:

EX: Given $1.3\overline{)1.56}$, multiply both the divisor and the dividend by 10.

$13\overline{)15.6}$

Now you may divide normally. Just remember to place the decimal in the quotient.

$$13\overline{)15.6} \quad \begin{array}{c} 1.2 \\ \end{array}$$

The decimal in the quotient is directly over the decimal in the dividend.

SECTION A

SECTION B

SECTION C

COMPREHENSIVE PRACTICE Test 1

COMPREHENSIVE PRACTICE Test 2

COMPREHENSIVE PRACTICE Test 3

Dividing Decimals by Powers of 10

There is a very useful shortcut worth knowing when it comes to dividing decimals by powers of 10 (10, 100, 1,000, etc.): Move the decimal point to the *left* in the dividend by the same number of places as there are zeros in the power of 10.

EX: Given $45.67 \div 100$, move the decimal point two places to the left: $45.67 \div 100 = 0.4567$.

Sometimes you have to add one or more zeros after the decimal.

EX: Given $23.45 \div 1,000$, move the decimal point three places to the left: $23.45 \div 1,000 = 0.02345$.

PERCENTAGES

A *percentage* is really a fraction with a denominator of 100. The percentage symbol (%) is another way of writing a denominator of 100.

EX:

25% is really $\frac{25}{100}$.

3% is really $\frac{3}{100}$.

Looking at percentages in this way, you can readily see that percentages less than 100% are really fractions less than 1 whole and that percentages greater than 100% are really fractions greater than 1 whole.

EX:

$10\% = \frac{10}{100}$, which is less than 1 whole.

$150\% = \frac{150}{100}$, which is greater than 1 whole.

Converting Between Decimals, Fractions, and Percentages

To convert a decimal to a percentage, multiply by 100.

EX: 0.426: $0.426 \times 100 = 42.6\%$

EX: 55, or 55.0: $55.0 \times 100 = 5,500\%$

To convert a percentage to a decimal, divide by 100.

EX: 45%: $45\% \div 100 = 0.45$

EX: 12.5%: $12.5\% \div 100 = 0.125$

To convert a fraction to a percentage:

1. Change the fraction to a decimal.

2. Change the decimal to a percentage.

EX: $\dfrac{2}{5} = 0.4 = 40\%$

EX: $\dfrac{9}{2} = 4.5 = 450\%$

To convert a percentage to a fraction:

1. Change the percentage to a fraction.

2. Reduce the fraction.

EX: $35\% = \dfrac{35}{100} = \dfrac{7}{20}$

EX: $6\% = \dfrac{6}{100} = \dfrac{3}{50}$

You should be familiar with the common fractional-to-decimal equivalents in the following list. If you learn these, you can convert quickly among many fractions, decimals, and percentages.

The bar over a digit (or digits) means that the decimal places repeat to infinity (e.g., 0.3 goes on forever: 0.33333 . . .).

Fraction	Decimal	Percentage
$\dfrac{1}{4}$	0.25	25%
$\dfrac{2}{4} = \dfrac{1}{2}$	0.5	50%
$\dfrac{3}{4}$	0.75	75%
$\dfrac{1}{3}$	0.3	33.3%
$\dfrac{2}{3}$	0.6	66.6%
$\dfrac{1}{5}$	0.2	20%
$\dfrac{2}{5}$	0.4	40%
$\dfrac{3}{5}$	0.6	60%

$\dfrac{4}{5}$	0.8	80%
$\dfrac{1}{8}$	0.125	12.5%
$\dfrac{3}{8}$	0.375	37.5%
$\dfrac{5}{8}$	0.625	62.5%
$\dfrac{7}{8}$	0.875	87.5%

Basic percentage problems have three components:

1. The percent.

2. The base.

3. The percentage.

 EX: Given that 25% of 200 is 50,

 25% = the percent,

 200 = the base, and

 50 = the percentage.

It often helps to turn a percentage problem into an equation, and you usually need to turn the percentage into a decimal (i.e., divide it by 100).

 EX: Given "25% of 200 is 50," change "of" to "multiply" ($\times$), and "is" to "equals" (=).

 $0.25 \times 200 = 50$

Basic Percentage Problems

 To find the percentage of a given number, multiply the percentage by the number.

 EX: What is 10% of 50?

 $x = 0.1 \times 50 = 5$

To find the base when you know the percent and the percentage, set up an equation and divide both sides by the percentage.

SECTION A

SECTION B

SECTION C

COMPREHENSIVE PRACTICE Test 1

COMPREHENSIVE PRACTICE Test 2

COMPREHENSIVE PRACTICE Test 3

EX: Five (the percentage) is 10% (the percent) of what number (the base)? In the following equation, the base is x.

$0.1 \times x = 5$

$$\frac{0.1x}{0.1} = \frac{5}{0.1}$$ Divide both sides by 0.1 to solve for x.

$x = 50$ This is your answer.

Find the percentage when you know the base and the percent.

EX: What percentage of 50 is 5? Make the percentage of 50 (x) the percentage of 50. Then divide both sides by 50.

$x\% \times 50 = 5$

$x = 0.1$

Then turn 0.1 into a percentage by multiplying by 100: $0.1 \times 100 = 10\%$.

Percentage Discount and Tax Increase

To find the amount of discount or increase when the percentage is known:

1. Change the percentage to a decimal (or fraction).

2. Multiply by the original cost.

3. Add or subtract accordingly.

EX: A $250 stereo is discounted 18%. Find the new sale price.

Convert 18% to a decimal by dividing by 100, and multiply the decimal (0.18) by $250.

$18\% \div 100 = 0.18$

$0.18 \times \$250 = \$45$

Then subtract $45 (the 18% decrease) from $250 (the original cost) to find the new cost.

$\$250 - \$45 = \$205$

You can also subtract 18% from 100% to find that the discounted price is 82% of the original price and then calculate 82% of $250 (0.82 \times \$250)$.

Percentage Increase and Decrease

Often the problem asks you to determine the percentage of increase or decrease. This type of problem is easily solved by making a fraction out of the information provided.

1. Write the amount of increase or decrease as the numerator.

2. Write the original amount as the denominator.

3. Change the fraction to a percentage.

EX: My little brother grew from 60 to 66 inches in the last year. What percentage increase is this?

The amount of increase is 6 inches. Make this the numerator, and make his original height (60 inches) the denominator. Then change the fraction to a percentage.

$$\frac{6}{60} = \frac{1}{10} = 0.1 = 10\%$$

My little brother's height increased by 10%.

RATIO AND PROPORTION

A *ratio* is a comparison of two numbers, usually by division.

EX: In a class of 15 people, there are 7 boys and 8 girls. The ratio of boys to girls is 7 to 8, or 7:8, or $\frac{7}{8}$.

A *rate* is a ratio made up of two different units of measurement or amounts.

EX: I can drive my car 250 mi on 10 gal of gas. This relationship can be expressed as a ratio of miles to gallons: 250 to 10, 250:10, or $\frac{250 \text{ mi}}{10 \text{ gal}} = \frac{25}{1}$, or 25 miles per gallon.

A *proportion* is an equation of two equal ratios. All proportion equations have a special property: *Cross products are equal.* When you multiply the numerator on the left side of the equation by the denominator on the other side and then multiply the left-side denominator by the right-side numerator, the products are equal to each other. This is called *cross-multiplying*.

EX: If my car gets 25 miles to the gallon, then how many gallons do I need to drive 125 miles?

Set up a proportion to solve this problem. Make sure you align your units correctly on both sides of the equation: in this case, miles across from miles and gallons across from gallons.

$$\frac{25 \text{ mi}}{1 \text{ gal}} = \frac{125 \text{ mi}}{x \text{ gal}}$$

Now cross-multiply:

$$25x = 125$$

Now divide both sides by 25 to solve for x.

$$x = 5$$

This is your answer in gallons. You need 5 gal to go 125 mi.

Use proportions when converting from one form of measurement to another.

EX: If 1 qt equals 0.9 L, how many liters equal 4.5 qt?

Set up a proportion. Again, be sure to align the units correctly: qt across from qt and L across from L.

$$\frac{1 \text{ qt}}{0.9 \text{ L}} = \frac{4.5 \text{ qt}}{x \text{ L}}$$

Cross-multiply to solve for x.

$$x = 4.5 \times 0.9$$
$$x = 4.05 \text{ L}$$

This is your answer in liters: 4.05 L equals 4.5 qt.

You may also use proportions when you are working with scaled measurements.

EX: The scale on a map is 1 cm for every 15 km. If the actual distance traveled is 78 km, how far is the same distance on the map?

Set up a proportion to solve this problem. Be sure to align cm across from cm, and km across from km.

$$\frac{1 \text{ cm}}{15 \text{ km}} = \frac{x \text{ cm}}{78 \text{ km}}$$

Cross-multiply, and divide both sides by 15 to solve for x.

$$15x = 78$$
$$x = 5.2$$

This is your answer in centimeters: 78 km equals 5.2 cm on the map.

BASIC ALGEBRA

Algebra makes use of letters and symbols (called *variables*) as well as numbers. All of the same rules you learned for arithmetic apply in algebra. However, algebra contains many new rules, and this review presents some of them.

Key Terms

First, learn the following terms:

variable	a symbol, usually a letter, that takes the place of a number (Very often you need to substitute a number for a letter in an expression or to solve an equation for a certain variable.)
algebraic expression	a collection of numbers and variables connected by signs and symbols

EX: $3x$, $2y^3 + 4$, $\sqrt{6x}$, $-5 + c$, $a-b$

term   an individual piece of an expression

EX: $3x$ $2y^3 + 4$ 5 $a-b+c$

    1 term   2 terms   1 term   3 terms

In the term "$3x$," 3 is the *numerical coefficient*. It is a number (or numeral), and it is also a factor (because 3 and x are being multiplied).

In the term "$2y^3 + 4$," 2 is the numerical coefficient (or just the coefficient).

like terms   terms with the same variables *and* same exponents

EX:	
Like terms:	x^2 and $3x^2$, and $2a^2b$ and $29ba^2$
Unlike terms:	$2x$ and $4y$, and x^3 and x^2
equation	two equal expressions
EX:	

$$2y - 8y^2 - 9 = 0$$

$$a^2 - b^2 = c^2$$

$$f + 7 = f^2 - 24$$

$$2(x - 4) + x^2 = 3x - 8$$

Evaluating Expressions and Order of Operations

To *evaluate* means to find the value of something. When you are asked to evaluate an algebraic expression, you need to substitute a number for a variable in the expression and then simplify the expression. To simplify the expression, you have to follow the *order of operations*, which is simply a set of rules guaranteeing that you perform operations (addition, multiplication, etc.) in the proper order:

1. Start from the innermost set of grouping symbols (parentheses, brackets, or braces) and perform the operations within. Once you have performed those operations, remove the grouping symbols.

2. Simplify all exponents or radicals.

3. Multiply or divide, moving from left to right.

4. Add or subtract, moving from left to right.

A mneumonic device to help remember the order of operations is, "Please Excuse My Dear Aunt Sally."

P = parentheses

E = exponents

M = multiplying left to right

D = dividing left to right

A = adding left to right

S = subtracting left to right

EX: Evaluate $6x^2 \times (4 + 3x) - 6 + (x^2 \div 2)$, when $x = 2$. First, substitute 2 for x.

Parentheses:	$6(2)^2 \times (4 + 3[2]) - 6 + (2^2 \div 2) =$
Parentheses:	$6(2)^2 \times (4 + 6) - 6 + (4 \div 2) =$
Parentheses:	$6(2)^2 \times 10 - 6 + 2 =$
Exponents:	$6(4) \times 10 - 6 + 2 =$

Multiply and divide: $24 \times 10 - 6 + 2 =$

Add and subtract: $240 - 6 + 2 = 236$

Distributive Property

A key concept in algebra is the *distributive property*, by which a term is distributed over (or multiplied by) two or more terms.

EX: In the equation $6(x + 3) = 6x + 18$, 6 is a factor that has been distributed (multiplied) over the x and the 3. Similarly,

$$-5(y - 2x) = -5y + 10x$$

$$-(4x + 7y) = -1(4x + 7y) = -4x - 7y$$

Property of Zero

Another key concept in algebra is the *property of zero*, which states that, in a multiplication problem, if one of the factors is zero, then the product must be zero. Another way of stating this rule is:

If $a \times b = 0$, then either $a = 0$ or $b = 0$

This property also works in reverse. That is, if you know that one (or more) of the factors in a multiplication problem is zero, then the product will be zero. Stated another way:

If $a = 0$ or $b = 0$, then $a \times b = 0$

This property is essential in solving equations involving squared terms.

Simplifying Expressions and Solving Equations

At the heart and soul of algebra is simplifying expressions and solving equations. If you learn to master these two skills, you are in good shape.

To *simplify expressions*, combine (i.e., add or subtract) like terms. You may not combine unlike terms. To combine like terms, add their numerical coefficients; the exponents remain unchanged.

EX: Simplify the following equation:

$6 + x^2 - 2x - 5x^2 + 6x + 9 + 5x^3$

Combine like terms.

$-4x^2 + 4x + 15 + 5x^3$

This is the simplified expression.

Solving Equations

You must remember two essential rules whenever you are solving equations:

1. The goal is to *isolate the variable*, that is, get it by itself on one side of the equals sign.

2. The method is to *do the same thing to both sides of the equation, using inverse operations*.

If you remember these two rules, you will be able to solve almost any equation!

EX: Solve for x:

$7x - 10 = 11$

First, isolate the variable x. Add 10 (the inverse of subtraction) to both sides.

$7x - 10 + 10 = 11 + 10$

$\qquad 7x = 21$

Next, divide (the inverse of multiply) both sides by 7.

$\dfrac{7x}{7} = \dfrac{21}{7}$

$\quad x = 3$

To check your answer, substitute 3 for x in the original equation and simplify it.

$\quad 7x - 10 = 11$

$7(3) - 10 = 11$

$\quad 21 - 10 = 11$

$\qquad 11 = 11$

If the left side equals the right side, you have done it right!

Sometimes you may need to combine like terms on one (or both sides) of the equation before you use inverse operations.

EX: Given $19z - 10 + 4z = 3z - 4$, combine $19z$ and $4z$ on the left side.

$23z - 10 = 3z - 4$

Add 10 to both sides.

$23z = 3z + 6$

Subtract $3z$ from both sides.

$20z = 6$

Divide both sides by 20 to solve for z.

$z = \dfrac{6}{20} = \dfrac{3}{10}$

This is your answer.

EX: Given $5(x + 3) + 9 = 3(x - 2) + 6$, distribute 5 and 3.

$5x + 15 + 9 = 3x - 6 + 6$

Combine like terms.

$5x + 24 = 3x$

Subtract $5x$ from both sides.

$24 = -2x$

SECTION A

SECTION B

SECTION C

COMPREHENSIVE PRACTICE Test 1

COMPREHENSIVE PRACTICE Test 2

COMPREHENSIVE PRACTICE Test 3

Divide both sides by -2.

$-12 = x$

This is your answer.

Clearing Fractions

If the equation contains fractions, you can change them to whole numbers. This is called *clearing fractions*. To clear the fractions, multiply each term in the equation by the LCD of the fractions.

EX: In the equation $\frac{3}{5}y + 2 = \frac{1}{2}y$, the LCD is 10, because both 5 and 2 are factors of 10. Multiply each fraction by a number that makes the denominator equal to the LCD.

$\frac{3}{5} \times \frac{2}{2} = \frac{6}{10}$ and $\frac{1}{2} \times \frac{5}{5} = \frac{5}{10}$ for $\frac{6}{10}y + 20 = \frac{5}{10}$

Reduce the fractions, by multiplying both sides by 10, to get whole numbers.

$6y + 20 = 5y$ or $5y = 6y + 20$

Subtract $6y$ from both sides.

$-y = 20$

Never leave the variable negative. Multiply both sides by -1.

$y = -20$

This is your answer.

Systems of Equations

A *system of equations* is merely two or more equations (with two or more of the same variables) that are worked on at the same time. To solve a system of equations with two variables, look for a pair of variables (i.e., values of x and y) that makes both equations true at the same time (i.e., makes each left side equal to the corresponding right side) at the same time. You can solve a system of equations by adding the equations together to eliminate either the x-terms or the y-terms. To eliminate either one, both need to have the same coefficient but be opposite in sign.

Ex: $2y$ and $-2y$

Here is an example.

EX: The following is a system of equations:

$x + 2y = 12$ and $7x - 2y = 4$

Add the equations.

$$
\begin{array}{r}
x + 2y = 12 \\
+\ 7x - 2y = 4 \\
\hline
8x = 16
\end{array}
$$

Divide both sides by 8 to solve for x.

$x = 2$

Now substitute 2 for x into either of the original equations to solve for y, subtract 2 from both sides, and divide both sides by 2.

$x + 2y = 12$

$2 + 2y = 12$

$2y = 10$

$y = 5$

So you now know that $x = 2$ and $y = 5$. This pair of values makes both equations true.

If the equations do not already have terms with the same coefficients but opposite signs, you must multiply the equations by the appropriate number. Make sure to multiply *each term* in the equation by the number you choose.

EX:

$5x - 2y = -25$ and $3x + y = -4$

Multiply both sides of the second equation by 2.

$2 \times (3x + y) = 2 \times -4$

$6x + 2y = -8$

Now the equations can be added together to eliminate the y-terms.

$5x - 2y = -25$

$6x + 2y = -8$

$11x = -33$

Divide both sides by 11.

$x = -3$

Now substitute -3 for x into either of the original equations to solve for y:

$3x + y = -4$

$3(-3) + y = -4$

Simplify.

$-9 + y = -4$

Add 9 to both sides.

$y = 5$

This pair of values ($x = -3$, $y = 5$) makes both equations true.

SECTION A

SECTION B

SECTION C

COMPREHENSIVE PRACTICE Test 1

COMPREHENSIVE PRACTICE Test 2

COMPREHENSIVE PRACTICE Test 3

Word Problems

Word problems are often described as everyone's least favorite topic in algebra, and yet solving word problems is the area in which algebra is most useful. Also true is that, of all the aspects of solving word problems, people find it most difficult to translate the words into equations. Once this is done, however, the rest is just algebra! Here are a few tips to help you solve word problems:

- Express the unknown quantity as a variable (or variables).

- Think "addition" when you hear "increased by," "more than," and "total."

- Think "subtraction" when you read "decreased by," "less than," or "less."

- "is" means "="

- Multiplication is usually the required function when you hear "of" (e.g., "one-fourth of 12").

- Recall the vocabulary words "sum," "difference," "product," and "quotient."

A note about the word "difference" is that, if the word problem says, "The difference of a number and 3 is 2," you may assume that the order of the subtraction equation is the same as the order of the word problem.

In this case, let x = a number that satisfies the equation $x - 3 = 2$.

EX: The sum of twice a number and the number is 36. Find the number.

There are clues in the wording that help you construct the equation.

The word "sum" tells you that you need to write an addition equation.

You may choose x to stand for the number by writing a so-called *let statement:* Let x = the number.

The word "is" tells you where to put the equals sign.

So, if the sum of twice a number and the number is 36, then the equation is

$2x + x = 36$

But what is the value x? To arrive at the answer, you have to guess at and try probable values. In this case, try 12.

$$2x + x = 36$$
$$2(12) + 12 = 36$$
$$3x = 36$$
$$24 + 12 = 36$$
$$36 = 36$$

So $x = 12$. This is your answer.

SECTION **A**

SECTION **B**

SECTION **C**

COMPREHENSIVE PRACTICE **Test 1**

COMPREHENSIVE PRACTICE **Test 2**

COMPREHENSIVE PRACTICE **Test 3**

Formulas

Formulas are special types of equations that express a relationship between variables.

EX: The formula $A = \dfrac{1}{2}bh$ is for the area of a triangle, where

A = area, b = base, and h = height.

Usually you are given values for all but one of the variables, and you need to solve the equation for that variable.

EX: Find the area of triangle with base of 10 cm and height of 15 cm. In the area formula, substitute 10 cm for b and 15 cm for h.

$$A = \frac{1}{2}bh$$

$$A = \frac{1}{2} \times 10 \times 15$$

Simplify.

$$A = 75 \text{ cm}^2$$

Inequalities

Earlier we defined an equation as two equal expressions. An *inequality* is two unequal expressions.

EX:

$$2x < 8$$

$$y^2 - 9 > 0$$

$$a^2 + b^2 \leq c$$

$$13x + 4 \geq 275$$

In the preceding inequalities:

- $<$ means "less than."
- $\leq$ is read "less than or equal to".
- $>$ is "greater than."
- $\geq$ is "greater than or equal to."

The rules for solving inequalities are the same as for solving equations, with one important difference. Your goal and method are still the same: to isolate the variable and to do the same thing to both sides of the inequality using inverse operations.

EX: Given the inequality $2x < 8$, divide both sides by 2 to solve for x.

$$x < 4$$

This is your answer. The variable x is equal to all values less than (but not including) 4.

Look at another example.

EX: In the inequality $8a - 7 > 17$, add 7 to both sides.

$8a > 24$

Divide both sides by 8.

$a > 3$

This is your answer.

Here is the crucial new rule that applies only to inequalities: When multiplying or dividing by a negative number, reverse the inequality sign.

EX: Given the inequality $-5y + 6 \geq 11$, subtract 6 from both sides.

$-5y \geq 5$

Now divide by -5. Here is where this new rule comes in!

$y \leq -1$

Notice that the sign reversed from $\geq$ to $\leq$. Don't forget it!

Exponent Rules

You must follow certain rules when working with variables and exponents.

1. When multiplying similar bases, *add the exponents.*

   EX: $J^3 \cdot J^4 = J^7$

2. When dividing similar bases, *subtract the exponents.*

   EX: $r^4 \div r^3 = r^{4-3} = r^1$

3. When raising a power to another power, *multiply the exponents.*

   EX: $(s^2)^3 = s^{2 \cdot 3} = s^6$

4. When the exponent is negative, *move its base to the denominator and make the exponent positive. Take care to move only the bases with negative exponents.*

EX: $d^{-2} = \dfrac{1}{d^2}$

Or: $mr^{-3} = \dfrac{m}{r^3}$

In this example, leave m in the numerator and move r to the denominator.

5. *Any base (except zero) to the zero power equals 1.*

EX:

$k^0 = 1$

$4^0 = 1$

Basic Geometry | 97

SECTION A

SECTION B

SECTION C

COMPREHENSIVE PRACTICE Test 1

COMPREHENSIVE PRACTICE Test 2

COMPREHENSIVE PRACTICE Test 3

Factoring

Factoring is the opposite of distributing. Recall that the distributive property involved multiplying factors to find a product. When factoring, then:

- Start with the product and try to find its *common factor* (the one found in all of the terms).

  EX: In $4y + 10 - 8x$, each term contains a 2.

- Divide all terms by the common factor.

  EX: In $4y + 10 - 8x$, divide each term by 2: $4y + 10 - 8x$ becomes $2(2y + 5 - 4x)$.

  Note that if you were to distribute the 2, you would arrive at the original expression. This means you have factored correctly!

Try another couple of examples.

  EX:

  In $24x + 72y + 8$, the common factor is 8. The factored form is $8(3x + 9y + 1)$.

  In $5x + 2x^2 + x^3$, the common factor is x. The factored form is $x(5 + 2x + x^2)$

Remember, when you divide like bases, you subtract exponents.

BASIC GEOMETRY

Geometry is the study of shapes and figures in two dimensions (*planar geometry*) and in three dimensions (*solid geometry*). The following table contains key formulas about area, perimeter, and volume.

Area of a circle	$A = \pi r^2$ $A = $ area $\pi = 3.14$ $r = $ radius	
Area of a rectangle	$A = lw$ $A = $ area $l = $ length $w = $ width	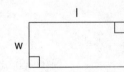
Area of a square	$A = s^2$ $A = $ area $s = $ side	
Area of a triangle	$A = \dfrac{1}{2} bh$ $A = $ area $b = $ base $h = $ height	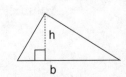

Circumference of a circle
(distance around outside)

$C = \pi d$
C = circumference
π = 3.14
d = diameter

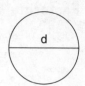

Perimeter of a rectangle
(length around outside)

$P = 2l + 2w$
P = perimeter
l = length
w = width

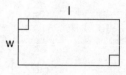

Perimeter of a square

$P = 4s$
P = perimeter
s = side

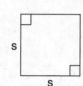

Perimeter of a triangle

$P = a + b + c$
P = perimeter
a, b, c = sides

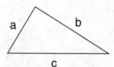

Pythagorean theorem
(applies only to
right triangles)

$a^2 + b^2 = c^2$
a, b = sides
c = hypotenuse

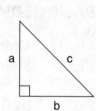

Surface area of a cube
(total area of all 6 faces)

$SA = 6s^2$
SA = surface area
s = side

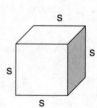

Surface area of a rectangular
solid (total area of all 6 faces)

$SA = 2lw + 2wh + 2lh$
SA = surface area
l = length
w = width
h = height

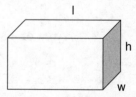

Volume of a cube

$V = s^3$
V = volume
s = side

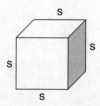

SECTION A

SECTION B

SECTION C

COMPREHENSIVE PRACTICE Test 1

COMPREHENSIVE PRACTICE Test 2

COMPREHENSIVE PRACTICE Test 3

Volume of a rectangular solid $V = lwh$
                                       V = volume
                                       l = length
                                       w = width
                                       h = height

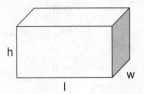

Measurements

English System

Linear	Capacity	Weight
inch (in)	ounce (oz)	ounce (oz)
foot (ft = 12 in)	pint (pt = 16 oz)	pound (lb = 16 oz)
yard (yd = 3 ft)	quart (qt = 2 pt)	ton (T = 2,000 lb)
	gallon (gal = 4 qt)	

Metric System

The metric system is based on powers of 10. This makes converting between different units of metric measurement quite simple: You need only multiply or divide by the correct power of 10 (10, 100, 1,000, and so on). The basic units are:

Linear	Capacity	Weight
meter	liter	gram

The following chart lists the metric prefixes and thus illustrates the relationship between metric units. You should be familiar with the prefixes, which always mean the same thing, regardless of whether you are working with linear, square, or cubic measurements.

milli	centi	deci	unit	deca	hecto	kilo
0.001	0.01	0.1	1	10	100	1,000

EX:

1 kilometer (km) = 10 hectometers (hm)

1 gram (g) = 1,000 milligrams (mg)

1 liter (L) = 10 deciliters (dL)

Points, Lines, and Planes

Points, lines, planes (and angles, the subject of the next section) are the basics of geometry—the building blocks for all else. As usual, we begin with basic terms.

line	always a straight line, extending in opposite directions to infinity (e.g., a beam of light or straight train tracks)
point	a self-evident definition (A line is composed of an infinite number of points.)
segment	a portion of a line, composed of a finite set of points

endpoints	the beginning and end points of the segment
ray	a portion of a line with only one endpoint, thus extending only in one direction to infinity
plane	a flat area that extends in two directions (length and width) to infinity (A tabletop and a blackboard are examples of portions of planes.)

In a plane, lines are either:

- *parallel lines*, or lines that never meet; parallel lines have no points in common.

EX: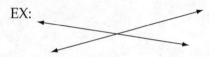

- *intersecting lines*, or lines that cross at one point; intersecting lines have one point in common.

EX: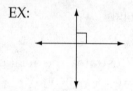

- *perpendicular lines*, or lines that intersect and form an angle of 90°; the small box (□) in the figure to the right indicates a right angle (90°).

EX:

Angles

Angles are two rays with a common endpoint. The endpoint is called the *vertex* of the angle, and the rays are called the *sides* of the angle. The size of an angle is measured in degrees (°).

acute angle	an angle greater than 0° and less than 90°
right angle	an angle that measures exactly 90°
obtuse angle	an angle greater than 90° and less than 180°
straight angle	an angle that measures exactly 180°
complementary angles	two or more angles whose sum is 90°
supplementary angles	two or more angles whose sum is 180°

Polygons

A *polygon* is a closed, two-dimensional figure that has more than two sides and that is composed of segments. Polygons are named by the number of sides they have. If all the sides of a polygon are the same length (such as an equilateral triangle or a square), it is called a *regular* polygon.

Triangles

A *triangle* is a polygon with three sides. Here are some key characteristics of triangles:

- The angles of a triangle always sum to 180°.

- If no two sides of a triangle are of the same length, then it is a *scalene* triangle. No two angles of a scalene triangle are equal to each other.

- If two sides of a triangle are of the same length, then it is an *isosceles* triangle. An isosceles triangle always has two equal angles.

- If all three sides of a triangle are the same length, then it is an *equilateral* triangle. All three angles of an equilateral triangle are 60°.

- If a triangle has a right angle, then it is a *right* triangle. The side opposite the right angle is the *hypotenuse*. The *Pythagorean theorem* applies to right triangles.

- If all three angles of a triangle are less than 90°, then it is an *acute* triangle.

- If one angle of the triangle is greater than 90°, then it is an *obtuse* triangle.

Quadilaterals

A *quadrilateral* is a polygon with four sides. Characteristics of quadrilaterals are as follows:

- The angles of a quadrilateral always sum to 360°.

- If a quadrilateral has four right angles, then it is a *rectangle*. In a rectangle, opposite sides are equal in length and are parallel.

- If all four sides of a rectangle are the same length, then it is a *square*.

Circles

A circle is actually not a polygon because it has an infinite number of sides. A *circle* is the set of all points equidistant (the same distance) from the center point. Refer to the diagram:

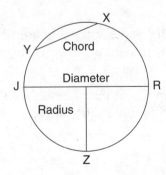

- The segment from *X* to *Y* is called a *chord*. It has both endpoints on the circle.

- The segment from *J* to *R* is called a *diameter*. All diameters are chords that pass through the center of the circle.

- The segment from the center to *Z* is called a *radius*. All radii are equal in length. A radius is always half the length of the diameter.

- Every circle contains 360°.

SECTION A

SECTION B

SECTION C

COMPREHENSIVE PRACTICE Test 1

COMPREHENSIVE PRACTICE Test 2

COMPREHENSIVE PRACTICE Test 3

Area

The *area* of a polygon is the space inside the polygon—the number of square units inside the polygon. Unlike linear, or straight-line, measurements (e.g., inches, meters), area is measured in square units (e.g., square yards, square centimeters). For important area formulas, refer to the chart of formulas at the beginning of this section on geometry. If you need to find the area of a figure for which you have no formula, you may subdivide the figure into polygons you recognize.

EX: To find the area of the following figure, introduce one perpendicular line, and find the total area of the resulting two figures: one triangle and one rectangle.

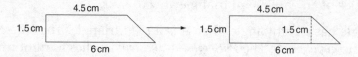

Area of rectangle: 1.5 cm × 4.5 cm = 6.75 cm².

Area of triangle: $\frac{1}{2}$ (1.5 cm × 1.5 cm) = 1.125 cm².

Area of figure: 6.75 cm² + 1.125 cm² = 7.875 cm².

Congruent polygons have the same size and the same shape. Polygons with the same area are not always congruent. The two rectangles in the diagram have the same area (0.75 in²), but they are not congruent.

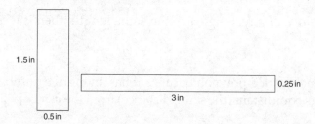

Similar polygons have the same shape but are not always the same size. The corresponding angles of similar polygons are equal to each other. The *ratios* of corresponding sides are equal to each other.

EX: The equilateral triangles in the diagram are similar. The corresponding sides in both triangles all have the same ratio, and the corresponding angles are all equal.

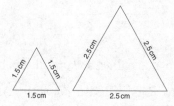

SECTION A

SECTION B

SECTION C

COMPREHENSIVE PRACTICE Test 1

COMPREHENSIVE PRACTICE Test 2

COMPREHENSIVE PRACTICE Test 3

I. Mathematics

45 Minutes

DIRECTIONS

The Mathematics Test section consists of four tests of 40 questions each. The questions are either computations or word problems. You should be able to answer all the questions in each test in 45 minutes. The correct answers with explanations of how they were solved will be found at the end of section B. **Work each problem carefully. You are not permitted to use a calculator to answer these questions.**

Each test question consists of an incomplete sentence or a question followed by four choices. Read each question carefully, then decide which choice is the correct answer. Your score will be the total number of correct answers. You may answer a question even if you are not completely sure of the correct response. Do not spend too much time on any one question. If you cannot answer a question, go on to the next question. Since it is important to be able to answer these questions in the allotted time, it is a good idea to use a timer.

1. 25% of 200 =
   a. 50
   b. 250
   c. 800
   d. 5000

2. 19% of $1,000 =
   a. $53
   b. $190
   c. $225
   d. $250

3. One inch equals 2.54 cm. How many centimeters tall is a 62-in woman?
   a. 24.41 cm
   b. 59.46 cm
   c. 64.54 cm
   d. 157.48 cm

4. $(3 \times 9) \div (5 \times 2) =$
   a. 0.27
   b. 0.37
   c. 2.7
   d. 7.5

5. Which of these numbers is a factor of 24?
   a. 8
   b. 16
   c. 32
   d. 48

6. A person buying a used car makes a down payment of $822.87 and 12 monthly payments of $91.43. What is the total amount paid?
   a. $914.30
   b. $1,097.16
   c. $1,188.59
   d. $1,920.03

7. What is the reciprocal of 3?
   a. $\frac{1}{9}$

   b. $\frac{1}{3}$

   c. $\frac{2}{3}$

   d. $1\frac{1}{3}$

8. If 1 km equals 0.625 mi, approximately how many miles will equal 4 km?
   a. 2.5 mi
   b. 3.375 mi
   c. 4.625 mi
   d. 6.4 mi

9. The sales tax in a large Eastern city is 8%. The cost of a $60.00 nursing encyclopedia, after the tax is added, is
   a. $68.00
   b. $67.50
   c. $64.80
   d. $60.80

10. In the number 978.92, the leftmost digit, 9, represents
    a. 9 ones.
    b. 9 tens.
    c. 9 hundreds.
    d. 9 thousands.

11. Which of these percentages is equal to 0.25?
    a. 0.0025%
    b. 0.25%
    c. 2.5%
    d. 25%

12. If hospital sheets are purchased in sets of 4 for $25.00 per set, and pillowcases are purchased in sets of 2 for $4.50 per set, what is the cost of 12 sheets and 24 pillowcases?
    a. $102
    b. $129
    c. $154
    d. $183

13. A room measures 12 ft by 15 ft by 8 ft. What is its volume?
    a. 216 ft^3
    b. 276 ft^3
    c. 1,360 ft^3
    d. 1,440 ft^3

14. If 1 dram equals 60 grains, how many drams are in 40 grains?
    a. $\dfrac{1}{3}$
    b. $\dfrac{2}{3}$
    c. $1\dfrac{1}{2}$
    d. 3

15. A vitamin capsule contained 2.3 mg riboflavin, but because of poor storage, 0.52 mg was lost. Find the number of milligrams left.
    a. 1.78 mg
    b. 1.82 mg
    c. 1.88 mg
    d. 2.22 mg

16. Which of these percentages equals 0.18?
    a. 0.18%
    b. 1.8%
    c. 18%
    d. 180%

17. At 12 noon the temperature was 68°F; at midnight it was 41°F. What was the average drop in temperature per hour?
    a. 2°
    b. 2.25°
    c. 13.5°
    d. 27°

18. A specific medication provides 3 mg of that medication per 5-mL dose. How many mL will be needed to provide 9 mg of the medication?
    a. 15 mL
    b. $5\dfrac{2}{3}$ mL
    c. 3 mL
    d. $1\dfrac{4}{5}$ mL

19. $\dfrac{3}{8} + \dfrac{1}{4} - \dfrac{1}{3} =$
    a. $\dfrac{7}{12}$
    b. $\dfrac{7}{24}$

SECTION A

SECTION B

SECTION C

COMPREHENSIVE PRACTICE Test 1

COMPREHENSIVE PRACTICE Test 2

COMPREHENSIVE PRACTICE Test 3

c. $\dfrac{1}{24}$

d. 0

20. During one winter season, the temperature ranged from a high of 33°F one day to a low of −20°F the next day. How many degrees Fahrenheit did the temperature fall?
    a. 7°
    b. 13°
    c. 17°
    d. 53°

21. A 3-ounce serving of corned beef hash supplies 155 calories. Approximately how many calories are supplied in a 5-ounce serving?
    a. 274 Cal
    b. 258 Cal
    c. 248 Cal
    d. 93 Cal

22. $8\dfrac{3}{4} - 5\dfrac{5}{12} =$

    a. $13\dfrac{1}{2}$

    b. $13\dfrac{3}{4}$

    c. $14\dfrac{1}{6}$

    d. $14\dfrac{2}{3}$

23. A hospital basketball team won 18 games and lost 12 games last season. What was the ratio of wins to losses?
    a. 5:4
    b. 3:2
    c. 2:3
    d. 3:5

24. The unit needs strips of adhesive tape that are $4\dfrac{1}{2}$ inches long. How many strips can be obtained from a 200-inch roll?
    a. 25
    b. 44
    c. 75
    d. 900

25. 45 is 60% of what number?
    a. 133.33
    b. 75
    c. 63
    d. 27

SECTION A

SECTION B

SECTION C

COMPREHENSIVE PRACTICE Test 1

COMPREHENSIVE PRACTICE Test 2

COMPREHENSIVE PRACTICE Test 3

26. $5a = 10b + 15$. If $b = 2$, then $a =$
   a. 3
   b. 5
   c. 7
   d. 35

27. Edna invests \$4,000 and receives yearly interest of \$200. What is the rate of interest on Edna's investment?
   a. 4%
   b. 5%
   c. 6%
   d. 8%

28. Fried's rule for computing an infant's dose of medication is:

   $$\text{infant's dose} = \frac{C}{150} \times \text{adult dose}$$

   where C = the child's age in months
   If the adult dose of medication is 25 mg, how much of that medication should be given to a 9-month-old infant?
   a. 0.06 mg
   b. 1.25 mg
   c. 1.5 mg
   d. 225 mg

29. A $\frac{1}{4}$-cup serving of cereal provides 96 calories. Approximately how many calories will be provided by a $\frac{7}{8}$-cup serving of this cereal?

   a. $67\frac{1}{5}$ Cal
   b. 84 Cal
   c. 336 Cal
   d. 384 Cal

30. $4 \times 5 \times 6 \times 0 =$
   a. 120
   b. 45
   c. 26
   d. 0

31. The recommended daily allowance for magnesium is 420 mg. Men ordinarily consume only 75% of this amount. How many mg of the recommended allowance is the average male missing each day?
   a. 105 mg
   b. 179 mg
   c. 315 mg
   d. 34 mg

32. Fourteen of the 42 students in a class are male. What portion of the class is female?

    a. $\dfrac{1}{3}$

    b. $\dfrac{1}{2}$

    c. $\dfrac{2}{3}$

    d. $\dfrac{3}{4}$

33. If $x = 46 + 0$, and $y = 64(0)$, then
    a. $x < y$
    b. $x = y$
    c. $x + y = 0$
    d. $x > y$

34. A student was billed $7.29 for a long-distance telephone call. The first 3 minutes cost $1.62, and 81 cents were charged for each additional minute. How long was the telephone call?
    a. 6 minutes
    b. 7 minutes
    c. 9 minutes
    d. 10 minutes

35. To make a pancake mix, $1\dfrac{1}{3}$ cups of nonfat milk are needed. You already have $\dfrac{3}{4}$ cup. How much more do you need?

    a. $\dfrac{7}{12}$ cup

    b. $\dfrac{5}{12}$ cup

    c. $\dfrac{2}{3}$ cup

    d. $\dfrac{5}{6}$ cup

36. If $x = 2$, then $x^3(x^2 - x) =$
    a. 16
    b. 12
    c. 6
    d. 0

37. If a person with an average daily total consumption of 3,000 Calories has 450 Calories for breakfast, what percentage of his total daily intake is consumed at breakfast?
    a. 7%
    b. 13.5%
    c. 15%
    d. 25%

38. $2.25 \div 0.15 =$
    a. 0.015
    b. 0.15
    c. 1.5
    d. 15

Questions 39 and 40 refer to the following figure.

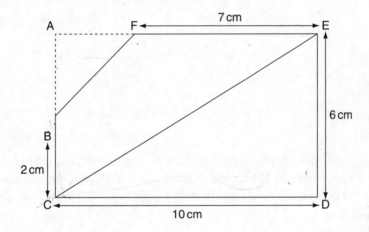

39. What is the area of triangle CED?
    a. 120 cm^2
    b. 60 cm^2
    c. 30 cm^2
    d. 16 cm^2

40. The triangle *BAF* is cut from the rectangle shown in the figure. What is the area of the remaining polygon *BCDEF*?
    a. 12 cm^2
    b. 48 cm^2
    c. 54 cm^2
    d. 60 cm^2

SECTION A

SECTION B

SECTION C

COMPREHENSIVE PRACTICE Test 1

COMPREHENSIVE PRACTICE Test 2

COMPREHENSIVE PRACTICE Test 3

II. Mathematics

Work each problem carefully. Use scrap paper to do your calculations. (The correct answers and explanations are at the end of Section B.)

1. $403 - 349 =$
   a. 54
   b. 55
   c. 154
   d. 256

2. According to Department of Agriculture guidelines, the acceptable range of weight for a 5'6" woman is 114 to 146 pounds. If a 5'6" woman weighs 160 pounds, how much is she over the maximum acceptable weight for her height?
   a. 14 lb
   b. 24 lb
   c. 32 lb
   d. 46 lb

3. $\dfrac{7}{8} - \dfrac{1}{3} =$
   a. $\dfrac{1}{3}$
   b. $\dfrac{13}{24}$
   c. $\dfrac{16}{11}$
   d. $\dfrac{5}{6}$

4. One teaspoon is equivalent to 60 drops. How many drops are in $1\dfrac{1}{4}$ teaspoons?
   a. 64
   b. 72
   c. 75
   d. 84

5. $8 + 4(5) =$
   a. 17
   b. 28
   c. 52
   d. 60

SECTION A

SECTION B

SECTION C

COMPREHENSIVE PRACTICE Test 1

COMPREHENSIVE PRACTICE Test 2

COMPREHENSIVE PRACTICE Test 3

6. A vial of penicillin contains 480,000 units. How many 80,000-unit doses can be made from the vial?
   a. 5
   b. 6
   c. 32
   d. 50

7. $\dfrac{3}{8} \times \dfrac{1}{4} =$

   a. $\dfrac{3}{2}$

   b. $\dfrac{3}{32}$

   c. $\dfrac{2}{3}$

   d. $\dfrac{13}{32}$

8. Frank has been taking 0.06-mL doses of medication. Which of these amounts represents a dose that is larger than Frank's dose?
   a. 0.009 mL
   b. 0.100 mL
   c. 0.006 mL
   d. 0.049 mL

9. $1.25 \div 0.05 =$
   a. 0.025
   b. 0.25
   c. 2.5
   d. 25

10. From a container holding $4\dfrac{1}{4}$ L of sterile water, $2\dfrac{1}{2}$ L were used. How many liters remain?

    a. $1\dfrac{3}{4}$ L

    b. $2\dfrac{1}{8}$ L

    c. $2\dfrac{1}{4}$ L

    d. $2\dfrac{3}{4}$ L

11. To get 1 as an answer, you must multiply $\dfrac{3}{4}$ by

    a. $\dfrac{3}{4}$

    b. 1

c. $\dfrac{4}{3}$

d. $1\dfrac{1}{4}$

12. A patient's cholesterol intake is 300 mg on Monday, 120 mg on Tuesday, 80 mg on Wednesday, and 100 mg on Thursday. What is her average cholesterol intake over the 4 days?
   a. 125 mg
   b. 150 mg
   c. 240 mg
   d. 600 mg

13. $3y = 2x + 9$. If $x = 6$, then $y =$
   a. 1
   b. 3
   c. 7
   d. 21

14. $1.63 \times 0.01 =$
   a. 0.0163
   b. 0.1630
   c. 1.0063
   d. 1.6301

15. In an experiment to relieve itching, patients were given 6 g of activated charcoal daily for 8 weeks. How many grams of charcoal did each patient take during the experiment?
   a. 48 g
   b. 294 g
   c. 326 g
   d. 336 g

16. $\dfrac{1}{40} =$
   a. 0.40
   b. 0.25
   c. 0.025
   d. 0.016

17. On a scale drawing of a hospital ward, 1 in represents 8 ft. How many ft are represented by $6\dfrac{3}{4}$ in?
   a. $48\dfrac{3}{8}$
   b. 51
   c. 54
   d. 60

18. The reciprocal of $\frac{1}{6}$ =

    a. $\frac{1}{36}$

    b. $\frac{1}{3}$

    c. $\frac{5}{6}$

    d. 6

19. 18% of 72 =
    a. 0.25
    b. 12.96
    c. 40
    d. 129.6

20. Plasma is $\frac{8}{10}$ water. How many mL of water are in 450 mL of plasma?

    a. 45 mL
    b. 360 mL
    c. 400 mL
    d. 405 mL

21. If $a = 5$ and $b = 3$, then $\frac{3b + a}{2a - b}$ =

    a. 2

    b. $\frac{3}{2}$

    c. $\frac{7}{4}$

    d. 6

Questions 22 to 24 refer to the following information: The children's clinic has a 30 × 40-foot rectangular playground.

22. How many square feet does the playground contain?
    a. 140 ft²
    b. 1,200 ft²
    c. 1,400 ft²
    d. 2,500 ft²

23. If fencing is placed around all four sides of the playground at a cost of $5.00 per foot, how much will the fencing cost?
    a. $350
    b. $600
    c. $700
    d. $800

SECTION A

SECTION B

SECTION C

COMPREHENSIVE PRACTICE Test 1

COMPREHENSIVE PRACTICE Test 2

COMPREHENSIVE PRACTICE Test 3

24. If the long side of the playground is reduced by 10 ft, what will the perimeter of the new yard be?
    a. 900 ft
    b. 130 ft
    c. 120 ft
    d. 100 ft

25. 140% =
    a. $\dfrac{7}{50}$

    b. $\dfrac{14}{25}$

    c. $1\dfrac{1}{7}$

    d. $1\dfrac{2}{3}$

26. A capsule that contains 240 mg of vitamin C supplies 400% of the U.S. Recommended Daily Allowance (USRDA) of that vitamin for adults. Find, to the nearest mg, the USRDA of vitamin C for adults.
    a. 60 mg
    b. 96 mg
    c. 167 mg
    d. 960 mg

27. What is the missing number in the series 2, 4, 8, 14, __, 32?
    a. 28
    b. 23
    c. 22
    d. 20

28. To amend the Constitution, $\dfrac{3}{4}$ of the states must approve an amendment. If 21 of the 50 states have approved an amendment, how many more states must do so before the Constitution can be amended?
    a. 17
    b. 22
    c. 29
    d. 38

29. 0.44 =
    a. $\dfrac{1}{44}$

    b. $\dfrac{2}{5}$

    c. $\dfrac{4}{11}$

    d. $\dfrac{11}{25}$

30. There are 75 g of a drug per 100 mL of solution. How many mL of solution are needed to provide 300 g of the drug?
    a. 40 mL
    b. 250 mL
    c. 400 mL
    d. 2250 mL

31. Which fraction is exactly halfway between $\frac{1}{2}$ and $\frac{1}{4}$?

    a. $\frac{1}{3}$

    b. $\frac{7}{16}$

    c. $\frac{5}{12}$

    d. $\frac{3}{8}$

32. If $x = 4$, then $x^3 =$
    a. 12
    b. 20
    c. 32
    d. 64

33. Fried's rule states that the drug dose for an infant is determined by the following formula:

    $$\text{infant's dose} = \frac{C}{150} \times \text{adult dose}$$

    where C = the child's age in months. If an infant is 10 months old, by what value should you multiply the adult dose?

    a. $\frac{1}{50}$

    b. $\frac{1}{15}$

    c. $\frac{1}{10}$

    d. $\frac{1}{3}$

34. If $5x - 7 = 2x + 8$, then $x =$

    a. $\frac{1}{3}$

    b. $\frac{15}{7}$

    c. 5
    d. 15

SECTION A

SECTION B

SECTION C

COMPREHENSIVE PRACTICE Test 1

COMPREHENSIVE PRACTICE Test 2

COMPREHENSIVE PRACTICE Test 3

35. There were 600% as many diabetics in 1978 as there were in 1935. For every 200 people with diabetes in 1935, how many diabetics were there in 1978?
    a. 12,000
    b. 1,200
    c. 320
    d. 260

36. In the spring of 1980, the interest on $10,000 United States Treasury bills was 15.7% annually. How much simple interest was earned in six months?
    a. $78.50
    b. $157
    c. $785
    d. $1,570

37. 16 percent of $x = 128$. What is the value of x?
    a. 20.48
    b. 800
    c. 1,250
    d. 2,048

38. A university study showed that 6.6% of men 55 to 57 years old had ventricular premature heartbeat. To the closest whole number, how many cases would be expected in a sample of 300 men who are 55 to 57 years old?
    a. 20
    b. 22
    c. 45
    d. 198

39. What percentage of 140 is 7?
    a. 5%
    b. 7%
    c. 9.8%
    d. 20%

40. A solution contains 8% alcohol. How many mL of solution can be made from 40 mL of alcohol?
    a. 132 mL
    b. 200 mL
    c. 320 mL
    d. 500 mL

SECTION **A**

SECTION **B**

SECTION **C**

COMPREHENSIVE PRACTICE **Test 1**

COMPREHENSIVE PRACTICE **Test 2**

COMPREHENSIVE PRACTICE **Test 3**

III. Mathematics

45 minutes

Work each problem carefully. Use scrap paper to do your calculations. (The correct answers are at the end of Section B.)

1. $68 \times 42 =$
    a. 2,546
    b. 2,856
    c. 2,956
    d. 3,256

2. Normal body temperature is 37°C. John's temperature is 35.8°C. How many degrees Celsius below normal is John's temperature?
    a. 1.2°
    b. 1.8°
    c. 2.2°
    d. 2.8°

3. $\dfrac{4}{5} + \dfrac{1}{4} =$
    a. $\dfrac{1}{5}$
    b. $\dfrac{5}{9}$
    c. $\dfrac{21}{20}$
    d. $\dfrac{17}{20}$

4. In apothecaries' measure, 60 grains are equal to 1 dram. How many grains are in 24 drams?
    a. 0.4 grain
    b. 2.5 grains
    c. 1,240 grains
    d. 1,440 grains

5. $? + 268 = 532$
    a. 264
    b. 274
    c. 336
    d. 800

117

6. A flask holds $3\frac{1}{2}$ oz of solution. How many oz of solution will 3 flasks hold?

   a. $10\frac{1}{2}$ oz

   b. $9\frac{1}{2}$ oz

   c. $8\frac{1}{2}$ oz

   d. $6\frac{1}{2}$ oz

7. $\dfrac{3}{2} \div \dfrac{2}{3} =$

   a. $\dfrac{1}{4}$

   b. $\dfrac{9}{16}$

   c. $\dfrac{16}{9}$

   d. 4

8. After exercise, Jim's pulse rate was 26 beats in 12 seconds. What was the rate in beats per minute?
   a. 104 beats per minute
   b. 130 beats per minute
   c. 156 beats per minute
   d. 312 beats per minute

9. $4.5 \times 2.05 =$
   a. 8.025
   b. 9.025
   c. 9.225
   d. 11.025

10. A storeroom is 12 m long, 10 m wide, and 9 m high. What is its volume?
    a. 325 m^3
    b. 636 m^3
    c. 961 m^3
    d. $1,080 \text{ m}^3$

11. $\dfrac{3}{5} =$

    a. 0.35
    b. 0.58
    c. 0.60
    d. 0.65

12. One liter = 1,000 mL. How many liters are equivalent to 200 mL?
    a. $\frac{1}{5}$ L
    b. 2 L
    c. 5 L
    d. 20 L

13. $4x = y + 16$. If $y = 20$, then $x =$
    a. 36
    b. 9
    c. 4
    d. 1

14. In a hospital survey, 15% of 660 patients said they were dissatisfied with the quality of patient care. How many patients were dissatisfied?
    a. 111 patients
    b. 99 patients
    c. 81 patients
    d. 44 patients

15. $24.68 \div 0.02 =$
    a. 0.1234
    b. 12.34
    c. 123.4
    d. 1,234

16. One ounce of fat supplies 270 Cal. How many ounces of fat are needed to supply 1,215 Cal?
    a. 45 oz
    b. 5.5 oz
    c. 4.8 oz
    d. 4.5 oz

17. 35% of 14 =
    a. 0.025
    b. 4.9
    c. 40
    d. 490

18. One ounce of a certain cereal contains 112 cal. One serving of this cereal contains $\frac{7}{8}$ oz. How many calories are there in one serving?
    a. 63 cal
    b. 96 cal
    c. 98 cal
    d. 128 cal

19. If $A < B$ and $C < B$, then the values of A, B, and C could be
    a. $A = 1, B = 2, C = 3$
    b. $A = 4, B = 1, C = 3$
    c. $A = 3, B = 4, C = 3$
    d. $A = 3, B = 4, C = 4$

SECTION A

SECTION B

SECTION C

COMPREHENSIVE PRACTICE Test 1

COMPREHENSIVE PRACTICE Test 2

COMPREHENSIVE PRACTICE Test 3

20. If you make 3 bandages, $5\frac{1}{4} \times 4$ in each, from fabric that is 20×4 in, the fabric that is left over will measure

    a. $2\frac{1}{2}$ in

    b. $3\frac{1}{2}$ in

    c. $4\frac{1}{4}$ in

    d. $14\frac{1}{2}$ in

21. $6 \times 5 \times 3 \times 0 =$
    a. 0
    b. 90
    c. 330
    d. 900

22. There are 40 grains of sodium bromide to 600 mL of solution. How many mL of solution are needed to provide 72 grains of sodium bromide?
    a. 1,080 mL
    b. 333.3 mL
    c. 108 mL
    d. 4.8 mL

23. If $a = 5$, $b = 3$, $c = 1$, then $\dfrac{a + b + c^2}{a - b + c^2} =$
    a. 1
    b. 3
    c. 9
    d. 81

24. About 1,700 quarts of blood flow to the kidneys each day. What is the average flow per hour to the nearest whole number?
    a. 170 qt/hr
    b. 142 qt/hr
    c. 85 qt/hr
    d. 71 qt/hr

25. $6.24\% =$
    a. 0.0624
    b. 0.624
    c. 6.24
    d. 62.40

26. Alcohol freezes at $-114°C$ and boils at $78°C$. What is the number of degrees between the boiling and freezing points of alcohol?
    a. 36°C
    b. 182°C

c. 184°C

d. 192°C

27. $(3 \div 9)(12 \div 2) =$

   a. $\dfrac{1}{18}$

   b. $\dfrac{1}{2}$

   c. 2

   d. 18

28. How many 3×3-in gauze pads can be made from a 24×24-in gauze square?

   a. 64

   b. 48

   c. 32

   d. 16

29. $0.65 =$

   a. $\dfrac{6}{11}$

   b. $\dfrac{13}{20}$

   c. $\dfrac{2}{3}$

   d. $\dfrac{1}{65}$

30. Eight doses of a medication require a total of 0.12 mL of drug X. For 10 doses, how many mL of drug X are needed?

   a. 0.96 mL

   b. 0.14 mL

   c. 0.15 mL

   d. 1.2 mL

31. If $x = 2$, then $x^3(x + 1) =$

   a. 11

   b. 17

   c. 18

   d. 24

32. The sodium content of three different jars of peanut butter was measured. Jar X contained 0.89 g, jar Y contained 1.2 g, and jar Z contained 0.004 g. Find, to the nearest 10th of a gram, the *average* amount of sodium contained in these jars.

   a. 0.6 g

   b. 0.7 g

   c. 0.8 g

   d. 2.1 g

SECTION A

SECTION B

SECTION C

COMPREHENSIVE PRACTICE Test 1

COMPREHENSIVE PRACTICE Test 2

COMPREHENSIVE PRACTICE Test 3

33. Which fraction is closest to $\frac{1}{3}$?

    a. $\frac{5}{12}$

    b. $\frac{7}{8}$

    c. $\frac{7}{24}$

    d. $\frac{2}{9}$

34. A solution containing 50 oz of water lost 32% of the water by evaporation. How many ounces of water were left?
    a. 34 oz
    b. 24 oz
    c. 18 oz
    d. 16 oz

35. 6 percent of which number is 150?
    a. 9
    b. 250
    c. 900
    d. 2,500

36. An 8-oz glass of orange juice contains 110 Cal. How many calories are in 1 gallon of orange juice?
    a. 440 cal
    b. 880 cal
    c. 1,320 cal
    d. 1,760 cal

37. If $8y + 6 = 40$, then $y =$
    a. $4\frac{1}{4}$
    b. 5
    c. 6
    d. 34

38. A circle graph is used to show the percentage of clinic funds spent on different items. How many degrees of the circle should be used to show that 25% of the funds are spent on rent?
    a. 25
    b. 45
    c. 70
    d. 90

39. What percentage of 96 is 12?
    a. 0.125%
    b. 11.52%

c. 12.5%
d. 800%

40. The relationship between Celsius (C) degrees and Kelvins (K) is expressed by the formula °C + 273 = K. Express 67°C on the Kelvin scale.
    a. −340K
    b. −206K
    c. 206K
    d. 340K

SECTION A

SECTION B

SECTION C

COMPREHENSIVE PRACTICE Test 1

COMPREHENSIVE PRACTICE Test 2

COMPREHENSIVE PRACTICE Test 3

IV. Mathematics

45 Minutes

Work each problem carefully. Use scrap paper to do your calculations. (The correct answers are at the end of Section B.)

1. $239.76 - 57.359 =$
   a. 182.411
   b. 182.401
   c. 192.401
   d. 297.119

2. $321 + 407 - 219 =$
   a. 509
   b. 511
   c. 517
   d. 947

3. A student spent $2.50 for lunch on Monday, $1.85 on Tuesday, and $2.25 on Wednesday. What was the average cost of lunch for the three days?
   a. $2.10
   b. $2.20
   c. $3.30
   d. $6.60

4. If $3y = 2x + 8$, and $x = 20$, then $y =$
   a. 48
   b. $18\dfrac{2}{3}$
   c. 16
   d. $9\dfrac{1}{3}$

5. $76.2 \times 1.04 =$
   a. 106.68
   b. 79.248
   c. 78.248
   d. 76.08

6. $3\frac{3}{4} + 1\frac{2}{5} =$

   a. $4\frac{3}{20}$

   b. $4\frac{3}{10}$

   c. $5\frac{5}{9}$

   d. $5\frac{3}{20}$

7. During a sale, a bookstore reduced the price of books 15%. The sale price of a $25.00 book was
   a. $10.00
   b. $21.25
   c. $23.50
   d. $24.85

8. A cube measures 12 cm by 15 cm by 8 cm. What is its volume?
   a. 1,440 cm^3
   b. 1,360 cm^3
   c. 1,584 cm^3
   d. 1,225 cm^3

9. $524 + (3 \times 5) =$
   a. 532
   b. 539
   c. 2,623
   d. 7,860

10. Which of the following fractions has the largest value?

    a. $\dfrac{1}{9 \times 3}$

    b. $\dfrac{1}{9 + 3}$

    c. $\dfrac{1}{9 - 3}$

    d. $\dfrac{1}{9 \div 3}$

11. If 1 cup of corn supplies 140 Cal, how many calories are in $\frac{5}{8}$ cup of corn?

    a. 17.5 cal
    b. 75 cal
    c. 87.5 cal
    d. 224 cal

SECTION A

SECTION B

SECTION C

COMPREHENSIVE PRACTICE Test 1

COMPREHENSIVE PRACTICE Test 2

COMPREHENSIVE PRACTICE Test 3

12. 3.45 ÷ 0.15 =
    a. 0.023
    b. 0.23
    c. 2.3
    d. 23

13. Fifteen grams of a mixture contain two substances: K = 7 g, and L = 8 g. If 21 g of K are available, how many g of L will be needed to make the same mixture?
    a. 20 g
    b. 22 g
    c. 24 g
    d. 45 g

14. To the nearest 3 decimal places, 367 ÷ 35 =
    a. 1.049
    b. 10.408
    c. 10.486
    d. 14.857

15. To allow a tape recorder in a class, school policy states that $\frac{2}{3}$ of the students in that class must request to use it. If 15 of 48 students have made that request, how many more must do so before a tape recorder will be allowed in the class?
    a. 16
    b. 17
    c. 32
    d. 33

16. One quart equals 0.9 liters. How many liters equal 3.6 quarts?
    a. 2.2
    b. 3.1
    c. 3.2
    d. 5.1

17. How many non-overlapping 2 × 3-in squares are contained in a 9 × 10-in rectangle?
    a. 9
    b. 12
    c. 15
    d. 18

18. If 3x < 4, then x could be
    a. 1
    b. $1\frac{1}{3}$
    c. 2
    d. 12

19. 250 mL of solution contain 30 mL of a medication. How many mL of this medication are in 100 mL of solution?
    a. 7.5 mL
    b. 12.0 mL

SECTION A
SECTION B
SECTION C
COMPREHENSIVE PRACTICE Test 1
COMPREHENSIVE PRACTICE Test 2
COMPREHENSIVE PRACTICE Test 3

c. 15.0 mL
d. 75.0 mL

20. At the start of a diet, Mr. Smith weighed 184 lbs. Eight days later, he weighed 179 lbs. What was his average weight loss per day?
a. 5 lbs
b. $\frac{3}{4}$ lb
c. $\frac{1}{2}$ lb
d. $\frac{5}{8}$ lb

21. $8a^3 \cdot 5a^4 =$
a. $40a^7$
b. $40a^{12}$
c. $13a^7$
d. $13a^{12}$

22. The amount of iron recommended for a typical adult woman is 18 mg daily. One woman's average daily diet supplies 75% of this amount. How much more iron should her daily diet contain to supply the recommended daily amount?
a. 13.5 mg
b. 10.5 mg
c. 4.5 mg
d. 3.5 mg

23. The 6% sales tax on textbooks was $3.54. How much did the textbooks themselves cost?
a. $3.75
b. $21.24
c. $55.46
d. $59.00

24. A feeding requires $1\frac{1}{3}$ cups of nonfat milk. A person already has $\frac{3}{4}$ cup. How much more is needed?
a. $\frac{7}{12}$ cup
b. $\frac{5}{12}$ cup
c. $\frac{2}{3}$ cup
d. $\frac{5}{6}$ cup

25. Factor $4a^2 - 49$ completely.
    a. $(2a - 7)$
    b. $\sqrt{4a^2 - 49}$
    c. $2a(2a - 7)$
    d. $(2a + 7)(2a - 7)$

26. How many degrees are in each of the two unmarked angles of the following parallelogram?

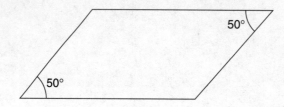

    a. 310°
    b. 260°
    c. 130°
    d. 80°

27. $\sqrt{45} =$
    a. $3\sqrt{5}$
    b. 9×5
    c. 15×3
    d. $5\sqrt{3}$

28. 3.4% of 260 =
    a. 7.65
    b. 8.84
    c. 86.67
    d. 88.4

29. Of 60 patients treated with a certain medication, 24 showed no improvement. What percentage of patients improved?
    a. 60%
    b. 40%
    c. 36%
    d. 24%

30. Which of the following decimals equals 3.7%?
    a. 0.037
    b. 0.370
    c. 3.070
    d. 3.700

SECTION A

SECTION B

SECTION C

COMPREHENSIVE PRACTICE Test 1

COMPREHENSIVE PRACTICE Test 2

COMPREHENSIVE PRACTICE Test 3

31. A baby drank an average of $7\frac{1}{4}$ oz during each of four feedings. If the baby drank $6\frac{3}{8}$ oz, $7\frac{1}{2}$ oz, and $7\frac{3}{8}$ oz in the first three feedings, how many ounces were taken during the fourth feeding?

   a. 29 oz

   b. $7\frac{1}{12}$ oz

   c. $7\frac{1}{4}$ oz

   d. $7\frac{3}{4}$ oz

32. $3\sqrt{36}$ =
   a. 9
   b. 18
   c. 54
   d. 108

33. Which of the following fractions equals 0.15?

   a. $\frac{1}{15}$

   b. $\frac{1}{5}$

   c. $\frac{1}{6}$

   d. $\frac{3}{20}$

34. If 30% of a number is 90, what is that number?
   a. 300
   b. 270
   c. 120
   d. 27

35. Which of the following values equals 0.35×10^4?
   a. 350,000
   b. 3,500
   c. 0.0035
   d. 0.000035

36. A circle graph is divided into three equal sections. How many degrees are in each section?
   a. 30°
   b. 60°

c. 90°
d. 120°

37. $3\frac{3}{8} \times 2\frac{1}{3} =$

    a. $6\frac{1}{8}$

    b. $6\frac{17}{24}$

    c. $7\frac{3}{4}$

    d. $7\frac{7}{8}$

38. Of the children coming into a clinic, 7.5% have a certain condition. For every 150 children who visit the clinic, how many are expected to have this condition?
    a. 112.5
    b. 20
    c. 11.25
    d. 1.125

39. If x% of 150 = 12, then x =
    a. 8
    b. 12.5
    c. 18
    d. 80

40. Which of the following equations illustrates the distributive property of multiplication?
    a. $3x + 4(a - 2) = 3x + 4a - 8$
    b. $3x + 4(a - 2) = 3x + 4a - 2$
    c. $3x + 4(a - 2) = (3x + 4)(a - 2)$
    d. $3x + 4(a - 2) = 4(a - 2) + 3x$

Answers

I. MATHEMATICS

1. **The answer is a.** Solve this problem in one of two ways:

   (a) Convert 25% into a decimal and multiply it by 200: $0.25 \times 200 = 50$.

   (b) Convert 25% into a fraction ($\frac{1}{4}$) and multiply it by 200:

   $$\frac{1}{4} \times \frac{200}{1} = \frac{200}{4} = 50.$$

2. **The answer is b.** Convert 19% into a decimal (0.19) and multiply the decimal by $1,000. The shortcut for multiplying decimals by a power of 10 (in this case, 1,000) is to move the decimal to the right by the same number of places as there are zeros in the power of 10. In this case, 1,000 has 3 zeros; so move the decimal 3 places to the right (0.19 becomes 190.0).

3. **The answer is d.** Set up a ratio to solve this problem. Make sure you keep the units properly aligned: inches across from inches, and centimeters across from centimeters.

   $$\frac{1 \text{ in}}{2.54 \text{ cm}} = \frac{62 \text{ in}}{x \text{ cm}}$$

   $$x = 157.48 \text{ cm}$$

   Once your proportion is set up, cross-multiply to solve for x.

   You can also solve this problem by multiplying 2.54 cm/in by 62 in to get 157.48 cm.

4. **The answer is c.** Follow the order of operations to solve this problem. First, multiply within the parentheses, then divide to obtain the answer:

   $(3 \times 9) \div (5 \times 2) =$

   $27 \div 10 = 2.7$

5. **The answer is a.** A factor is a number that divides evenly into a certain number. Answer b, 16, does not divide into 24 evenly, and 32 and 48 are both too large to be factors of 24. In fact, 48 is a multiple of 24, because 24 divides evenly into it. Only 8 divides into 24 evenly—three times.

6. **The answer is d.** This problem asks you to find the total amount paid for the car. This means you have to add different amounts. If a person made 12 monthly payments of $91.43 each, then multiply 12 by $91.43 to find out how much the person paid during that period.

   $91.43 \times 12 = 1,097.16$

SECTION A

SECTION B

SECTION C

COMPREHENSIVE PRACTICE Test 1

COMPREHENSIVE PRACTICE Test 2

COMPREHENSIVE PRACTICE Test 3

Add the down payment, $822.87, to the monthly amount, to arrive at your answer:

$1,097.16 + $822.87 = $1,920.03

7. **The answer is b.** The reciprocal of a fraction is the inverse of the fraction (the fraction turned upside down). Because 3 can be rewritten as $\frac{3}{1}$, its reciprocal is $\frac{1}{3}$.

8. **The answer is a.** Just as in question 3, set up a proportion to solve this problem. Make sure you keep the units properly aligned: km across from km and miles across from miles.

$$\frac{1 \text{ km}}{0.625 \text{ mi}} = \frac{4 \text{ km}}{x}$$

Cross-multiply to solve for x.

$x = 0.625 \times 4$

$1x = 2.5 \text{ mi}$

You may also think of this problem in this way: If each kilometer equals 0.625 miles, then 4 kilometers must equal 4 km $\times$ 0.625 mi/km = 2.5 mi.

9. **The answer is c.** Calculate the 8% sales tax on $60.00, and add this amount to the pretax amount ($60.00) to find your final answer. Convert 8% into a decimal by dividing by 100:

8% = 0.08.

Then multiply $60.00 by 0.08 to find the sales tax: $4.80. Finally, add $4.80 to the pretax amount, $60.00:

$60.00 + $4.80 = $64.80

10. **The answer is c.** Recall place values to answer this question.

Moving to the *left* from the decimal point, the places are:	Moving to the *right* from the decimal point, the places are:
ones	tenths
tens	hundredths
hundreds	thousandths
thousands	ten-thousandths
ten-thousands	hundred-thousandths
hundred-thousands	millionths
millions	

$\vdots$ $\vdots$

11. **The answer is d.** To change a decimal to a percentage, multiply by 100, and tack on the percentage sign.

    $0.25 \times 100 = 25\%$

12. **The answer is b.** The sheets cost $25.00 per set, and each set contains 4 sheets. If you want to buy 12 sheets, you need 3 sets. This costs $75.00 ($3 \times \$25.00$).
    The pillowcases cost $4.50 per set, and each set contains 2 pillowcases. If you want to buy 24 pillowcases, you will need 12 sets. This will cost $54.00 ($12 \times 4.50$). Your total cost is $75.00 + $54.00 = $129.00.

13. **The answer is d.** To find the volume of a rectangular solid (a box), multiply the length by the width by the height: $12 \text{ ft} \times 15 \text{ ft} \times 8 \text{ ft} = 1{,}440 \text{ ft}^3$. Volume is a cubic measurement, and therefore your answer must be in cubic units, in this case, cubic feet.

14. **The answer is b.** Just as in 3 and 8, set up a proportion to solve this problem. Make sure you keep the units properly aligned: drams across from drams and grains across from grains. Then cross-multiply and divide both sides by 60 to solve for x.

    $$\frac{1 \text{ drams}}{60 \text{ grains}} = \frac{x}{40 \text{ grains}}$$

    $$60x = 40$$

    $$x = \frac{2}{3} \text{ dram}$$

15. **The answer is a.** Subtract the amount lost from the original amount. Be sure to line up the decimals.

    $2.30 \text{ mg} - 0.52 \text{ mg} = 1.78 \text{ mg}$

16. **The answer is c.** To change a decimal to a percentage, multiply by 100, and tack on the percentage sign (%).

    $0.18 \times 100 = 18\%$

17. **The answer is b.** To find the average drop in temperature per hour, you must first find two things:

    (1) Calculate the total drop in temperature:

    $68° - 41° = 27°$

    (2) The difference from 12 noon to midnight is 12 hours.

    Divide the decrease in temperature by the number of hours:

    $$\frac{27°}{12 \text{ hours}} = 2.25° \text{ per hour}$$

18. **The answer is a.** Set up a proportion to solve this problem. Make sure you align the units correctly: mg across from mg, and mL across from mL. Then cross-multiply and divide both sides by 3 to solve for x.

    $$\frac{3 \text{ mg}}{5 \text{ mL}} = \frac{9 \text{ mg}}{x}$$

SECTION A
SECTION B
SECTION C
COMPREHENSIVE PRACTICE Test 1
COMPREHENSIVE PRACTICE Test 2
COMPREHENSIVE PRACTICE Test 3

$$3x = 45$$

$$x = 15\text{mL}$$

You can also recognize that 9 is 3×3; therefore you would need three times the volume or $5 \times 3 = 15$.

19. **The answer is b.** Find the least common denominator of the three fractions, and then change them all to equivalent fractions with the new denominator. The common denominator is 24, because all three denominators are factors of 24. Write the equivalent fractions:

$$\frac{3}{8} = \frac{9}{24}, \frac{1}{4} = \frac{6}{24}, \text{ and } \frac{1}{3} = \frac{8}{24}$$

The original problem becomes:

$$\frac{9}{24} + \frac{6}{24} - \frac{8}{24} = \frac{7}{24}$$

20. **The answer is d.** To find the drop in temperature, subtract the low from the high.

$$33° - (-20°) = 33 + 20 = 53°$$

21. **The answer is b.** Set up a proportion to solve this problem. Make sure you keep the units properly aligned: oz across from oz and Cal across from Cal. Then cross-multiply and divide both sides by 3 to solve for x.

$$\frac{3 \text{ ounces}}{155 \text{ Calories}} = \frac{5 \text{ ounces}}{x}$$

$$3x = 755$$

$$x = 258.3 \approx 258 \text{ Cal}$$

The question asks for an approximate answer, so 258 is the correct choice.

22. **The answer is c.** The common denominator in this problem is 12. Change both fractional parts of the mixed numbers to equivalent fractions with denominators of 12, and then add the mixed numbers. Remember to reduce your answer.

$$8\frac{3}{4} = 8\frac{9}{12}$$

$$8\frac{9}{12} + 5\frac{5}{12} = 13\frac{14}{12}$$

$$13\frac{14}{12} = 14\frac{2}{12} = 14\frac{1}{6}$$

23. **The answer is b.** To find the ratio of wins to losses, make a fraction of the wins and losses:

$$\frac{18 \text{ wins}}{12 \text{ losses}} = \frac{3}{2}, \text{ or } 3:2.$$

24. **The answer is b.** You need to find out how many units of $4\frac{1}{2}$ there are in 200. This is a division problem:

$$200 \div 4\frac{1}{2}$$

Change $4\frac{1}{2}$ to a mixed number.

$$\frac{200}{1} \div \frac{9}{2}$$

Invert the mixed number and multiply. Ignore the fraction, and round the answer down to a whole number.

$$\frac{200}{1} \times \frac{2}{9} = \frac{400}{9} = 44\frac{1}{9} \approx 44 \text{ strips}$$

25. **The answer is b.** Change this problem into an equation, and solve for x.

$$45 = 0.6x$$

$$75 = x$$

You may also set up a proportion, cross-multiply, and divide each side by 60 to solve for x.

$$\frac{45}{x} = \frac{60}{100}$$

$$60x = 4{,}500$$

$$x = 75$$

26. **The answer is c.** In the problem, substitute 2 for b.

$$5a = 10(2) + 15$$

Then simplify, combine like terms, and divide both sides by 5 to solve for x.

$$5a = 20 + 15$$

$$5a = 35$$

$$a = 7$$

27. **The answer is b.** Edna's investment is \$4,000, and the \$200 interest she receives is a part, or percentage, of that amount. To find out how much of a percentage, write a fraction, change the fraction to a decimal, and change the decimal to a percentage.

$$\frac{200}{4{,}000} = \frac{2}{40} = \frac{1}{20} = 0.05$$

$$0.05 \times 100 = 5\%$$

SECTION A

SECTION B

SECTION C

COMPREHENSIVE PRACTICE Test 1

COMPREHENSIVE PRACTICE Test 2

COMPREHENSIVE PRACTICE Test 3

28. **The answer is c.** If the infant's dose should be equal to the child's age in mo/150 × adult dose, then substitute 25 mg for the adult dose and 9 months for the infant's age. Then simplify:

$$\frac{9 \text{ mo}}{150} \times 25 \text{ mg} = \text{child's dose}$$

Change 25 to a fraction, multiply, and convert to a decimal to find your answer.

$$\frac{9}{150} \times \frac{25}{1} = \text{child's dose}$$

$$\frac{225}{150} = \frac{3}{2} = 1.5 \text{ mg}$$

29. **The answer is c.** You may set up a proportion to solve this problem. As always, make sure to align your units correctly: cups across from cups and Cal across from Cal. Then cross-multiply, simplify, and multiply both sides by 4 to solve for x.

$$\frac{\frac{1}{4} \text{ cup}}{96 \text{ Cal}} = \frac{\frac{7}{8} \text{ cup}}{x}$$

$$\frac{1}{4}x = 96 \times \frac{7}{8}$$

$$\frac{1}{4}x = 84$$

$$x = 336 \text{ Cal}$$

30. **The answer is d.** Any number multiplied by 0 is 0. It does not matter what $4 \times 5 \times 6$ comes out to because the product is ultimately multiplied by 0, making the final product 0.

31. **The answer is a.** If men ordinarily consume 75% of the recommended daily allowance of 420 mg of magnesium, then they *do not* consume the remaining 25%. This 25% is the amount the average male is missing. To calculate this amount, convert 25% into a decimal and multiply.

$$25\% = 0.25$$

$$0.25(420) = 105 \text{ mg}$$

32. **The answer is c.** Fourteen of the 42 students are male. The remaining 28 students must be female. To find what portion of the total students is female, set up a fraction and reduce.

$$\frac{28}{42} = \frac{2}{3}$$

SECTION A

SECTION B

SECTION C

COMPREHENSIVE PRACTICE Test 1

COMPREHENSIVE PRACTICE Test 2

COMPREHENSIVE PRACTICE Test 3

33. **The answer is d.**

$x = 46 + 0$

$x = 46$

$y = (64)(0)$

$y = 0$

Therefore, $x > y$.

34. **The answer is d.** The trick is to make the connection between cost per minute and the length of the call. The first 3 minutes of the call cost \$1.62. So:

$\$7.29 - \$1.62 = \$5.67$

This amount represents the cost for the remaining minutes of the call, with each minute costing \$0.81. Divide the remaining cost by the cost per minute, and you have the time for cost remaining: 7 min.

$$\frac{\$5.67}{\$0.81/\text{min}} = 7 \text{ min}$$

Finally, add these 7 min to the first 3 min of the call: 3 min + 7 minutes = 10 min.

35. **The answer is a.** Since $1\frac{1}{3}$ is the total, subtract $\frac{3}{4}$ from $1\frac{1}{3}$ to find out how much more is needed. Before you subtract, change $1\frac{1}{3}$ to an improper fraction, and find the LCD, which is 12.

$$1\frac{1}{3} = \frac{4}{3} = \frac{16}{12} \text{ and } \frac{3}{4} = \frac{9}{12}$$

$$\frac{16}{12} - \frac{9}{12} = \frac{7}{12}$$

36. **The answer is a.** Substitute 2 for x and simplify the expression as follows:

$x^3(x^2 - x) =$

$2^3(2^2 - 2) =$

$8(4 - 2) =$

$8(2) = 16$

37. **The answer is c.** The total daily consumption is 3,000 Cal, and 450 Cal are a portion, or percentage, of the total. Change this information to a fraction. Then, to calculate this percentage, divide the part by the whole, and multiply by 100 to convert the decimal into a percentage.

$$\frac{450}{3,000} = 0.15$$

$0.15 = 15\%$

38. **The answer is d.** To divide decimals, make sure the divisor (the number outside the box) is a whole number. In this case, move the decimal two places to the right to change 0.15 into 15. You must move the decimal two places to the right in the dividend as well.

$$0.15\overline{)2.25} \rightarrow 15\overline{)225} \rightarrow 15\overline{)225}^{\,15}$$

39. **The answer is c.** The area of a triangle can be found using the following formula, and, from the figure, substituting the appropriate dimensions.

$$A = \frac{1}{2}\,(bh)$$

$$A = \frac{1}{2}\,(10\ \text{cm})(6\ \text{cm})$$

$$A = \frac{1}{2}\,(60\ \text{cm}^2)$$

$$A = 30\ \text{cm}^2$$

40. **The answer is c.** To find the area of the irregularly shaped polygon *BCDEF*, you can subtract the area of the small triangle *BAF* from the area of the large rectangle *CDEA*.

To find the area of triangle *BAF*, you need the base and the height, which are missing from the diagram. However, because opposite sides of a rectangle are the same length, you can determine the missing measurements through subtraction:

Because *CD* = *AE*, it is true that *AE* − *FE* = *AF*: 10 − 7 = 3 cm

Because *DE* = *CA*, it is true that *CA* − *CB* = *BA*: 6 − 2 = 4 cm

Now that you have the height (*h*) and base (*b*), you can find the area of triangle *BAF*, using the area formula and substituting the appropriate dimensions:

$$A = \frac{1}{2}\,(bh)$$

$$A = \frac{1}{2}\,(3\ \text{cm})(4\ \text{cm})$$

$$A = \frac{1}{2}\,(12\ \text{cm}^2)$$

$$A = 6\ \text{cm}^2$$

This is the area of the triangle.

The area of a rectangle can be found using the following formula and substituting the appropriate dimensions:

$A = lw$

$A = (10 \text{ cm})(6 \text{ cm})$

$A = 60 \text{ cm}^2$

This is the area of the rectangle.

Finally, because all values are in square centimeters, simply subtract 6 (the triangle's area) from 60 (the rectangle's area) to get 54, the area of polygon *BCDEF* in square centimeters.

SECTION

A

SECTION

B

SECTION

C

COMPREHENSIVE PRACTICE

Test 1

COMPREHENSIVE PRACTICE

Test 2

COMPREHENSIVE PRACTICE

Test 3

II. Mathematics

1. **The answer is a.** This problem requires you to borrow twice: $403 - 349 = 54$.

2. **The answer is a.** The upper limit is 146 lbs. To calculate by how much 160 lbs. exceeds this maximum, subtract 146 from 160: $160 - 146 = 14$ lbs.

3. **The answer is b.** Find the lowest common denominator (LCD) for both fractions, and then change them to equivalent fractions. The LCD is 24, because both 8 and 3 are factors of 24.

$$\frac{7}{8} = \frac{21}{24} \quad \text{and} \quad \frac{1}{3} = \frac{8}{24}$$

Once you have a common denominator, subtract the numerators.

$$\frac{21}{24} - \frac{8}{24} = \frac{13}{24}$$

4. **The answer is c.** You may set up a proportion to solve this problem. Make sure you align the units properly: teaspoons across from teaspoons and drops across from drops.

$$\frac{1\,t}{60 \text{ drops}} = \frac{1\frac{1}{4}\,t}{x}$$

Cross-multiply. (You may turn $1\frac{1}{4}$ into 1.25 if you choose.)

$$1x = (60)(1.25)$$

$$x = 75 \text{ drops}$$

You can also solve by multiplying 1.25 teaspoons by 60 drops per teaspoon.

5. **The answer is b.** Following the order of operations, you must multiply 4 by 5 first, and then add 8.

$$8 + 4(5) =$$

$$8 + 20 = 28$$

6. **The answer is b.** There is a total of 480,000 units, and the question asks how many groups (doses) of 80,000 you can make from this total. This is what division is all about: determining how many same-size groups are contained within a larger group.

$$\frac{480,000}{80,000} = \frac{48}{8} = 6 \text{ doses}$$

SECTION A

SECTION B

SECTION C

COMPREHENSIVE PRACTICE Test 1

COMPREHENSIVE PRACTICE Test 2

COMPREHENSIVE PRACTICE Test 3

7. **The answer is b.** To multiply fractions, multiply the numerators, and multiply the denominators.

$$\frac{3}{8} \times \frac{1}{4} = \frac{3}{32}$$

8. **The answer is b.** To find the largest dose, compare the decimals. Start with the digit in the tenths place. Because 0.100 has a 1 in the tenths place, it is larger than all of the other choices, because they all have a 0 in the tenths place.

9. **The answer is d.** To divide decimals, you must make sure the divisor (the number outside the box) is a whole number. In this case, move the decimal two places to the right to make 0.05 into 5. You must move the decimal two places to the right in the dividend as well.

$$0.05\overline{)1.25}$$

$$5\overline{)125}^{\;25}$$

10. **The answer is a.** To subtract mixed numbers, find a common denominator, and then write equivalent fractions. Notice, however, that when you make the equivalent fractions in this problem, $\frac{1}{4}$ is smaller than $\frac{2}{4}$. This means you have to borrow 1 whole ($\frac{4}{4}$) from the whole number part of the mixed number, and add it to the fraction part of the mixed number. This makes the fraction large enough to subtract from.

$$4\frac{1}{4} = 3\frac{5}{4} \text{ and } 2\frac{1}{2} = 2\frac{2}{4}$$

$$3\frac{5}{4} - 2\frac{2}{4} = 1\frac{3}{4} L$$

11. **The answer is c.** The fraction $\frac{4}{3}$ is known as the *reciprocal* of $\frac{3}{4}$, and it is defined as the number needed to multiply by in order to obtain a product of 1.

$$\frac{3}{4} \times \frac{4}{3} = \frac{12}{12} = 1$$

12. **The answer is b.** To find the *average* cholesterol intake over 4 days, you must first find the total amount of cholesterol intake over those 4 days.

300 mg	Monday
120 mg	Tuesday
80 mg	Wednesday
+ 100 mg	Thursday
600 mg	

Next, divide this total by 4, to find the average intake over 4 days.

$$\frac{600 \text{ mg}}{4 \text{ day}} = 150 \text{ mg/day}$$

13. **The answer is c.** Substitute 6 for x in the equation, simplify, combine like terms, and divide both sides by 3 to solve for y.

    $3y = 2x + 9$

    $3y = 2(6) + 9$

    $3y = 12 + 9$

    $3y = 21$

    $y = 7$

14. **The answer is a.** To multiply decimals, multiply the numbers as you would whole numbers, ignoring the decimals. Then count the number of decimal places in both numbers and count that many places in from the right.

       1.63   2 decimal places

     $\times$ 0.01   2 decimal places

       0.0163   4 decimal places

15. **The answer is d.** First calculate how many grams patients received in 1 week.

    6 g/day $\times$ 7 days/week = 42 g/week

    Then calculate how many grams patients received in 8 weeks.

    42 g/week $\times$ 8 weeks = 336 g

16. **The answer is c.** Divide 40 into 1.

    $$\begin{array}{r} 0.025 \\ 40\overline{)1.00} \end{array}$$

17. **The answer is c.** You may set up a proportion to solve this problem. Make sure you align the units properly: in across from in and ft across from ft.

    $$\frac{1 \text{ in}}{8 \text{ ft}} = \frac{6\frac{3}{4} \text{ in}}{x}$$

    Then cross-multiply, convert the mixed number to an improper fraction, multiply the fractions, and simplify the improper fraction.

    $$1x = (8)(6\frac{3}{4})$$

    $$x = \frac{8}{1} \times \frac{27}{4}$$

    $$x = \frac{216}{4} = 54 \text{ ft}$$

You can also solve this problem by multiplying $6\frac{3}{4}$ in by 8 ft/in = 54 ft.

18. **The answer is d.** The reciprocal of any number is the number you multiply by in order to obtain a product of 1.

$$\frac{1}{6} \times \frac{6}{1} = \frac{6}{6} = 1$$

Put another way, you can obtain the reciprocal of a number by switcing the numerator and denominator. In our example, to find the reciprocal of $\frac{1}{6}$, switch the 1 and the 6 to get $\frac{6}{1}$, or 6.

19. **The answer is b.** Change 18% to a decimal by dividing by 100.

$$18\% \div 100 = 0.18$$

Then multiply the numbers, and make sure your answer has the correct number of decimal places.

$$0.18 \times 72 = 12.96$$

20. **The answer is b.** Plasma is $\frac{8}{10}$ water. If you have 450 mL of plasma, then $\frac{8}{10}$ of that is water. To find the amount of water, multiple the total by $\frac{8}{10}$.

$$\frac{450}{1} \times \frac{8}{10} = \frac{3,600}{10} = 360\,\text{mL}$$

21. **The answer is a.** Substitute the values given for a and b, and simplify:

$$\frac{3b + a}{2a - b} \rightarrow \frac{3(3) + 5}{2(5) - 3} = \frac{9 + 5}{10 - 3} = \frac{14}{7} = 2$$

22. **The answer is b.** The area (A) of a rectangle (whether in square footage, square meters, or any unit of measurement) is found by using the following formula:

$$A = lw$$

where l = length and w = width.

$$A = (30 \text{ ft})(40 \text{ ft})$$

$$A = 1,200 \text{ ft}^2$$

23. **The answer is c.** You need to find the perimeter of the rectangular playground. The perimeter of a rectangle can be found using the following formula:

$$P = 2l + 2w$$

where l = length and w = width. Substitute 30 ft for l and 40 ft for w.

$$P = 2(30 \text{ ft}) + 2(40 \text{ ft})$$

$$P = 60 + 80 = 140 \text{ ft}$$

SECTION A

SECTION B

SECTION C

COMPREHENSIVE PRACTICE Test 1

COMPREHENSIVE PRACTICE Test 2

COMPREHENSIVE PRACTICE Test 3

If fencing costs $5.00 per foot, multiply 140 ft by this amount to find the total cost for fencing.

140 feet × $5/foot = $700

24. **The answer is c.** Reducing the long side of the rectangle makes each side 30 feet and turns the rectangle into a square. The perimeter of a square may be found using the following formula:

$P = 4s$

where s = a side of the square. Substitute 30 ft for s.

$P = 4(30) = 120$ ft

25. **The answer is d.** To change 140% to a mixed number, first convert it to a decimal by dividing by 100.

140% ÷ 100 = 1.4

Change the decimal part into a fraction and reduce the fraction.

$$1.4 = 1\frac{4}{10}$$

$$1\frac{1}{10} = 1\frac{2}{5}$$

26. **The answer is a.** If 240 mg represent 400% of, or 4 times, the USRDA, divide 240 by 4 to find 100% of the USRDA.

$$\frac{240}{4} = 60\,\text{mg}$$

27. **The answer is c.** The number you add to move from one number to the next increases by 2 each time.

2 + 2 = 4

4 + 4 = 8

8 + 6 = 14

14 + 8 = 22

22 + 10 = 32

28. **The answer is a.** First, determine how many states make up $\frac{3}{4}$ of the 50 total.

$$\frac{3}{4} \times \frac{50}{1} = \frac{150}{4} = 37.5 \approx 38$$

So 38 states are needed to make up $\frac{3}{4}$ of 50. Next, subtract 21 from 38 to find out how many more are needed.

38 − 21 = 17

SECTION A

SECTION B

SECTION C

COMPREHENSIVE PRACTICE Test 1

COMPREHENSIVE PRACTICE Test 2

COMPREHENSIVE PRACTICE Test 3

29. **The answer is d.** Because 0.44 ends in the hundredths place, turn it into a fraction with 100 in the denominator, and then reduce the fraction.

$$\frac{44}{100} = \frac{11}{25}$$

30. **The answer is c.** Set up a proportion to solve this problem. Be sure to align the units correctly: g across from g and mL across from mL. Then cross-multiply and divide both sides by 75 to solve for x.

$$\frac{75 \text{ g}}{100 \text{ mL}} = \frac{300 \text{ g}}{x}$$

$$75x = 30,000$$

$$x = 400 \text{ mL}$$

31. **The answer is d.** To find the fraction halfway between $\frac{1}{2}$ and $\frac{1}{4}$, find the *average* of $\frac{1}{2}$ and $\frac{1}{4}$. First, create like fractions, and add them:

$$\frac{1}{2} = \frac{2}{4}$$

$$\frac{2}{4} + \frac{1}{4} = \frac{3}{4}$$

Divide by 2 to find the average.

$$\frac{3}{4} \div 2 = \frac{3}{4} \times \frac{1}{2} = \frac{3}{8}$$

Alternatively, if you recognize that $\frac{1}{2} = \frac{4}{8}$ and $\frac{1}{4} = \frac{2}{8}$, then $\frac{3}{8}$ is halfway between $\frac{2}{8}$ and $\frac{4}{8}$.

32. **The answer is d.** Substitute 4 for x, and simplify.

$$x^3 = 4^3 = 4 \times 4 \times 4 = 64$$

33. **The answer is b.** Substitute 10 months for the age of the infant in the formula, and simplify.

$$\frac{10 \text{ months}}{150} \times \text{adult dose} = \frac{1}{15} \times \text{adult dose}$$

34. **The answer is c.** To eliminate x from one side of the equation, subtract 2x from both sides of the equation.

$$5x - 7 = 2x + 8$$

$$\underline{-2x \qquad -2x}$$

$$3x - 7 = 8$$

Then add 7 to both sides of the equation, and divide both sides by 3 to solve for x.

$3x - 7 = 8$

$+7 \quad\quad +7$

$3x = 15$

$\div 3 \ \div 3$

$x = 5$

35. **The answer is b.** The wording "600% as many diabetics" means the same thing as "6 times as many." For example, if there was 1 diabetic in 1935, then 600% more in 1978 would be 6 workers. As a result, for every 200 workers in 1935, there would be 6×200, or 1,200 workers in 1978.

36. **The answer is c.** On $10,000, an annual interest rate of 15.7% will yield $1,570 in interest *in one year*.

$0.157 \times 10,000 = \$1,570$

However, the question asks for the interest *in 6 months*. Divide $1,570 by 2 to reach the correct answer: $785.

37. **The answer is b.** To solve this problem, turn it into an equation, converting the phrase "of what" into x, and divide both sides by 0.16 to solve for x.

$16\% \times x = 128$

$0.16x = 128$

$x = 800$

38. **The answer is a.** This problem calls for three steps.

First: Change 6.6% to a decimal by dividing by 100: 0.066.

Second: To find 6.6% of 300, multiply 300 by 0.066: 19.8.

Third: Because the question asks for your answer to the "closest whole number," round 19.8 up to 20.

39. **The answer is a.** To solve this problem, turn it into an equation, converting the phrase "What percentage" into x, divide both sides by 140 to solve for x, and convert the value for x into a percentage at the end of the problem.

$x \cdot 140 = 7$

$140x = 7$

$x = 0.05$

Change 0.05 to a percentage by multiplying by 100: 5% is your answer.

40. **The answer is d.** If every solution you make contains 8% alcohol, then the question is really asking how many groups of 8% solution you can make from 40 mL of

alcohol. In other words, how many 8% units are there in 40? You should recognize this as division. Change 8% to a decimal by dividing by 100.

$40 \div 8\% =$

$40 \div 0.08 = 500 \text{ mL}$

To avoid the decimal, you could also convert 40 to 4,000: $4,000 \div 8 = 500 \text{ mL}$.

SECTION A

SECTION B

SECTION C

COMPREHENSIVE PRACTICE Test 1

COMPREHENSIVE PRACTICE Test 2

COMPREHENSIVE PRACTICE Test 3

III. Mathematics

1. **The answer is b.** $68 \times 42 = 2{,}856$

2. **The answer is a.** To find our how far 35.8 is below 37, subtract. (It is OK to add the decimal point and a zero to 37.)

   $37.0^\circ - 35.8^\circ = 1.2^\circ$

3. **The answer is c.**

   $$\frac{4}{5} = \frac{16}{20} \text{ and } \frac{1}{4} = \frac{5}{20}$$

   $$\frac{16}{20} + \frac{5}{20} = \frac{21}{20}$$

4. **The answer is d.** You may set up a proportion to solve this problem. Remember to align the units correctly: grains across from grains and drams across from drams. Then cross-multiply to solve for x.

   $$\frac{60 \text{ grains}}{1 \text{ dram}} = \frac{x}{24 \text{ drams}}, \; x = 1{,}440 \text{ grains.}$$ You can also solve as 60 grains/dram $\times$ 24 drams = 1,440 grains.

5. **The answer is a.** Substitute x for ?, and subtract 268 from both sides of the equation.

   $$x + 268 = 532$$
   $$ -268 -268$$
   $$ x = 264$$

6. **The answer is a.** If 1 flask holds $3\frac{1}{2}$ oz, then 3 flasks (each with $3\frac{1}{2}$ oz) will hold:

   $$3\frac{1}{2} \times 3 = 9\frac{3}{2} = 10\frac{1}{2}$$

7. **The answer is b.** Invert the second fraction and multiply.

   $$\frac{3}{2} \div \frac{2}{3} = \frac{3}{2} \times \frac{3}{2} = \frac{9}{4}$$

8. **The answer is b.** You may set up a proportion to solve this problem. Remember to align the units correctly: beats across from beats and seconds across from seconds. Use 60 seconds instead of 1 minute for the second ratio. Then just cross-multiply, and divide both sides by 12 to solve for x.

   $$\frac{26 \text{ beats}}{12 \text{ sec}} = \frac{x}{60 \text{ sec}}$$

   $$12x = 1{,}560$$

148

$x = 130$

You can also solve this by dividing 26 beats by 12 seconds to find 2.16 beats per second. Then multiply 2.16 beats/sec by 60 seconds to arrive at 130 beats.

9. **The answer is c.** Multiply, ignoring the decimal places; count the number of decimal places in both numbers, and count in from the right.

2.05	2 decimal places
$\times\ 4.5$	1 decimal place
9.225	3 decimal places total

10. **The answer is d.** Use the following formula to find the volume of a rectangular solid (like a storeroom), and substitute the given values.

$V = lwh$

where l = length, w = width, and h = height.

$V = 12\ \text{m} \times 10\ \text{m} \times 9\ \text{m}$

$V = 1,080\ \text{m}^3$

11. **The answer is c.** Divide 3 by 5 to find the decimal equivalent of $\frac{3}{5}$.

$$\frac{3}{5} = 5\overline{)3}^{\,0.6}$$

12. **The answer is a.** You may set up a proportion to solve this problem. Remember to align the units properly: liters across from liters and mL across from mL. Then cross-multiply, and divide both sides by 1,000 to solve for x.

$$\frac{1\text{L}}{1,000\ \text{mL}} = \frac{x}{200\ \text{mL}}$$

$1,000x = 200$

$$x = \frac{200}{1,000} = \frac{1}{5}$$

You can also solve this by dividing 200 mL by 1,000 mL = 0.2 L = $\frac{2}{10} = \frac{1}{5}$.

13. **The answer is b.** Substitute 20 for y, combine like terms, and divide both sides by 4 to solve for x.

$4x = y + 16$

$4x = 20 + 16$

$4x = 36$

$x = 9$

14. **The answer is b.** To find 15% of 660, first convert 15% to a decimal by dividing by 100: 15% = 0.15. Then multiply 0.15 by 660. (Ignore the decimal places, then

count the total places in both numbers and count places in from the right in your answer.)

600   0 decimal places

$\times$ 0.15   2 decimal places

99.00   2 decimal places

15. **The answer is d.** Multiply both the dividend and the divisor by 100, and perform the division.

$0.02\overline{)24.68}$

$2\overline{)2,468}$

$\dfrac{1,234}{2\overline{)2,468}}$

16. **The answer is d.** You may set up a proportion to solve this problem. Remember to align your units correctly: oz across from oz and cal across from cal. Then cross-multiply, and divide both sides by 270 to solve for x.

$$\frac{1\ oz}{270\ cal} = \frac{x}{1,215\ Cal}$$

$270x = 1,215$

$x = 4.5\ oz$

Another way of solving this is to divide 1,215 cal by 270 calories/oz = 4.5 oz.

17. **The answer is b.** To find 35% of 14, change 35% to a decimal by dividing by 100: 35% = 0.35. Then multiply 0.35 by 14.

$0.35 \times 14 = 4.90$

Because 0.35 has 2 decimal places and 14 has none, the answer has 2 decimal places.

18. **The answer is c.** You may set up a proportion to solve this problem. As always, remember to align the units properly: oz across from oz and Cal across from Cal. Cross multiply to solve for x.

$$\frac{1\ oz}{112\ Cal} = \frac{\frac{7}{8}\ oz}{x}$$

$$x = \frac{7}{8} \times 112$$

$$x = \frac{7}{8} \times \frac{112}{1} = \frac{784}{8} = 98\ Cal$$

You can also solve this by multiplying 112 Cal/oz times $\frac{7}{8}$ oz = 98 Cal.

III. Mathematics Answers | 151

SECTION A
SECTION B
SECTION C
COMPREHENSIVE PRACTICE Test 1
COMPREHENSIVE PRACTICE Test 2
COMPREHENSIVE PRACTICE Test 3

19. **The answer is c.** If $A < B$ and $C < B$, then *both* A and C must be less than B. Looking at the answers, only one choice has both A and C less than B: choice c.

20. **The answer is c.** The width of each bandage is the same as the width of the fabric: 4 in. So multiply:

$$5\frac{1}{4} \text{ in} \times 3 = 15\frac{3}{4} \text{ in}$$

Then subtract:

$$20 \text{ in} - 15\frac{3}{4} \text{ in} = 4\frac{1}{4} \text{ in}$$

The remaining fabric $= 4\frac{1}{4} \times 4$ in.

21. **The answer is a.** There is a property of zero that states, for any two numbers a and b, if $ab = 0$, then either $a = 0$ or $b = 0$. This property can be applied to this problem (in reverse), even though four numbers are being multiplied. Because one of those numbers is zero, the product has to be zero. You do not need to do any multiplication to solve this one!

22. **The answer is a.** You may set up a proportion to solve this problem. As always, be sure to align your units correctly: grains across from grains and mL across from mL. Then cross-multiply, and divide both sides by 40 to solve for x.

$$\frac{40 \text{ grains}}{600 \text{ mL}} = \frac{72 \text{ grains}}{x}$$

$$40x = 43{,}200$$

$$x = 1{,}080 \text{ mL}$$

23. **The answer is b.** To solve this problem, plug in the values for a, b, and c, and simplify.

$$\frac{a + b + c^2}{a - b + c^2} = \frac{5 + 3 + 1^2}{5 - 3 + 1^2} = \frac{9}{3} = 3$$

24. **The answer is d.** If 1,700 quarts of blood flow to the kidneys each day (or every 24 hours), then the average hourly flow is:

$$24\overline{)1{,}700} \approx 71 \text{ quarts/hour} \quad (70.83)$$

We round up to 71 because 0.83 is greater than 0.5

25. **The answer is a.** To change a percentage to a decimal, divide by 100 and drop the percentage (%) sign.

$$6.24\% \div 100 = 0.0624$$

Recall the shortcut for dividing by 10, 100, 1,000, and so on: Move the decimal point to the left the same number of places as there are zeros in the divisor.

26. **The answer is d.** To find the number of degrees between −114°C and 78°C, subtract one from the other.

78° − (−114°) =

78° + 114° = 192°

In other words, just add the amounts above and below zero, ignoring signs: 78° (above zero) + 114° (below zero) = 192°. Either method is OK, because you are looking only for the *number* of degrees between −114° and 78°; the sign of your answer does not matter. In this case, there are 192° of difference.

27. **The answer is c.** Simplify each expression within the parentheses, change 6 to a fraction, and multiply.

$(3 \div 9) \times (12 \div 2) =$

$\frac{1}{3} \times 6 = \frac{1}{3} \times \frac{6}{1} = \frac{6}{3} = 2$

28. **The answer is a.** Use the following formula to find the area of a square:

$A = l \times w$

where l = length and w = width. First find the area of the gauze square.

$A = 24 \times 24 = 576$ square in

Use the same formula to find the area of each gauze pad.

$A = 3 \times 3 = 9$ in^2

To find out how many little gauze pads can be made from the large gauze square, divide 576 square in by 9 square in: 64 pads is your answer.

29. **The answer is b.** Because 0.65 ends in the hundredths place, you may turn it into a fraction by placing 65 over 100 and then reduce the fraction.

$\frac{65}{100} = \frac{65 \div 5}{100 \div 5} = \frac{13}{20}$

30. **The answer is c.** You may set up a proportion to solve this problem. As always, make sure to align the units correctly: doses across from doses and mL across from mL. Cross-multiply, and divide both sides by 8 to solve for x.

$\frac{8 \text{ doses}}{0.12 \text{ mL}} = \frac{10 \text{ doses}}{x}$

$8x = 1.2$

$x = 0.15$ mL

You can also solve this by dividing 0.12 mL by 8 doses to find 0.015 mL/dose and then multiplying by 10 doses to arrive at 0.15 mL.

31. **The answer is d.** Substitute 2 for x, simplify the expression inside the parentheses, and then simplify the expression outside the parentheses.

$$x^3(x + 1) =$$

$$2^3(2 + 1) =$$

$$2^3(3) =$$

$$8(3) = 24$$

32. **The answer is b.** First, add all three amounts of sodium. Remember to line up the decimal points. It is OK to add zeros to the right of the decimal point so that they line up.

0.890 gram + 1.200 grams + 0.004 gram = 2.094 grams

Divide this by 3, because there are three samples.

$$\frac{2.094}{3} = 3\overline{)2.094}^{0.698} \approx 0.7 \text{ grams}$$

33. **The answer is c.** An easy way to compare fractions is to convert them all to decimals, that is, divide the denominator into the numerator.

$$\frac{1}{3} = 0.33$$

Compare this to:

$$\frac{5}{12} = 0.42$$

$$\frac{7}{18} = 0.38$$

$$\frac{7}{24} = 0.29$$

$$\frac{2}{9} = 0.22$$

When you compare the decimal equivalents, you find that $\frac{1}{3}$ is closest to $\frac{7}{24}$.

34. **The answer is a.** First, convert 32% to a decimal by dividing by 100.

$$32\% \div 100 = 0.32$$

Then calculate 32% of 50 by multiplying.

0.32	2 decimal places
×50	0 decimal places
16.00	2 decimal places

SECTION A

SECTION B

SECTION C

COMPREHENSIVE PRACTICE Test 1

COMPREHENSIVE PRACTICE Test 2

COMPREHENSIVE PRACTICE Test 3

Finally, subtract 16 from 50 to find out how many ounces of water remain.

$50 - 16 = 34$ oz

35. **The answer is d.** First, convert 6% to a decimal by dividing by 100:

$6\% \div 100 = 0.06$

Now translate the problem into an equation, substituting x for the phrase "of which" and dividing both sides by 0.06 to solve for x.

$0.06x = 150$

$\div 0.06 \quad \div 0.06$

$x = 2,500$

Note: To divide 0.06 into 150, multiply by 100 to make your divisor a whole number, and divide.

$0.06\overline{)150} =$

$6\overline{)15,000}^{\,2,500}$

36. **The answer is d.** Before you solve this problem, you need to convert gallons into ounces. Here some conversions you should become familiar with:

1 pint	16 fluid ounces	
2 pints	32 fluid ounces	1 quart
4 pints	128 fluid ounces	1 gallon

You may set up a proportion to solve this problem. As usual, make sure you align your units properly. Cross-multiply, and then divide both sides by 8 to solve for x.

$$\frac{8 \text{ oz}}{110 \text{ Cal}} = \frac{128 \text{ oz}}{x}$$

$$8x = 14,080$$

$$x = 1,760 \text{ Cal}$$

You can also solve this problem by finding cal/oz and multiplying by 128 oz.

$$\frac{110 \text{ Cal}}{8 \text{ oz}} = 13.75 \text{ Cal/oz}$$

13.75 Cal/oz $\times 128$ oz $= 1,760$ Cal

37. **The answer is a.** Subtract 6 from both sides of the equation, and divide both sides of the equation by 8 to solve for x.

$8y + 6 = 40$

$\quad -6 = -6$

$\quad 8y = 34$

$$y = \frac{34}{8} = 4\frac{2}{8} = 4\frac{1}{4}$$

38. **The answer is d.** The entire circle contains 360 degrees. If you want to represent 25%, or $\frac{1}{4}$, of the circle as rent, find 25%, or $\frac{1}{4}$ of 360°.

$$\frac{1}{4} \times \frac{360°}{1} = \frac{360°}{4} = 90°$$

Ninety degrees of the circle represent 25%, or $\frac{1}{4}$.

39. **The answer is c.** Convert the question into an equation, replacing the phrase "What percentage of" with x%.

$12 = x$% of 96, or

$12 = x(96)$

(We will deal with x being a percentage at the end of the problem.) Divide both sides of the equation by 96, and convert the result into a percentage by multiplying it by 100.

$12 = 96x$

$$\frac{12}{96} = \frac{96x}{96} = \frac{1}{8} = x$$

$x = 0.125$

$x = 0.125 \times 100 = 12.5\%$

40. **The answer is d.** Plug in 67° for °C, and simplify.

°C + 273 = K

67° + 273 = 340K

IV. Mathematics

1. **The answer is b.** Remember to line up the decimal points.

   $239.760 - 57.359 = 182.401$

2. **The answer is a.** Work this problem left to right. Add first.

   $321 + 407 = 728$

   Then subtract.

   $728 - 219 = 509$

3. **The answer is b.** First, find the total cost for three days. Then divide this total by 3 to get the average cost.

   $\$2.50 + \$1.85 + \$2.25 = \$6.60$

   $$\$6.60 \div 3 = \$2.20/\text{day}$$

4. **The answer is c.** Substitute 20 for x and simplify. Then combine like terms, and divide both sides of the equation by 3 to solve for y.

   $3y = 2x + 8$

   $3y = 2(20) + 8$

   $3y = 40 + 8$

   $3y = 48$

   $y = 16$

5. **The answer is b.** You don't have to worry about lining up the decimal places in this problem. Just multiply as you normally would.

   76.2 1 decimal place

   $\underline{\times 1.04}$ 2 decimal places

   79.248

   Make sure your answer has three decimal places.

6. **The answer is d.** First, find a common denominator for the two fractions. The LCD is 20, because both 4 and 5 are factors of 20. Write equivalent fractions, and add them.

   $$3\frac{3}{4} = 3\frac{15}{20} \text{ and } 1\frac{2}{5} = 1\frac{8}{20}$$

   $$3\frac{15}{20} + 1\frac{8}{20} = 4\frac{23}{20} = 5\frac{3}{20}$$

7. **The answer is b.** To find the sale price of a regularly priced book, you must do two things. First, find 15% of $25.00. Do this by multiplying $25 by 0.15.

   $0.15\ (\$25) = \$3.75$

156

Second, subtract $3.75 from $25.00 to get the sale price.

$25.00 − $3.75 = $21.25

8. **The answer is a.** Use the following formula to find the volume (V) of a cube, and plug in the values given in the problem.

$V = hwl$

where h = height, w = width, and l = length.

$V = 12 \text{ cm} \times 15 \text{ cm} \times 8 \text{ cm} = 1{,}440 \text{ cm}^3$

9. **The answer is b.** Solve this problem in two steps. First, multiply inside the parentheses.

$524 + (3 \times 5) =$

Second, add the two remaining numbers.

$524 + 15 = 539$

10. **The answer is d.** If you are comparing fractions with the same numerator (as in our example), then the fraction with the *smallest* denominator has the *largest* value. In this case, $9 \div 3$ yields the smallest number. So the fraction with this denominator has the largest value.

11. **The answer is c.** You may set up a proportion to solve this problem. Be sure to align the units correctly: cups across from cups and Cal across from Cal. Then cross-multiply, and change the fraction to a decimal.

$$\frac{1 \text{ cup}}{140 \text{ Calories}} = \frac{\frac{5}{8} \text{ cup}}{x}$$

$$x = 140 \times \frac{5}{8} = \frac{700}{8} = 87.5 \text{ Cal}$$

You can also solve by multiplying 140 Cal/cup by $\frac{5}{8}$ cup to arrive at 87.5 Cal.

12. **The answer is d.** To divide decimals, you must make sure the divisor (the number outside the box) is a whole number. In this case, move the decimal two places to the right to turn 0.15 into 15. Move the decimal two places to the right in the dividend as well.

$3.45 \div 0.15 = 23$

Here is the method of division:

$$0.15\overline{)3.45}$$

$$\begin{array}{r} 23 \\ 15\overline{)345} \end{array}$$

SECTION A

SECTION B

SECTION C

COMPREHENSIVE PRACTICE Test 1

COMPREHENSIVE PRACTICE Test 2

COMPREHENSIVE PRACTICE Test 3

13. **The answer is c.** First, use the information given to write the following proportion. Make sure you align the units correctly: substance K across from substance K and L across from L. The cross-multiply, and divide both sides of the equation by 7 to solve for x.

$$\frac{K}{L} = \frac{K}{L}$$

$$\frac{7\,g}{8\,g} = \frac{21\,g}{x}$$

$$7x = 168\,g$$

$$x = 24\,g$$

14. **The answer is c.** Divide using long division. Because the question asks for an answer to the "nearest 3 decimal places," you must divide out to the fourth decimal place (to round the answer properly).

$$\begin{array}{r} 10.4857 \\ 35\overline{)367.000} \end{array}$$

Stop dividing once you reach the fourth decimal place. Because the digit in the fourth decimal place is 5 or bigger, round the digit in the third decimal place up by 1. This makes your answer 10.486.

15. **The answer is b.** First find out what $\frac{2}{3}$ of 48 is:

$$\frac{2}{3} \cdot \frac{48}{1} = \frac{96}{3} = 32$$

There need to be 32 students who request tape recorders. Because 15 have already requested them, then $32 - 15$, or 17 more students, need to make the request to allow them in class.

16. **The answer is c.** You may set up a proportion to solve this problem. Be sure to align the units correctly: quarts across from quarts and liters across from liters. Then cross-multiply to solve for x, and make sure your answer has enough decimal places.

$$\frac{1\,qt}{0.9\,L} = \frac{3.6\,qt}{x}$$

$$x = (3.6)(0.9)$$

$$x = 3.24\,L$$

You can also solve this problem by multiplying 0.9 L/qt by 3.6 qt to get 3.24 L.

17. **The answer is c.** The area of the rectangle is $9 \times 10 = 90$ in^2. This is the number of 1×1-in squares, each with an area of 1 in^2. But the problem asks for 2×3-in squares, each with an area 6 in^2. To find out how many 6 in^2 squares fit in 90 in^2, divide 90 by 6, to get 15.

SECTION A

SECTION B

SECTION C

COMPREHENSIVE PRACTICE Test 1

COMPREHENSIVE PRACTICE Test 2

COMPREHENSIVE PRACTICE Test 3

18. **The answer is a.** Divide both sides by 3.

$3x < 4$

$x < \dfrac{4}{3}$

Because x is smaller than $\dfrac{4}{3}$, or $1\,\dfrac{1}{3}$, the only answer you can choose is 1.

19. **The answer is b.** You may set up a proportion to solve this problem. Be sure to align the units correctly: mL of solution across from mL of solution and mL of medication across from mL of medication. Then cross-multiply, and divide both sides by 250 to solve for x.

$\dfrac{30\ \text{mL}}{250\ \text{mL}} = \dfrac{x}{100\ \text{mL}}\,2$

$250x = 3{,}000$

$x = 12\ \text{mL}$

20. **The answer is d.** Solve this problem in two steps. First, subtract 179 from 184 to find the total weight loss: 184 lbs − 179 lbs = 5 lbs. Second, divide the 5 lbs by the 8 days it took to lose this weight:

$\dfrac{5}{8}$ lb/day = average weight loss

21. **The answer is a.** The rule for multiplying similar bases with exponents is to *add* the exponents.

$8a^3 \cdot 5a^4 = 40a^7$

22. **The answer is c.** First, you must find out what 75% of 18 mg is equal to:

$0.75 \times 18\ \text{mg} = 13.5\ \text{mg}$

Next, subtract 13.5 mg from 18 mg to find out how many more mg of iron are needed.

$18\ \text{mg} - 13.5\ \text{mg} = 4.5\ \text{mg}$

23. **The answer is d.** To solve this problem, turn it into an equation, making x equal to the cost of the textbooks, and divide both sides by 0.06 to solve for x.

6% of *the original cost* = $3.54

$0.06x = \$3.54$

$x = \$59.00$

24. **The answer is a.** First, convert $1\,\dfrac{1}{3}$ into $\dfrac{4}{3}$. Next, find a common denominator for 3 and 4.

$\dfrac{4}{3} = \dfrac{16}{12}$ and $\dfrac{3}{4} = \dfrac{9}{12}$

$$\frac{16}{12} = \frac{9}{12} = \frac{7}{12} \text{ cup}$$

25. **The answer is d.** The product $4a^2 - 49$ is known as a difference of two squares, because both the first and last terms are perfect squares and one is being subtracted from the other. There is a shortcut for factoring such a product. Knowing that your answer will be two binomials, you may assume that the first term of each will be the square root of $4a^2$, that the second term will be the square root of 49, and that the second term will also be opposite in sign. The signs must be opposite so that, when multiplied, their terms will cancel each other out. Thus

    $$4a^2 - 49 = (2a + 7)(2a - 7)$$

26. **The answer is c.** You must know two things about parallelograms to solve this problem. (1) There are 360° in the angles of a parallelogram. (2) Opposite angles in a parallelogram are equal. Once you recall these facts, the rest is simple. Subtract 100° (50° + 50°) from 360° to calculate how many degrees the two unmarked angles have in total. Divide this amount (260°) in half, because the two angles are equal; 260° ÷ 2 = 130°.

27. **The answer is a.** Split 45 into factors, and assign each factor its own radical sign. Then simplify.

    $$\sqrt{45} =$$
    $$\sqrt{9 \times 5} =$$
    $$\sqrt{9} \times \sqrt{5}$$
    $$3 \times \sqrt{5} = 3\sqrt{5}$$

28. **The answer is b.** Convert 3.4% into a decimal by dividing by 100, and then multiply it by 260.

    $$0.034 \times 260 = 8.840$$

29. **The answer is a.**

    $$60 - 24 = 36 \text{ patients improved}$$

    $$\frac{36}{60} = \frac{3}{5} = 0.6$$

    $$0.6 \times 100 = 60\%$$

30. **The answer is a.** To change a percentage to a decimal, divide the percentage by 100, and drop the % sign.

    $$3.7\% \div 100 = 0.037$$

31. **The answer is d.** Solve this problem in three steps. First, multiply the average feeding by the total number of days.

    $$7\frac{1}{4} \text{ oz} \times 4 \text{ feedings} = 29 \text{ oz}$$

SECTION A

SECTION B

SECTION C

COMPREHENSIVE PRACTICE Test 1

COMPREHENSIVE PRACTICE Test 2

COMPREHENSIVE PRACTICE Test 3

Then, subtract each of the 3 feedings from this total. You need to find a common denominator, which is 8.

$$7\frac{1}{2} = 7\frac{4}{8}$$

Third, add the three feedings.

$$6\frac{3}{8} \text{ oz} + 7\frac{4}{8} \text{ oz} + 7\frac{3}{8} \text{ oz} = 21\frac{2}{8} \text{ oz}$$

Finally, subtract $21\frac{2}{8}$ oz from the average of 29 oz.

$$29 \text{ oz} = 28\frac{8}{8} \text{ oz}$$

$$28\frac{8}{8} - 21\frac{2}{8} = 7\frac{6}{8} = 7\frac{3}{4} \text{ oz}$$

32. **The answer is b.**

$$3\sqrt{36} = 3 \times 6 = 18$$

33. **The answer is d.** Because 0.15 ends in the hundredths place, change it to a fraction by placing 15 over 100, and reducing the fraction.

$$\frac{15}{100} = \frac{3}{20}$$

34. **The answer is a.** To solve this problem, turn it into an equation.

30% of a number is 90

0.3 of x = 90

Convert 30% to a decimal, and divide both sides of the equation by 0.3 to solve for x.

$$0.3x = 90$$

$$x = 300$$

35. **The answer is b.**

$$10^4 = 10,000$$

$$10,000 \times 0.35 = 3,500$$

The shortcut for multiplying decimals by a power of 10 is to move the decimal to the *right* by the same number of places as there are zeros in the power of 10. Following this rule, 0.35 becomes 3,500!

36. **The answer is d.** Every circle contains 360°; so if the circle graph is divided into three equal sections, we can find the number of degrees in each section by dividing 360° by 3.

$$\frac{360°}{3°} = 120°$$

37. **The answer is d.** Convert each mixed number into an improper fraction, and then multiply them.

$$3\frac{3}{8} = \frac{27}{8} \text{ and } 2\frac{1}{3} = \frac{7}{3}$$

$$\frac{27}{8} \times \frac{7}{3} = \frac{189}{24} = 7\frac{7}{8}$$

38. **The answer is c.** Convert 7.5% into a decimal by dividing by 100: 7.5% ÷ 100 = 0.075. Then multiply 0.075 by 150 to find your answer.

$$0.075 \times 150 = 11.250$$

39. **The answer is a.** Deal with x being a percentage at the end of the problem.

x% of 150 = 12, or

$$150x = 12$$

Divide both sides by 150, and turn 0.08 into a percentage by multiplying by 100.

$$x = 0.08 \times 100 = 8\%$$

40. **The answer is a.** The distributive property of multiplication allows you to distribute across a sum or difference. This is easier shown than explained.

EX: The expression $3 \times (4 + 5)$ means that the 3 is distributed across $4 + 5$. Each addend (4 and 5) in the parentheses is multiplied by 3.

$(3 \times 4) + (3 \times 5)$

$12 + 15$

27

The only answer that illustrates this property is choice a:

$3x + 4(a - 2) = 3x + 4a - 8$

On the right side of the equation, 4 has been distributed across a and -2.

BIBLIOGRAPHY

Burton, Grace M., and Evan M. Maletsky. *Math Advantage*. New York: Harcourt/Brace, 1999.

Dolciani, Mary P., Richard A. Swanson, and John A. Graham. *Algebra*. Boston: Houghton Mifflin, 1992.

Fair, Jan, and Sadie Chavis Bragg. *Algebra I*. Upper Saddle River, NJ: Prentice Hall, 1990.

Foster, Alan G., Gell, Joan M., and Gordon, Berchie W. *Merrill Algebra I*. Philadelphia, PA: Glencoe, 1995.

Jurgensen, Ray C., Richard G. Brown, and John W. Jurgensen. *Geometry*. Boston: Houghton Mifflin, 1988.

Lowry, David W., Earl G. Ockenga, and Walter E. Rucker. *Pre-Algebra*. Lexington, MA: D. C. Heath and Company, 1986.

Moise, Floyd L., and Edwin E. Downs. *Geometry*. Reading, MA: Addison-Wesley, 1991.

Smith, Charles, Mervin Keedy, Marvin Bittinger, and Lucy J. Orfan. *Algebra*. Reading, MA: Addison-Wesley, 1988.

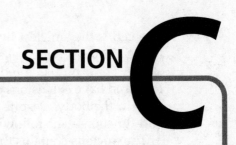

Science Content Review

General Biology

CELL STRUCTURE AND FUNCTION

Terms to Be Defined

cell
nucleus
DNA
plasma (cell) membrane
interstitial fluid
selectively permeable
  (semipermeable)
cytoplasm
organelles

mitochondria
ribosome
endoplasmic reticulum
  (ER)
Golgi complex
lysosome
cell wall
chloroplast
vacuole

chromatin
chromosomes
mitosis
semipermeable membrane
zygote
meiosis
ATP
RNA

The **cell** is the smallest living unit and the basic unit of function and structure for all living things. Living cells average approximately 60% water and vary in size and shape. For example, a red blood cell is disk-shaped, whereas nerve cells can be very long and have extensions on their main body. Cells also vary in terms of the roles they play in the body. Despite their differences, cells have a number of common features and functions. The following description is that of a general animal cell.

The **nucleus** contains the genetic information, or **DNA** (deoxyribonucleic acid), and controls the activities of the cell. The **plasma** (or **cell**) **membrane** is what is known as a **semipermeable membrane** that separates the contents of the cell from the surrounding fluid, the **interstitial fluid.** The interstitial fluid contains substances such as amino acids, sugars, fatty acids, hormones, neurotransmitters, and salts. The term **selectively permeable (semipermeable)** refers to the selective nature of the plasma membrane. It contains pores and channels that allow only particles of the right size or the right chemical nature to pass through. Additionally, the plasma membrane contains receptors that bind with specific substances. Thus it allows for special entry or signals the cell to perform a certain activity.

The **cytoplasm** is the fluid matrix found between the plasma membrane and the nucleus that acts as scaffolding for the organelles. **Organelles**, or "little organs," are specialized units in the cell that perform certain functions. The **mitochondria** are the locations for cellular respiration, that is, the conversion of food to energy at the cellular level. Thus the mitochondria are the sites of energy production and of most of its **ATP** (adenosine triphosphate), which is a chemical the cell uses to transfer energy within the cell. **Ribosomes** are the sites of protein synthesis in the cell and contain **RNA.** Some ribosomes float freely, whereas others are attached to the **endoplasmic reticulum (ER).** The ER serves as a means for transport within the cell and is made up of many channels. Rough ER, named for the fact that it has ribosomes on its surface, serves to store and deliver the proteins made by the attached ribosomes. Smooth ER is free of ribosomes and is found in a variety of cells. It performs varying functions in different cells, including the storage of enzymes and minerals and the folding of proteins, among other things. It is thought to be involved in the detoxification of chemicals and the metabolism of fats. The **Golgi complex** modifies and packages proteins destined either for use in the cell or for export from the cell. **Lysosomes** are sacs that contain strong digestive enzymes. These sacs are responsible for digesting cell structures that are no longer living or that are malfunctioning, and for digesting waste.

Plant cells can be distinguished by the facts that they are surrounded by a **cell wall** and that they contain chloroplasts. The cell wall is essential for protection of the cell, the maintenance of the shape, and water balance. **Chloroplasts** contain chlorophyll, which is necessary for photosynthesis. Plant cells also often have large **vacuoles**, which are compartments in the cytoplasm that act as places for secretion, excretion, and storage. (See Figure 1.)

Cells divide for a number of reasons: growth, repair, and the production of gametes (sperm or egg cells). The most important result of cell division is that the genetic material, DNA, is transmitted to the offspring. DNA is found in the nucleus in the form of chromatin and chromosomes. When a cell is not dividing, DNA is found in the form of loosely structured **chromatin**, but when a cell is dividing, the DNA is seen in condensed rod-shaped bodies called **chromosomes.**

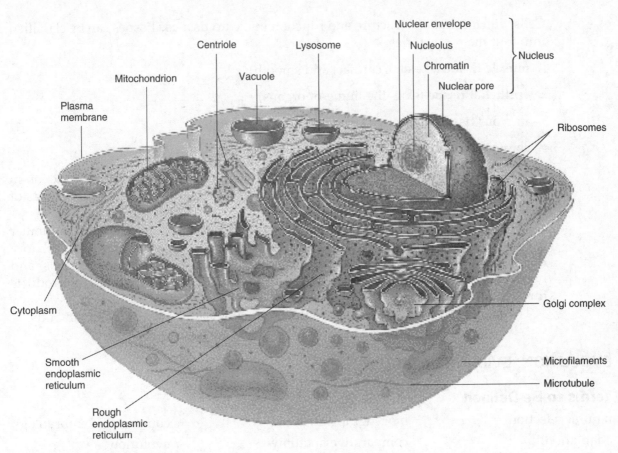

Figure 1. Structure of a Cell

When cells divide, the appropriate amount of genetic material must be passed on to the new, or so-called daughter, cells. In somatic (nonreproductive) cells, the new cells are identical copies of the parent cells. This is achieved by a doubling of the chromosomes prior to division. This type of cell division is referred to as **mitosis**, and it is useful in the growth and repair of our bodies. Another type of division takes place in the production of gametes. These reproductive cells contain half of the normal number of chromosomes so that the **zygote**, the cell created by the union of a sperm and egg, contains a full set of chromosomes, half from each parent. This type of division, or **meiosis**, consists first of a doubling of chromosomes and then two subsequent divisions. Thus the products are four daughter cells, each with half the normal number of chromosomes.

LEVELS OF ORGANIZATION

Terms to Be Defined

tissue

muscle tissue

epithelial tissue

nervous tissue

connective tissue

organ

organ system

organism

SECTION A

SECTION B

SECTION C

COMPREHENSIVE PRACTICE Test 1

COMPREHENSIVE PRACTICE Test 2

COMPREHENSIVE PRACTICE Test 3

Cells with a common structure and function make up **tissues.** Tissues can be classified into four main categories:

1. **muscle tissue** (skeletal, cardiac, and smooth)

2. **epithelial tissue** (skin, the lining of organs)

3. **nervous tissue** (neurons)

4. **connective tissue** (cartilage, blood, fat, bone)

Various tissues are combined into an **organ**, which performs a specialized function in the body. For instance, an organ involved in digestion and made up of three types of tissue is the stomach.

The next level of organization is the **organ system**, which is made up of a number of organs working together to carry out a major function. For example, the circulatory system includes many organs, such as the heart, blood vessels, spleen, tonsils, and lymph nodes. These organs work together to circulate and deliver necessary products throughout the body.

The highest level of organization is the **organism** itself, such as the human body.

EVOLUTION: EVIDENCE AND THEORIES

Terms to Be Defined

natural selection	biogeography	comparative embryology
adaptation	comparative anatomy	evolution
fossil record	molecular biology	

In 1859 Charles Darwin published *On the Origin of Species by Means of Natural Selection*, which presented evidence for evolution. **Evolution** is a theory regarding the processes that have produced the biological diversity we see today. Darwin's two main arguments were that:

1. the present species evolved from ancestral ones, and

2. evolution occurs by means of **natural selection**, the process by which the traits that promote or enhance an organism's ability to survive and reproduce are passed on to following generations.

For natural selection to occur, organisms must have variations, some of which give the individuals having them an advantage in the struggle for survival. The struggle for survival occurs because each generation of a species produces more offspring than can survive. In this struggle, the individuals best suited to their environment survive ("survival of the fittest") and pass on the traits to their offspring. This is called **adaptation**, and we say that these organisms are best adapted to their environments.

There is evidence supporting the theory of evolution, such as the **fossil record**, which consists of remnants or traces of organisms from past geologic ages. Fossils that have been dated show a time line for the appearance of different organisms in the following order: fish, then amphibians, then reptiles, and finally mammals and birds. This finding supports Darwin's first evolutionary argument and contradicts the theory that all species were created at the same time. Many other types of evidence have been found through the studies of:

- **biogeography** (the geographical distribution of plants and animals),

- **comparative anatomy** (the comparison of organisms' structures),

- **comparative embryology** (the comparison of organisms' embryos), and

- **molecular biology** (biology at the molecular level). We also see evolution occurring today. For example, the development of resistant strains of bacteria is an example of evolution occurring today.

EVOLUTION: CLASSIFICATION OF ORGANISMS

Terms to Be Defined

taxonomy	protist	family
kingdom	fungi	genus
animal	phylum	species
plant	class	
monera	order	

Due to the great biological diversity on our planet, a system was needed to organize the many species into groups. In **taxonomy** (the study of scientific classification), taxonomists group species according to their similarities and differences. There are many levels of classification, and each level is more specific than the one above it. The broadest units of classification are the **kingdoms**, of which there are five: **animal, plant, monera** (bacteria), **protist** (protozoa, algae, and some molds), and **fungi** (molds, mushrooms, yeasts, and the like). The next six classifications become increasingly specific: **phylum, class, order, family, genus,** and **species**. The scientific name of an organism is always the genus and the species of the organism, with the genus capitalized and the species not; for example, *Escherichia coli (E.coli)*, the well-nown bacterium found in the colons of warm-blooded animals, is of the genus *Escherichia* and the specis *coli*.

DIFFUSION AND OSMOSIS

Terms to Be Defined

active transport	osmosis	hypertonic
passive transport	isotonic	filtration
diffusion	hypotonic	

The plasma membrane controls entry to and exit from the cell by means of either passive or active mechanisms. **Active transport** involves the use of energy in the form of ATP to move substances across the membrane. **Passive transport** does not require energy and makes use of diffusion and filtration. In **diffusion**, particles move in a random manner, spreading evenly throughout an available space and moving from regions of high concentration to those of low concentration. For instance, if you open a perfume bottle at the front of the room, after a while the people in the back of the room smell the scent.

A specific type of diffusion is that of water, or **osmosis**. Water moves from an area of high water concentration (or low particle concentration) to an area of low water concentration (high particle concentration). For example, assume that red blood cells are

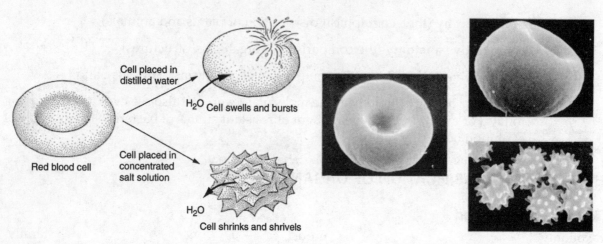

Figure 2. Osmosis and Red Blood Cells

in water containing a certain concentration of a solute. (See Figure 2.) When the solute concentration of the water is the same as that inside the cell, the solution is said to be **isotonic**. Thus, the amount of water that leaves the cell and the amount that enters it are equal. When the solute is more concentrated outside the cell than inside it, the solution is **hypertonic**. Water leaves the cell due to osmosis; it moves from the high-water/low-particle concentration to low-water/high-particle concentration. As a result, the cell shrinks. If the solute concentration outside the cell is lower than that inside the cell, the solution is **hypotonic**. Water flows into the cell (again high-water/low-particle concentration to low-water/high-particle concentration). If the flow continues long enough, the cell bursts.

Filtration is the movement of water and solutes through the membrane by fluid, or hydrostatic, pressure.

ECOLOGY: INTERRELATIONSHIPS

Terms to Be Defined

autotroph	food chain	mutualism
heterotroph	food web	biosphere
primary consumer	decomposer	biome
herbivore	biotic	deserts
omnivore	abiotic	tropical rain forest
secondary consumer	predator	deciduous forest
carnivore	prey	coniferous forest
tertiary consumer	symbiosis	tundra
trophic level	parasitism	
ecosystem	commensalism	

Autotrophs are organisms that produce their own food from inorganic substances. Plants are autotrophs. **Heterotrophs**, on the other hand, obtain their food by consuming plants or other animals. They are also referred to as consumers. **Primary**

consumers may be **herbivores** (plant eaters) or **omnivores** (plant and meat eaters). **Secondary consumers** are **carnivores** (meat eaters) or omnivores that eat herbivores. **Tertiary consumers** are carnivores that eat other carnivores or omnivores.

These divisions, which are made on the basis of how the organism meets its nutritional needs, make up the **trophic levels** of an **ecosystem**. The autotrophs are the most important trophic level in the ecosystem and are known as producers; the other levels are made up of the different types of consumers. The path along which food is transferred from level to level is called a **food chain**, and the interrelationship of many food chains is called a **food web**. An important role in an ecosystem is played by the **decomposers**, such as bacteria and fungi, which consume nonliving organic material and release inorganic material. Thus material is recycled through the ecosystem, and inorganic material is made available to the plants. Factors that affect an ecosystem are classified as biotic or abiotic. **Biotic** factors include the living parts of the ecosystem, and **abiotic** factors are nonliving influences, such as temperature, humidity, or soil composition. Within an ecosystem are many interrelationships among species, such as between **predator** and **prey**. Separate species living together (**symbiosis**) include **parasitism** (in which one species benefits and one species is harmed, such as a tapeworm in a human host), **commensalism** (in which one species benefits and one is unaffected, such as a remora and shark), and **mutualism** (in which both species benefit, such as lichen, which is made up of a fungus and an alga living together).

On a larger scale, a **biosphere** is the entire portion of our planet that is inhabited by living things in a variety of ecosystems and communities. Within the biosphere are groups of ecosystems that are common to the various types of geographical areas. These geographical areas are called **biomes**. Many of the terrestrial biomes are classified according to differences in climate. Some of the most familiar terrestrial biomes are as follows:

- **Deserts** have little precipitation and are more arid than all of the other biomes.

- **Tropical rain forests** typically have a relatively constant temperature (68°F–90°F), constant daylight length throughout the year, high humidity, and abundant rain (200–400 cm/year). These forests are known for their biodiversity, having more species than any other area of the world. Trees grow very tall and there is great competition for light. Little light reaches the forest floor.

- **Deciduous forests** are usually found in the temperate, midlatitude regions of the world, where the air contains enough moisture to support the growth of large trees. Deciduous trees, such as oaks and maples, are ones that drop their leaves during the dry months. The temperatures in this biome can range widely from season to season.

- **Coniferous forests** (taigas) are found at high and cool elevations, where the seasons consist of short summers and long, chilly winters. These areas are characterized by conifers, such as pines and firs, which do not shed their leaves in the cold, dry months.

- **Tundras** are characterized by very cold temperatures and high altitude. Here the conditions allow shrubs and bushes to grow, but no trees.

Aquatic biomes are abundant as well. Some familiar ones include swamps, wetlands, rivers and streams, coral reefs, and estuaries. Marine biomes occupy the oceans and are classified according to their water depth and proximity to the shoreline.

PLANTS AND PHOTOSYNTHESIS

Terms to Be Defined

photosynthesis	petal	style
chlorophyll	stamen	ovary
cuticle	filament	ovule
stomate	anther	seed
sepal	pistil	fruit
angiosperms	stigma	

All organisms obtain the organic substances they need by either autotrophic or heterotrophic means. To produce their own organic molecules from inorganic molecules in the environment, autotrophs use the process called **photosynthesis**. In this process, the green pigment **chlorophyll**, which is located in the chloroplasts of plant cells, absorbs light energy. This energy, in turn, drives the synthesis of food molecules:

$$6CO_2 + 6H_2O + \text{light energy} \rightarrow C_6H_{12}O_6 + 6O_2, \text{ or}$$

$$\text{carbon dioxide + water + light energy} \rightarrow \text{carbohydrates + oxygen}$$

Plants have acquired unique characteristics to help them survive in a terrestrial environment. The stems and leaves of most plants are covered by a **cuticle**, which is a waxy layer that helps prevent water loss through evaporation. Additionally, the leaves have **stomates**, which are pores on the lower surface of the leaves that allow carbon dioxide to enter and oxygen to be released during photosynthesis without losing too much water. The flower in flowering plants, or **angiosperms**, is responsible for reproduction. (See Figure 3.) The **sepals** encase the flower before it blooms, and the **petals** are useful in attracting pollinators. In the center of the petals are the stamen and pistils. The **stamen** consists of the **filament**, which supports the **anther**, where pollen is produced. The **pistil** consists of the **stigma** (which receives pollen), the **style** (which leads to the ovary), and the **ovary** (which contains the **ovules** and where fertilization occurs). After fertilization, the ovules within the ovary develop into **seeds**. After fertilization, the walls of the ovary thicken to protect the seed, and this thick, fleshy, protective layer is what we know and love as **fruit**.

GENETICS

Terms to Be Defined

gene	heterozygote	deoxyribose
allele	homozygote	phosphate group
dominance	sex-linked traits	nitrogenous base
segregation	autosome	transcription
independent assortment	genotype	messenger RNA (m-RNA)
codominance	phenotype	transfer RNA (t-RNA)
linkage	replication	uracil
double helix	nucleotide	amino acid

SECTION A
SECTION B
SECTION C
COMPREHENSIVE PRACTICE Test 1
COMPREHENSIVE PRACTICE Test 2
COMPREHENSIVE PRACTICE Test 3

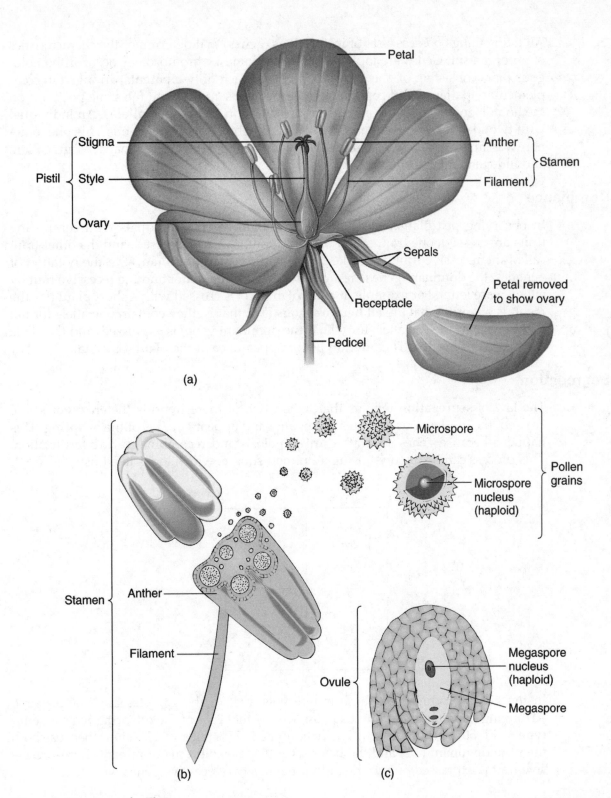

Figure 3. Structure of a Flower

All living things possess a set of instructions (**genes**) that determines the characteristics of an organism. Genes are located on chromosomes. Chromosomes occur in homologous pairs consisting of one chromosome from each of two parents, arranged in complementary patterns, and containing genes for the same traits at the same positions on the homologous pairs. Similarly, genes are found in pairs called **alleles**. An individual with two identical genes for a trait is called purebred, or **homozygous** This phenomenon was first explained by Gregor Mendel with his laws of dominance, segregation, and independent assortment.

Dominance

In observing pea plants, Mendel observed that, when individuals with contrasting traits are crossed, one trait, called the dominant trait, is expressed, and the other trait, called the recessive trait, is masked. This is the law of **dominance**. In the notation of genetics, the dominant gene is represented by a capital letter and the recessive trait by a lowercase letter. For example, if a tall plant (TT) is crossed with a short plant (tt), the result is offspring that are all **heterozygous** (Tt); that is, they contain one allele for tall and one for short. The allele for tall (T, the dominant gene) is expressed, and the allele for short (t) is hidden. The **phenotype**, or appearance of the plants, is all tall.

Segregation

The law of **segregation** tells us that, when two of these hybrids (heterozygotes) are crossed, the hidden trait becomes segregated and appears in 25% of the offspring. This happens because genes separate during meiosis and recombine during fertilization. This process can be pictured using a Punnett square, which looks like this:

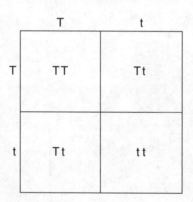

In the genes produced by these individuals, half of the gametes are T and half t. Arranging them on the Punnett square, we see that 25% of the offspring have a **genotype** of TT, 50% Tt, and 25% tt. The phenotype is 75% tall and 25% short, because both the pure dominant (TT) and the heterozygote (Tt) exhibit the dominant trait. A recessive trait is expressed only if the individual has two recessive genes.

Independent Assortment

The law of **independent assortment** tells us that genes on different chromosomes are inherited independently of each other. When genes for different traits are on the same chromosome, the traits are **linked**. Some traits do not show a pattern of dominance and the heterozygote for such a trait expresses a mixture of the two traits. This is called **codominance**.

Humans have 46 chromosomes, or 23 homologous pairs, of which 22 pairs are **auto-somes** (nonsex chromosomes) and one pair consists of the sex chromosomes (XX or XY). An individual with two X chromosomes is a female, and an individual with an X chromosome and a Y chromosome is a male. For some traits, the genes are found only on the X chromosome, but not on the Y, and these traits are called **sex-linked traits**. A male need inherit only one gene for such a trait from his mother for it to be expressed, but a female has to inherit two, one from each parent. Examples of sex-linked traits are color blindness and hemophilia.

DNA

Deoxyribonucleic acid (DNA) is what we have been calling the gene. The model explaining the structure of DNA was first proposed by James Watson and Francis Crick. (See Figure 4.) To understand the role of DNA in genetics, we must understand the structure of DNA, which is made up of thousands of units called **nucleotides**. Each nucleotide is composed of a **phosphate group (PO$_4$)**, a five-carbon sugar called **deoxyribose**, and a **nitrogenous base** (either adenine, cytosine, guanine, or thymine). The nucleotides form long chains, which are joined to form a **double helix**. Two strands of nucleotides are joined by nitrogenous bases connected to each other with hydrogen bonds. If you think of a DNA molecule as a ladder, the sugar and phosphate units form the uprights, and the pairs of nitrogenous bases are the rungs of the ladder. The bases can bond only in certain combinations: guanine (G) to cytosine (C) and adenine (A) to thymine (T), thus providing a series of four possible pairings: G-C, C-G, A-T, T-A.

Just as chromosomes replicate during cell division, DNA strands also replicate, that is, make exact copies of each themselves. During **replication**, the DNA strand opens, or unzips so to speak, at the base pairs. Free (or unattached) nucleotides are incorporated into the unzipped portion of the DNA, so that complementary base pairs join to form to exact duplicates. For example, if an unzipped strand has a sequence of ATCGA, it attracts nucleotides TAGCT. The result is two replicated DNA molecules that are identical to each other and to the original DNA.

DNA also serves as a template for the production of **messenger RNA (m-RNA)**. RNA differs from DNA in that it is single stranded, has the sugar ribose in place of deoxyribose, and replaces thymine with **uracil**. The process of forming m-RNA according to the information contained in the DNA molecule is called **transcription**. As in replication, the DNA strand opens but in this case acts as a template for the production of RNA. And, as in replication, the base sequence of the DNA strand determines the nucleotide order in the RNA strand. For example, if the DNA sequence is GCTTAA, the RNA strand is CGAAUU.

A molecule of m-RNA, which is made in the nucleus, moves out of the nucleus and is attached to a ribosome. At the ribosome, **transfer RNA (t-RNA)** molecules, which are coded for specific **amino acids**, line up along the RNA molecule at the ribosome. In so doing, they align their amino acids according to the code in the m-RNA and form them into proteins. This mechanism produces proteins according to the information coded in the original DNA molecule.

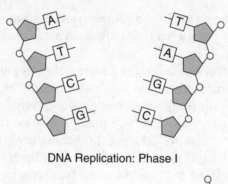

DNA Replication: Phase I

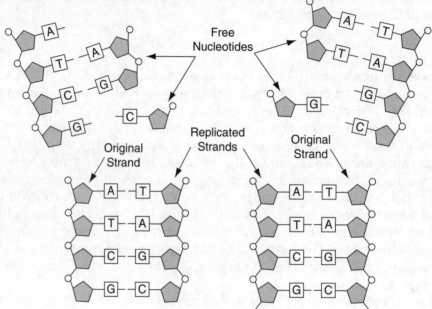

DNA Replication: Phase II

Figure 4. DNA Replication

Gene mutations are changes in the DNA nitrogenous base sequence, causing a change in the protein formed. There are also chromosomal mutations, in which either the structure or the number of chromosomes changes, resulting in such conditions as polyploidy (in which a full set of chromosomes fails to separate resulting in an individual that could be 3n) or nondisjunction in which one pair fails to separate, such as happens in Down's syndrome.

RESEARCH PROCEDURES

Terms to Be Defined

light microscope	variable	constant
electron microscope	independent variable	controlled experiment
data	dependent variable	

Microscopes greatly affected the progress of science, allowing scientists to see cells when they were introduced in the seventeenth century. In a **light microscope**, light is first passed through a specimen and then through a glass lens, which bends light in such a manner that an image is magnified. However, many internal structures of the cell are too small to be seen even through the light microscope, and thus the invention of the electron microscope in the 1950s greatly enhanced the study of cell biology. The **electron microscope**, which sends a beam of electrons through a specimen, can be used to examine structures that are too small to be seen through the light microscope. The light microscope can magnify specimens up to 2,000 times, whereas the electron microscope can magnify up to 2 million times. The compound microscopes you may have used in school usually magnify approximately 400 times under high power. The quality of the lenses determines the resolution of the microscope.

In science, we collect a good deal of **data**. During an experiment, we are often looking for data on **variables**, which are measurable factors or qualities that change during an experiment. Variables are classified as independent and dependent. An **independent variable** is one that is changed by the experimenter. The variable that changes in response to the independent variable is called the **dependent variable**. Factors that do not change are called **constants**. For example, suppose we performed an experiment to determine the effect of pressure on the volume of a gas. We would vary the pressure (the independent variable), record the change in volume caused by the pressure change (the dependent variable), and keep the temperature constant. We call such an experiment a **controlled experiment** because we are seeking data on only one independent variable. If we allowed temperature and pressure to vary together, we would not know whether the volume changed because of pressure or temperature.

Having collected data, it is important to represent it in ways that help us to analyze it and draw conclusions. One way of representing data is in the form of a graph, which often helps us to see correlations. When we represent data in the form of a graph, the independent variable is always plotted on the *x*-axis and the dependent variable on the *y*-axis. For example, Figure 5 shows the effect of pressure on the volume of a gas.

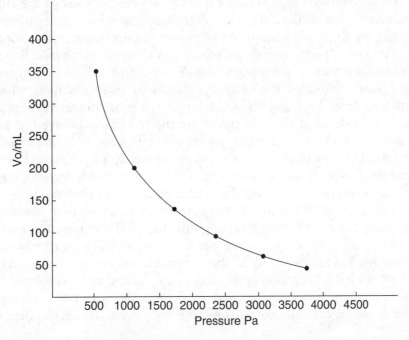

Figure 5. Effect of Pressure on the Volume of a Gas

Human Anatomy and Physiology

DIGESTION

Terms to Be Defined

mechanical digestion

chemical digestion

hydrolysis

enzymes

anus

alimentary canal

accessory organs

surface area

salivary glands

amylase

pharynx

esophagus

epiglottis

stomach

peristalsis

gastric juice

protease

chyme

small intestine

pyloric sphincter

liver

bile

gallbladder

pancreas

villi

large intestine (colon)

rectum

egestion

Digestion is the breaking down of nutrients into small, soluble molecules that can be absorbed into the blood. This is accomplished by **mechanical digestion** (breaking food into smaller pieces) and **chemical digestion** (breaking nutrients into small molecules). The process by which chemical digestion occurs is called **hydrolysis** (splitting molecules by adding water). Chemical digestion is sped up by the action of digestive **enzymes** (hydrolases). Humans, as opposed to simpler animals such as jellyfish, have a digestive system that is composed of a tube that extends between two openings: the mouth and the **anus**. (See Figure 6.) This tube, called the **alimentary canal**, is organized into specialized regions that carry out specific phases of the digestive process, e.g., mechanical digestion, chemical digestion, absorption. In addition to the alimentary canal, the digestive system has **accessory organs** (liver, gallbladder, and pancreas).

Food enters through the mouth, where it is chewed (mechanical digestion), increasing the **surface area**, which makes it easier to both swallow and digest. The presence of food also stimulates the **salivary glands** to release saliva, which contains the enzyme amylase. **Amylase** breaks down starch into smaller carbohydrate molecules (monosaccharides and disaccharides). As the food is swallowed, it is pushed by the tongue into the **pharynx** (throat), which splits, leading to both the windpipe and the **esophagus**. During swallowing, the top of the windpipe is covered by the **epiglottis** to prevent food from entering the respiratory system. From the esophagus, the food is passed to the **stomach** by muscular contractions called **peristalsis**.

The lining of the stomach releases **gastric juice**, which is made up of hydrochloric acid and **proteases** (protein digesting enzymes). The environment of the stomach is acidic, having a pH of approximately 2, because gastric enzymes work best in this environment. Fortunately, cells in the stomach lining secrete mucus, which protects the stomach wall from the action of the very acidic gastric juice. The smooth muscles of the stomach mix the partially digested food, and the result is a liquid called **chyme**. Chyme is released to the **small intestine**, in a series of small portions, through the

SECTION A

SECTION B

SECTION C

COMPREHENSIVE PRACTICE Test 1

COMPREHENSIVE PRACTICE Test 2

COMPREHENSIVE PRACTICE Test 3

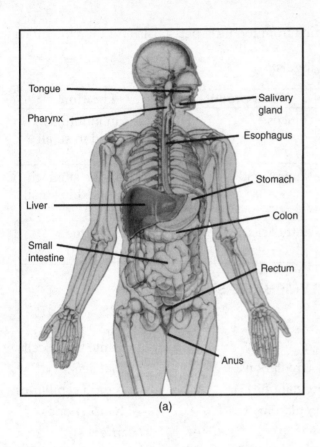

(a)

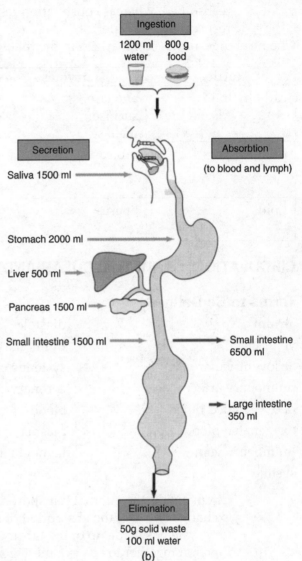

(b)

Figure 6. Digestive System

pyloric sphincter. Most of the digestion of food takes place in the small intestine, which can be up to 6 meters long in humans.

The small intestine is the major site not only for digestion but also for the absorption of nutrients into the bloodstream. Digestive enzymes are secreted by intestinal glands. Also contributing to digestion are the liver, the pancreas, and the gallbladder. The **liver** produces **bile**, a substance stored in the **gallbladder**, which helps in the breakdown of fats. The **pancreas** supplies a number of enzymes needed for digestion. To facilitate absorption, the small intestine is lined with **villi**, which greatly increase the intestinal surface area for the absorption of the end products of digestion into the blood and lymph. Undigested food is moved to the **large intestine**, or **colon**, which is responsible for reabsorbing water that has entered the alimentary canal. Thus the waste, or feces, that moves along the colon by peristalsis becomes increasingly solidified and is ultimately stored in the **rectum** until **egestion** (elimination from the body). Diarrhea is a result of peristalsis moving feces through the colon too quickly so that water is not reabsorbed, whereas constipation results from too little peristalsis and thus too much reabsorption of water.

Chemical digestion is summarized in the following list:

Nutrient	Enzymes	End product	Location
carbohydrate	amylase, sucrase, maltase	glucose	starts in mouth, is completed in small intestine
protein	proteases	amino acids	starts in the stomach, is completed in small intestine
lipids	lipases	fatty acid and glycerol	small intestine

CIRCULATION: CARDIOVASCULAR AND LYMPHATIC SYSTEMS

Terms to Be Defined

atrium	diastole	white blood cells
ventricle	pulmonary circulation	platelets
atrioventricular valve	systemic circulation	lymph capillaries
pulmonary artery	coronary circulation	lymph nodes
deoxygenated blood	blood	arteries
oxygenated blood	plasma	veins
pulmonary vein	hemoglobin	capillaries
systole		

Circulation is the internal transport of fluid throughout the body, which allows for the exchange of gases, the absorption of nutrients, and the disposal of waste. The circulatory system is made up of the cardiovascular system and the lymphatic system, which function together to achieve these goals.

The cardiovascular system in humans is made up of the heart, blood vessels, and blood. The heart consists of four chambers: two **atria** (singular: **atrium**), which receive blood, and two **ventricles**, which pump blood to the body. (See Figure 7.) The pathway of blood through the heart and lungs, beginning at the vena cava, is as follows:

- Blood enters the right atrium from the upper and lower body through veins called the superior vena cava and the inferior vena cava.

- From there it passes through an **atrioventricular valve** into the right ventricle. (The purpose of valves is to prevent backflow when the ventricles contract.)

- The right ventricle pumps blood through the semilunar valve into the **pulmonary arteries**, which carry the blood to the lungs. This blood is **deoxygenated** and becomes **oxygenated** in the lungs, where the gas exchange occurs.

- Newly oxygenated blood leaves the lungs via the **pulmonary veins**, which returns blood to the left atrium.

- From there it passes through another atrioventricular valve to the left ventricle.

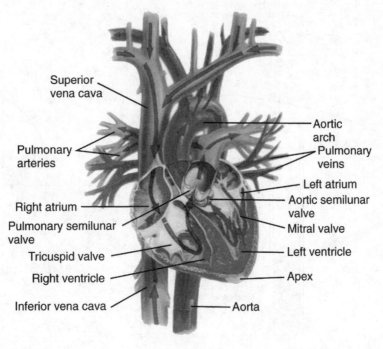

Figure 7. Human Heart

- Muscular contractions of the left ventricle pump blood through the aorta to all parts of the body.

Blood pressure from the pumping action of the heart forces blood to circulate. When the heart contracts, the pressure increases (**systole**), and when the heart relaxes, the pressure is lowered (**diastole**). The circulation of blood to the heart is called **coronary circulation**. The circulation of blood through the lungs is known as **pulmonary circulation**, and circulation throughout the body is known as **systemic circulation**.

Interestingly, **blood** is considered a type of connective tissue that is made up of a variety of cells suspended in liquid called **plasma**. (See Figure 8.) Red blood cells, white blood cells, and platelets make up 45% of whole blood, whereas plasma, which contains proteins, ions, hormones, and gases, makes up the other 55%. Red blood cells, or erythrocytes, are responsible for transporting oxygen, and they do not have nuclei or mitochondria. To suit their main function of transporting oxygen, red blood cells are small and thin (to allow for diffusion), and each cell contains approximately 270 million molecules of **hemoglobin**, which is an oxygen carrier.

Hemoglobin is an iron-rich compound, which explains the need for iron in our diets. **White blood cells**, or leukocytes, are less abundant than red blood cells and are involved in host immune defense. Not surprisingly, an infection is indicated when the number of white blood cells exceeds the normal concentration. **Platelets**, also found in plasma, are pieces of cells that are important in blood clotting.

As blood passes through the vessels of the circulatory system, fluid and proteins can leak out. This lost fluid diffuses into **lymph capillaries**, which are found throughout the cardiovascular system, and it thus enters the lymphatic system. (See Figure 9.) Inside the lymphatic system, the fluid, or lymph, returns to the circulatory system. **Lymph nodes** are special pockets in the lymphatic system where the lymph is filtered. White blood cells are present in these nodes to attack bacteria and viruses that may

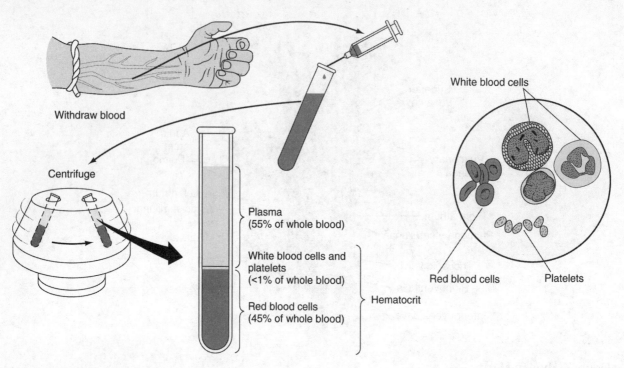

Figure 8. Blood Composition

be present in the fluid. This is why swollen and tender lymph nodes are a sign of an infection.

There are three kinds of blood vessels: arteries, veins, and capillaries. **Arteries** transport blood away from the heart. Because they carry blood at relatively high pressure, they are muscular. We feel a pulse in the arteries. **Veins** transport blood to the heart, and they contain valves to prevent the backflow of blood as it returns to the heart. **Capillaries** are tiny blood vessels that connect arteries and veins. Through the capillary walls (only one cell thick), materials enter and leave the blood.

RESPIRATION

Terms to Be Defined

pharynx	bronchioles	aerobic respiration
larynx	alveoli	anaerobic respiration
bronchi	diaphragm	lactic acid

Air enters the respiratory system through the nasal cavities, which lead to the **pharynx**. (See Figure 10.) Here, the glottis remains open, and the air travels to the **larynx** (the voice box). From the larynx, the air travels to the trachea, or windpipe, which branches into two **bronchi**, which lead to the lungs. Inside each lung, the branching continues, creating thinner and thinner tubes, called **bronchioles**. Finally, at the end of each bronchiole is an air sac called an **alveolus (pl. alveoli)**. These thin and permeable air sacs are the functional units of the lung.

The deoxygenated blood arrives at the lung via the pulmonary arteries from the right ventricle. The arteries branch into smaller and smaller vessels and finally become capillaries, which surround the alveoli. At the point where the capillaries and alveoli

Human Anatomy and Physiology

181

SECTION **A**

SECTION **B**

SECTION **C**

COMPREHENSIVE PRACTICE **Test 1**

COMPREHENSIVE PRACTICE **Test 2**

COMPREHENSIVE PRACTICE **Test 3**

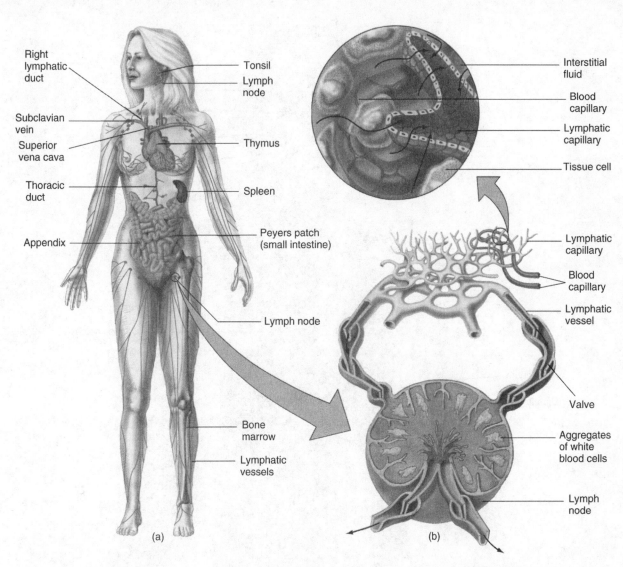

Figure 9. Lymphatic System

are in contact, an exchange occurs across the alveolar membrane via diffusion: The blood picks up oxygen, which is carried back to the heart, and it releases carbon dioxide, which is exhaled.

Breathing is the process by which air is moved into and out of the lungs. (See Figure 11.) This involves the muscular movement of the **diaphragm** (a sheet of muscle lining the bottom of the thoracic cavity) and of the rib cage, which raises and lowers the pressure in the chest cavity. Lowering pressure in the chest forces outside air into the lungs, and increasing pressure forces exhaled air out of the lungs. Exhaled air has a higher concentration of carbon dioxide (CO_2) and water than inhaled air. The rate of breathing is controlled by the nervous system, in response to CO_2 levels in the blood.

Cellular Respiration

Cellular respiration is the process by which we get energy from the food that we eat. Cellular respiration can be anaerobic or aerobic. **Aerobic respiration** occurs when oxygen

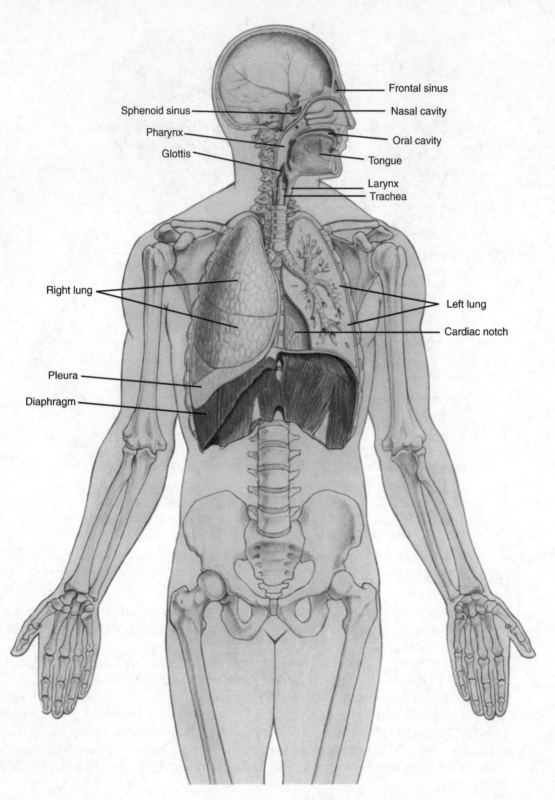

Figure 10. Respiratory System

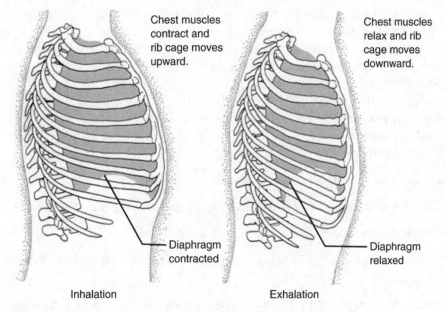

Figure 11. Inhalation and Exhalation

is present, and it is the opposite process to that of photosynthesis. During photosynthesis, a plant uses energy to convert water and carbon dioxide to glucose. In aerobic respiration, we use glucose, at a cellular level, to obtain energy. Its formula is:

$$C_6H_{12}O_6 + 6O_2 \rightarrow 6CO_2 + 6H_2O + energy$$

$$glucose + oxygen \rightarrow carbon\ dioxide + water + energy$$

Aerobic respiration, a very efficient process, begins in the cytoplasm of the cell and ends in the mitochondria, where the energy from glucose is stored in the form of ATP. If oxygen is not present, **anaerobic respiration** occurs, which is less efficient, producing a lower amount of ATP. **Lactic acid**, which is produced during anaerobic respiration, is a cause of sore muscles after strenuous exercise. Anaerobic respiration in yeast is called fermentation, producing ethanol rather than lactic acid.

REGULATION: NERVOUS SYSTEM

Terms to Be Defined

neuron	synapse	somatic
sodium	sensory neuron	autonomic
potassium	interneuron	reflex arc
impulse	motor neuron	spinal cord
dendrite	nerve	brain
cell body	central nervous system	cerebrum
axon	(CNS)	cerebellum
axon terminal	peripheral nervous	brain stem
neurotransmitter	system (PNS)	medulla

SECTION A

SECTION B

SECTION C

COMPREHENSIVE PRACTICE Test 1

COMPREHENSIVE PRACTICE Test 2

COMPREHENSIVE PRACTICE Test 3

The nervous system directly regulates body functions and responds to environmental stimuli. The functional unit of the nervous system is the **neuron**. (See Figure 12.) At rest, neurons have an electrical potential due to differences in **sodium** and **potassium** ion concentrations across the cell membrane. Generally, an **impulse** is generated when the **dendrites** of a neuron are stimulated by the environment or by another neuron. The stimulus results in a moving electrical charge. The impulse travels from the **cell body** along the **axon** until it reaches the ends, or **axon terminals**. This triggers the release of **neurotransmitters**, which travel across **synapses** and may trigger other neurons or muscles. Axons may have myelin sheaths, which help transmit impulses faster.

There are three main types of neurons:

1. **Sensory neurons** transmit impulses from sense organs and receptors.

2. **Interneurons** make up the brain and spinal cord.

3. **Motor neurons** carry impulses from interneurons to skeletal and visceral muscles and glands.

Nerves are groups, or bundles, of the axons of sensory and/or motor neurons. The nervous system includes other types of cells that nourish and support the neurons.

The nervous system is usually divided into two subsystems:

1. The **central nervous system (CNS)** includes the brain and spinal cord.

2. The **peripheral nervous system (PNS)** includes the nerves and sense receptors.

The PNS is responsible for transmitting information to and from the CNS, which is responsible for processing information. The PNS is further divided into two branches: the **somatic** branch is concerned with the external environment, and the **autonomic** branch is concerned with the internal environment.

A **reflex arc** carries out simple, quick, and automatic responses to certain stimuli. Reflex actions are commonly defensive and do not necessarily involve the brain. Examples of reflex actions include the reaction to stepping on a sharp object or touching a hot stove.

The **spinal cord** extends from the brain downward and is enclosed by the bones of the vertebral column, or spine. Openings between the vertebrae allow nerves to join with the spinal cord. The spinal cord passes messages to and from the brain, and acts

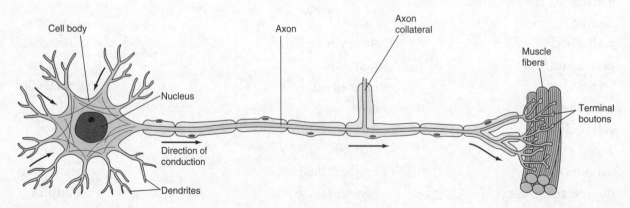

Figure 12. Neuron

Human Anatomy and Physiology   185

SECTION A

SECTION B

SECTION C

COMPREHENSIVE PRACTICE Test 1

COMPREHENSIVE PRACTICE Test 2

COMPREHENSIVE PRACTICE Test 3

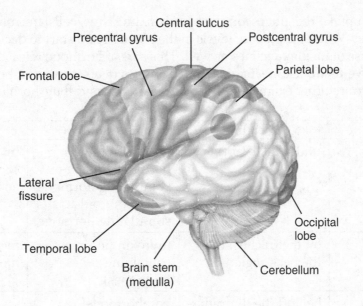

Figure 13. The Brain

as the center for reflex actions. Damage to the spinal cord may result in paralysis and may be permanent.

The **brain** is protected and enclosed within the cranium and is divided into three areas. (See Figure 13.)

1. The **cerebrum** makes up the largest portion of the human brain and is the site of complex and high-level thinking. Conscious and voluntary actions are controlled here, as are other functions such as speech, vision, hearing, and memory.

2. The **cerebellum** is located below and behind the cerebrum. It is responsible for muscular coordination and balance.

3. The **brain stem**, or **medulla**, controls basic homeostatic functions such as body temperature, blood pressure, and breathing. (Homeostasis is explained in the next section.)

REGULATION: ENDOCRINE SYSTEM

Terms to Be Defined

homeostasis   hormone   negative-feedback mechanism

An important function of the endocrine system is to maintain **homeostasis**, which is the body's way of keeping its internal environment stable by means of secretions from the endocrine glands. These glands are also called ductless glands because they secrete hormones directly into the bloodstream. **Hormones** are chemicals that act as messengers and that help control the important processes of growth, metabolism, reproduction, osmotic balance, and development. Most hormones work by binding to a specific type of cell by means of a receptor and influencing the activity of the cell. Hormones are usually activated by some type of stimulus. One example is the hormone insulin. When we ingest a meal, the food is broken down by our digestive system, and glucose is released from starches into our bloodstream. The presence of glucose triggers the release of insulin from the pancreas, and insulin binds to cells in the body, causing them to uptake the glucose in the bloodstream. Thus, cells are able to use this glucose for energy. When the glucose levels in the bloodstream start to decline, the stimulus for the release of insulin declines as well. This sort of hormone release regulation is called a **negative-feedback mechanism** and prevents oversecretion of hormones.

Here are other examples of endocrine glands and their hormones:

Gland	Location	Hormone(s)	Function
pituitary gland	under the brain	growth-stimulating hormone, follicle-stimulating hormone (FSH), thyroid-stimulating hormone	master gland, controls other endocrine glands
thyroid gland	on the trachea, in the neck region	thyroxin (iodine-containing hormones)	regulates metabolism
parathyroid gland	behind the thyroid gland	parahormone	regulates calcium metabolism
adrenal gland	on the kidneys	Adrenaline, steroids (cortisone)	so-called fight-or-flight hormone; regulate water balance, blood pressure, joint articulation
Isles of Langerhans	pancreas	insulin, glucagon	control storage of sugar in liver and blood level of sugar
testes (male gonad)	in scrotum	testosterone	male secondary sex characteristics
ovaries (female gonad)	pelvic region	estrogen and progesterone	female secondary sex characteristics, menstrual cycle

SUPPORT AND MOVEMENT: THE MUSCULOSKELETAL SYSTEM

Terms to Be Defined

red marrow	ligament	cardiac muscle
osteocytes	tendon	smooth muscle
skeleton	cartilage	skeletal (striated) muscle
axial	osteoarthritis	flexor
appendicular	rheumatoid arthritis	extensor
joints	osteoporosis	

The musculoskeletal system is composed of bones, connective tissue, and muscle. The system's functions are the support and protection of the internal organs, and movement.

In addition, blood cells are made in the **red marrow** of the long bones. (See Figure 14.) Bone contains **osteocytes**, which produce a hard, calcium-rich extracellular matrix. Blood vessels extend through bone, providing nutrients and oxygen and taking away wastes.

Bones

More than 200 bones make up the human **skeleton**. (See Figure 15.) The **axial** portion of the skeleton consists of the skull, vertebrae, ribs, and sternum. The **appendicular** skeleton is made up of the bones of the shoulders, arms, pelvis, and legs.

Joints connect the bones of the skeleton. Sutures are immovable joints that join the bones of the skull, permitting growth but no movement. Other types of joints are movable, allowing muscles to move bones at a point of articulation (where the bones meet). The shoulders and hips have ball-and-socket joints, the elbows and knees have hinge joints, and sliding or gliding joints are found at the wrists.

Diseases affecting the skeletal system are:

- **Osteoarthritis** (a degenerative bone and joint disease)

- **Rheumatoid arthritis** (a degenerative joint disease caused by an autoimmune response)

- **Osteoporosis** (a disease caused by calcium loss often found in older people, especially postmenopausal women)

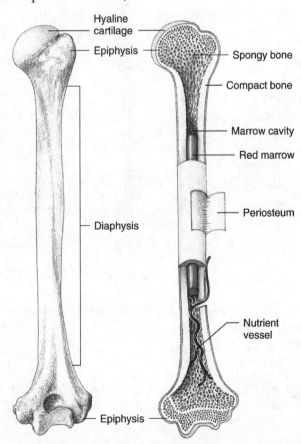

Figure 14. Bone Structure

SECTION A

SECTION B

SECTION C

COMPREHENSIVE PRACTICE Test 1

COMPREHENSIVE PRACTICE Test 2

COMPREHENSIVE PRACTICE Test 3

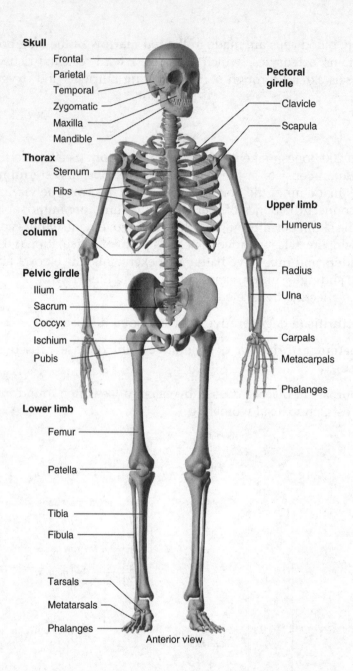

Skull
Frontal
Parietal
Temporal
Zygomatic
Maxilla
Mandible

Pectoral girdle
Clavicle
Scapula

Thorax
Sternum
Ribs

Upper limb
Humerus

Vertebral column

Radius
Ulna

Pelvic girdle
Ilium
Sacrum
Coccyx
Ischium
Pubis

Carpals
Metacarpals
Phalanges

Lower limb
Femur

Patella

Tibia
Fibula

Tarsals
Metatarsals
Phalanges

Anterior view

Figure 15. Skeleton

Connective Tissue

Ligaments connect bones to other bones. **Tendons** connect muscles to bones. **Cartilage** cushions bones at the joints.

Muscles

Muscle cells are among the most active in the body, using an enormous amount of energy in the form of ATP. The human body has three types of muscle:

1. **Cardiac** muscle is found only in the heart and is involuntary.

2. **Smooth muscle**, also involuntary, is found in the internal organs of the digestive tract and in blood vessels.

3. **Skeletal** muscle is also called **striated muscle** due to the microscopic appearance of the individual muscle cells, or fibers. Skeletal muscles move bones and are responsible for voluntary movements. Skeletal muscles, attached to bones by tendons, move the bones when they contract and thereby shorten.

Many skeletal muscles are found in opposing pairs. In such a pair, one muscle, the **flexor**, bends or moves a limb away from anatomical position. The other muscle, the **extensor**, returns the limb to the anatomical position. The biceps muscle (a flexor) and the triceps muscle (an extensor) of the upper arm are good examples of this.

Thus, the musculoskeletal system can be thought of as a system of levers (bones), moving around fulcrums (joints), with the forces provided by the muscles.

EXCRETION

Terms to Be Defined

kidney	loop of Henle	urethra
nephron	distal convoluted tubule	sweat glands
glomerulus	ureter	liver
Bowman's capsule	urine	
proximal convoluted tubule	urinary bladder	

The **kidneys** are the principal excretory organs of the body. (See Figure 16.) The outer portion of the kidneys is the renal cortex, and the inner portion is called the renal medulla. The functional unit of the kidney is the **nephron**, which consists of the **glomerulus**, **Bowman's capsule**, the **proximal convoluted tubule**, the **loop of Henle**, and the **distal convoluted tubule**. Blood, under pressure, enters the capillaries of the glomerulus, which is located inside the cup-shaped Bowman's capsule. Materials in the blood, such as water, soluble salts, urea, and soluble nutrients, diffuse out of the blood into Bowman's capsule. The kidneys also absorb any small soluble particles that are in high concentration from the blood, thus helping to maintain homeostasis. As this filtrate passes through the tubules of the nephron, the water, nutrients, and ions are reabsorbed into the blood by diffusion, osmosis, or active transport through the capillaries surrounding the tubules.

The concentrated mixture of wastes that is left in the tubules forms **urine**, which enters the collecting tubules to the **ureters**. The ureters transport urine to the **urinary bladder** for storage. Urine is excreted through the **urethra**, which is near the vagina in females and through the penis in males.

In addition to the kidneys, the **sweat glands**, lungs, and **liver** function in excretion.

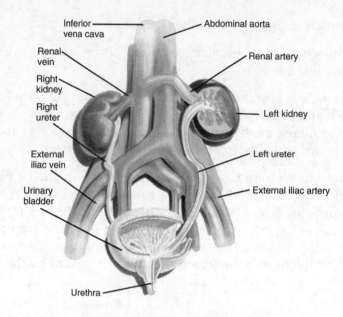

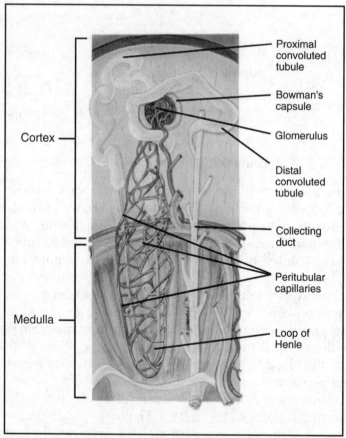

Figure 16. Urinary System and Cross Section of the Kidney

REPRODUCTION

Terms to Be Defined

gamete	interstitial cells	ovulation
sperm	testosterone	fallopian tubes
egg	epididymis	uterus
zygote	vas deferens	endometrium
monoploid	ejaculatory duct	menstruation
diploid	urethra	placenta
penis	ovaries	fetus
scrotum	progesterone	umbilical cord
testes	estrogen	
seminiferous tubules	oocyte	

Sexual reproduction starts with the fusion of two **gametes** (**sperm** and **egg**) to form a **zygote** (the united sperm and egg). Each gamete is **monoploid** (or haploid), meaning it contains half the normal complement of chromosomes. Thus, since the zygote is created from the union of a sperm and an egg, it contains the full complement of chromosomes and is thus called **diploid**.

In the male, the genitalia, or the external reproductive organs, are the **penis** and the **scrotum**. (See Figure 17.) The internal reproductive organs consist of the **testes**, the primary male reproductive organs. The testes contain **seminiferous tubules**, where sperm form, and **interstitial cells**, which produce male sex hormones such as **testosterone**. When sperm is produced in the seminiferous tubules, it then travels into the **epididymis**, which is made of coiled tubes that store sperm while they mature. The sperm are sent through the epididymis during ejaculation into the **vas deferens** to the **ejaculatory duct** to the **urethra**. The urethra, which runs the length of the penis and opens to the external environment, is common to both the reproductive and urinary systems.

In the female, the primary reproductive organs are the **ovaries**, which produce both eggs and the hormones **progesterone** and **estrogen**. (See Figure 18.) Inside the ovaries are ovarian follicles, each of which contains an immature egg called an **oocyte**. As the egg develops, the follicle also matures and enlarges. When fully mature, the follicle releases the egg in the stage called **ovulation**, which occurs approximately every 28 days. The egg then travels through the **fallopian tubes**, where it can be fertilized. If fertilized, the egg travels to the **uterus**, where it becomes implanted in the uterine lining, the **endometrium**, and remains there for the rest of its development. If the egg is not fertilized (i.e., the woman is not pregnant), the endometrial lining is shed, and it thickens again in preparation for the possibility of implantation in the next cycle. The shedding is a process known as **menstruation**.

If fertilization occurs, the developing embryo implants itself in the uterus, where it develops during its gestation period of nine months. Tissues of the embryo and the mother grow together to form the **placenta**. The blood of the embryo and mother are never directly connected, but nutrients and oxygen from the mother and wastes from the embryo are exchanged through the placenta. The **fetus** is connected to the placenta by the **umbilical cord**.

SECTION A

SECTION B

SECTION C

COMPREHENSIVE PRACTICE Test 1

COMPREHENSIVE PRACTICE Test 2

COMPREHENSIVE PRACTICE Test 3

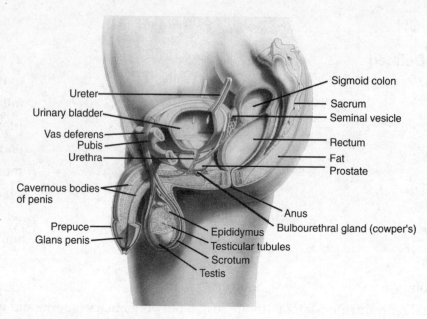

Figure 17. Male Reproductive System

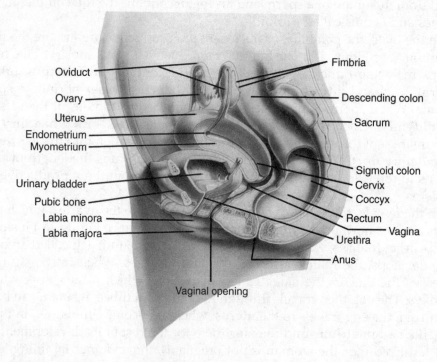

Figure 18. Female Reproductive System

SENSES

Terms to Be Defined

cornea	optic nerve	incus
iris	outer ear	stapes
pupil	tympanic membrane	Eustachian tube

retina
rod cells
cone cells

middle ear
malleus
lens

inner ear
cochlea

Sight

At the front of the eyeball, the transparent **cornea** allows light to enter the eye. (See Figure 19.) Behind the cornea is the **iris**, which not only gives our eyes color but also changes in size, regulating how much light is allowed to enter the **pupil**, which is in the middle of the iris. The **lens** focuses light onto the retina, its shape being changed by attached muscles. The **retina** is the innermost layer of the eyeball and contains two types of photoreceptor cells. **Rod cells** are sensitive to light, distinguish between black and white, and allow us to see at night. **Cone cells** allow us to distinguish colors in the day. When they are stimulated by light, the photoreceptor cells transmit the information along the **optic nerve** to the brain.

Hearing

The ear is responsible not only for hearing but for balance as well. (See Figure 20.) Its anatomy can be divided into three regions: the **outer ear**, the **middle ear**, and the **inner ear**.

1. The **outer ear** collects sounds and transmits them to the **tympanic membrane**, which separates the outer ear from the middle ear.

2. In the **middle ear**, the vibrations produced by sound are transmitted through three small bones (ossicles): the **malleus, incus,** and **stapes.** As the vibrations pass through the oval window, they enter the inner ear. The middle ear is also connected to the **Eustachian tube**, which opens into the pharynx. This tube equalizes the pressure between the middle ear and the atmosphere, sometimes making your ears "pop."

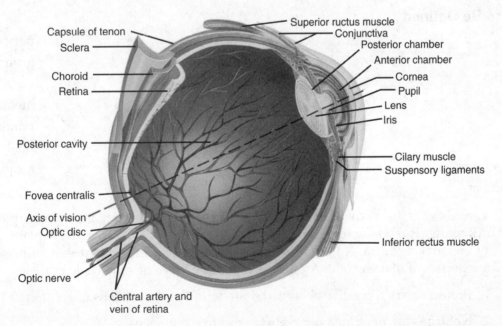

Capsule of tenon
Sclera
Choroid
Retina
Posterior cavity
Fovea centralis
Axis of vision
Optic disc
Optic nerve
Central artery and vein of retina

Superior ructus muscle
Conjunctiva
Posterior chamber
Anterior chamber
Cornea
Pupil
Lens
Iris
Cilary muscle
Suspensory ligaments
Inferior rectus muscle

Figure 19. Structure of the Eye

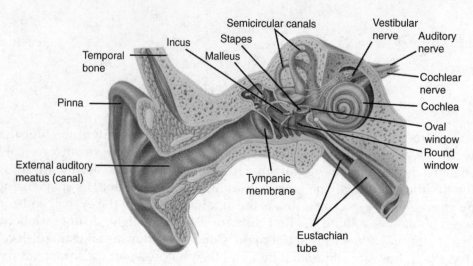

Figure 20. Structure of the Ear

3. The **inner ear** has many channels containing fluid that moves in response to your movement or to sound. Sound coming into the inner ear moves the fluid, causing the **cochlea**, a part of the inner ear, to transduce (or convert) the movement into signals or action potentials. Movement of the small hairs in a portion of the cochlea influences the signals sent from sensory neurons to the brain. The semicircular canals are involved in balance.

Basic Chemistry

ATOMIC STRUCTURE, ISOTOPES, IONS, AND THE PERIODIC TABLE

Terms to Be Defined

matter	isotope	period
atom	atomic mass	group
proton	ion	metal
neutron	cation	metalloid
electron	anion	nonmetal
element	valence electron	noble gas
atomic number	periodic table	radio-isotope
mass number	nucleons	

Chemistry is the study of **matter**, which is anything that has mass and occupies space. All matter is made up of atoms, and the properties of matter can be explained by the atoms making it up. An **atom** is the smallest unit of an element that still retains the properties of that element. Atoms contain three types of subatomic particles:

1. **Protons** carry a positive charge and are found in the nucleus of an atom.

2. **Neutrons** are neutral and are also found in the nucleus.

3. **Electrons** carry a negative charge and are found outside the nucleus and arranged according to their energy level.

An **element** is identified by its symbol and its atomic number. In Figure 21, for example, the upper left corner of the periodic table shows "3/Li." The "3" is the atomic number, and "Li" is the symbol for lithium. The **atomic number** is equal to the number of protons found in the nucleus of each of its atoms; lithium has three protons in its nucleus. The **mass number** of an atom is equal to the number of **nucleons** (protons and neutrons) in its nucleus. To find the number of protons in an atom, just look at its atomic number. For the atom to be neutral, the number of electrons in an atom must equal the number of protons. To find the number of neutrons in an atom, subtract the atomic number from the mass number of the element. For example, in Figure 21, the element carbon (C) has an atomic number of 6, indicating 6 protons. We can infer that the number of electrons is also 6, because carbon carries no charge; it is neutral. Therefore, the mass number of carbon, or the sum of the number of protons and neutrons, is 12, and the number of neutrons in carbon is 6 (12 – 6).

Sometimes atoms of the same element can be found with different mass numbers and therefore with different numbers of neutrons. (The number of protons never changes because that would make the atom a different element. For example, nitrogen always has 5 protons, and carbon always has 6 protons.) Atoms of the same element (with the same number of protons) that contain a different number of neutrons are called **isotopes**. An example is ^{14}C (carbon-14). The notation "14" before the element symbol is the mass number of the isotope; it equals the number of protons and neutrons. Since carbon has 6 protons, carbon-14 has 8 neutrons (14 – 8). The **atomic mass** of an element is a weighted average of the mass numbers of all naturally occurring isotopes of the element. Some isotopes are radioactive, these are called **radio-isotopes**. For example, a treatment of thyroid cancer uses ^{131}I (iodine-131), a radio-isotope. Iodine is transported to the thyroid gland.

The number of electrons can change as well because an atom can gain or lose electrons. When the number of electrons does not equal the number of protons, the atom carries a charge. Charged atoms are called **ions**. For instance, a neutral sodium atom

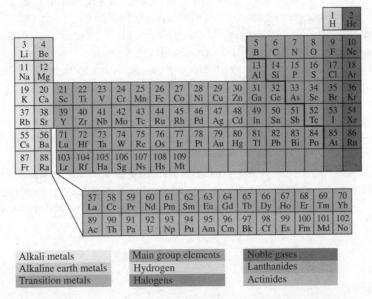

Figure 21. The Periodic Table

has 23 protons and 23 electrons. However, a sodium ion (Na^+), which forms by losing an electron, has 23 (positively charged) protons and 22 (negatively charged) electrons. Losing an electron is the same as losing one unit of negative charge. The sodium ion therefore has a plus sign after it: Na^+. An ion with a positive charge, like this one, is called a **cation**. An ion with a negative charge is called an **anion**; it has more electrons than protons.

Electrons are found at different energy levels of an atom. Electrons found in the outermost energy level are called **valence electrons**. Elements with small atomic numbers may have a maximum of two valence electrons; all other elements may have a maximum of eight valence electrons.

The **periodic table** (Figure 21) contains all the known elements, arranged in horizontal rows called **periods**, in order of increasing atomic number. The columns, or **groups**, on the table contain elements with similar properties because of their similar electron configurations. From left to right across a period, the elements move from **metals** on the left-hand side of the chart to **metalloids** and finally to **nonmetals** on the right-hand side. The last group on the right is the **noble gases**, which have full valence shells and are inert. There are many more metals than nonmetals.

BONDING

Terms to Be Defined

octet rule	covalent bond	polar covalent bond
ionic bond	nonpolar covalent bond	dipole
Lewis electron dot diagram		

An atom becomes more stable as its electron configuration becomes like that of a noble gas. This means 2 valence electrons for small atoms and 8 valence electrons for all others. The **octet rule** states that atoms tend to combine in such a way that they each have 8 electrons in their valence shells, giving them the same electronic configuration as a noble gas. Atoms can achieve this stable configuration by gaining, losing, or sharing electrons. When an atom loses electrons, it becomes a positive ion. When an atom gains electrons, it becomes a negative ion. Positive and negative ions attract each other, forming an **ionic bond**. We can represent the valence shell of atoms using **Lewis electron dot diagrams**. (See Figure 22.) In the figure, sodium (Na) loses an electron to form a sodium ion (Na^+), and chlorine gains an electron from sodium to form a chloride ion (Cl^-).

Sodium and chloride ions attract each other, forming a sodium chloride crystal. Ionic compounds have high melting and boiling points, but dissolve in polar solvents such as water. Some atoms form molecules by sharing pairs of electrons, forming what is known as a **covalent bond**. In Figure 23, two chlorine atoms share electrons.

When two atoms share electrons equally, as in Cl_2, we say the bond is a **nonpolar covalent bond**. If, however, two different atoms form a **polar covalent bond**, they share electrons unequally, the electrons being held closer to one atom than to the other. HCl is an example; the shared electrons are held closer to chlorine than to hydrogen.

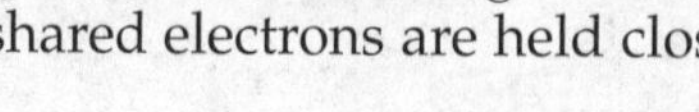

$$Na \cdot \; \overset{\times\times}{\underset{\times\times}{Cl}} \times \longrightarrow Na^+ \; + \; \overset{\times\times}{\underset{\times\times}{:Cl:}} \times$$

Figure 22. Lewis Electron Dot Diagram

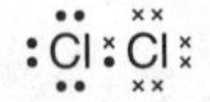

$$:\ddot{Cl}{\times}^{\times\times}_{\times\times}Cl{\times}$$

Figure 23a. Covalent Bond: Cl_2

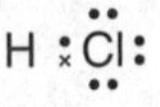

$$H:\ddot{Cl}:$$

Figure 23b. Polar Covalent Bond: HCl

Compounds can have single, double, or triple covalent bonds. If a molecule has polar covalent bonds and the distribution of charge is unequal, so that the molecule has a positive and a negative end, the molecule is called a **dipole** (two poles). Dipoles attract each other, other dipoles, and ions, and they have higher melting and boiling points than nonpolar molecules. A special type of dipole attraction is the hydrogen bond. Polar solvents, which we mentioned earlier, are solvents that are dipoles.

ELEMENTS, COMPOUNDS, AND STATES OF MATTER

Terms to Be Defined

element	solid	freezing
compound	melting	sublimation
gas	evaporation	substance
liquid	condensation	

A **substance** is something that has the same composition and properties. An **element** is a simple substance, made up of one type of atom. A **compound** is a substance made up of different atoms bonded together. An element cannot be broken down into anything simpler; a compound can be broken down into elements. Both forms of matter are substances because their composition and properties do not vary.

Matter can be found in different phases:

- In the **gas** form, the attractions between the atoms or molecules are weak, and the particles move around in a random and erratic manner. If placed in a container, a gas takes the shape of its container and spreads to fill its volume.

- A **liquid** has more attraction between its particles. It takes the shape of the container it is in, but it does not vary in its volume.

- A **solid** does not take the shape of the container it is in and does not flow, and its particles have very little movement.

The process that takes a solid to a liquid is **melting**, and the process that turns a liquid to a gas is **evaporation**. In reverse, the gas-to-liquid conversion is called **condensation**, and a liquid turns into a solid by **freezing**. The direct change between the solid phase and the gaseous phase without an apparent liquid phase is called **sublimation**; for example, iodine undergoes sublimation when heated, and dry ice does the same when exposed to the room temperature.

During a phase change, the amount of heat that is input or extracted from the substance changes, but the temperature remains the same. (See Figure 24.) This is because

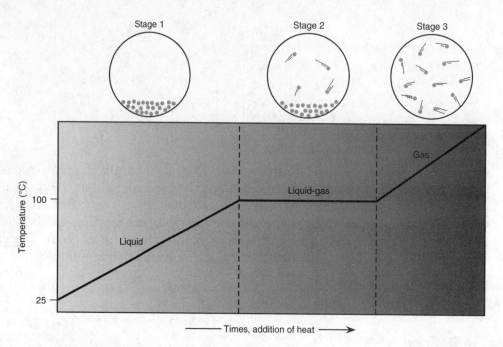

Figure 24. Liquid-to-Gas Phase Change

all of the heat is being used to change the phase of the substance, not the temperature. Thus, the evaporating and condensing points of water are both 100°C. All liquids tend to evaporate and all gases tend to condense, eventually reaching equilibrium. The evaporated gas above a liquid exerts a pressure called vapor pressure, which is specific for each liquid and for each temperature. For a liquid to boil, its vapor pressure must be equal to the pressure on it. At high altitudes where the barometric pressure is lower, liquids boil at lower temperatures.

MIXTURES, SOLUTIONS, TINCTURES, AND EMULSIONS

Terms to Be Defined

homogeneous mixture	solute	emulsion
solution	tincture	solubility
solvent	heterogeneous mixture	

A mixture differs from a substance in that its composition may vary from one sample to the next. Soil, air, and seawater are examples of mixtures. A **homogeneous mixture** is one in which the composition does not vary within the sample. A good example of a homogeneous mixture is a **solution**, such as a tablespoon of sugar thoroughly dissolved in a cup of hot water. In this solution, each sample of the water should contain an equal amount of dissolved sugar. In a solution, the substance that does the dissolving is called the **solvent**, and the substance being dissolved is the **solute**. A **tincture** is a solution in which the solvent is alcohol. For instance, a tincture of iodine contains iodine dissolved in alcohol.

A **heterogeneous mixture** is one in which the composition may vary within a sample; everyday examples are trail mix or granite. An **emulsion**, for example, refers to a liquid dispersed in another liquid in which it is not soluble (**solubility** is the ability of a solute to dissolve in a particular solvent). Take, for instance, oil and vinegar. Oil remains suspended as droplets in vinegar, in which it is not soluble. The addition of certain substances, called emulsifiers, stabilize emulsions. For instance, adding an egg to oil and vinegar makes mayonnaise, which is uniform throughout.

CHEMICAL VERSUS PHYSICAL CHANGES

Terms to Be Defined

chemical change	synthesis (combination) reactions	acid
physical change	single replacement reactions	base
reaction	double displacement reactions	pH scale
reactant	acid-base reaction	indicator
product	neutralization reaction	decomposition reactions

Iron left exposed to the environment reacts with oxygen in the air. The result is a new compound, iron oxide. This type of change, in which a substance changes into a new and different substance, is a **chemical change**. Now take, for instance, the melting of a cup of ice cubes. The result is a glass of water. A change has occurred, but the substance remains the same. This is a **physical change**, a change in which the substance undergoing the change remains the same. Ice and the resultant substance after melting are both water; therefore melting is a physical change.

Many types of chemical changes, or chemical **reactions**, may be shown with chemical equations. The substances that react with each other are written on the left side of the equation, and they are called the **reactants**. The substances that are the end products of the reaction are written on the right side of the equation, and they are called the **products**. The law of conservation of mass tells us that matter is neither created nor destroyed. So the same number of atoms of each element must be present on each side of an equation. The equation is balanced using coefficients, the numbers placed in front of the each substance. For example, two hydrogen molecules are indicated as $2H_2$.

In this section we review four main categories of reactions:

1. synthesis or combination reactions

2. single replacement reactions

3. double displacement reactions

4. decomposition reactions

When we look at chemical reactions, we think of substances combining in quantities called moles. A mole is equal to 6.02×10^{23} particles. You can think of it as a quantity, sort of like a dozen or a gross.

Synthesis, or Combination, Reactions

Synthesis, or **combination**, **reactions** involve two or more reactants that combine to create a new product. For example:

$$2H_2 + O_2 \rightarrow 2H_2O$$

SECTION A

SECTION B

SECTION C

COMPREHENSIVE PRACTICE Test 1

COMPREHENSIVE PRACTICE Test 2

COMPREHENSIVE PRACTICE Test 3

In this reaction, two moles of hydrogen react with one mole of oxygen to produce two moles of water. As you can see, there are 4 atoms of hydrogen and 2 atoms of oxygen on each side. This is a balanced equation for a synthesis reaction.

Single Replacement Reactions

Single replacement reactions involve an element reacting with a compound. During this reaction, an atom of the single element replaces an element in the compound. For example:

$$Cl_2 + 2NaBr \rightarrow 2NaCl + Br_2$$

Chlorine replaces bromine in the compound.

Double Displacement Reactions

Double displacement reactions involve two ionic compounds. The positive ions, or metal, in each compound switch positions. A common type of double displacement reaction is an **acid-base reaction**. The products are always a salt and water. Since the products are neutral (neither acidic nor basic), these specific types of displacement reactions are called **neutralization reactions**. For example:

$$NaOH + HCl \rightarrow NaCl + H_2O$$

Sodium hydroxide reacts with hydrogen chloride to form sodium chloride (a salt) and water.

Remember that, in an aqueous solution, an **acid** donates hydrogen ions (H^+) and a **base** donates hydroxide ions (OH^-). Another way of defining acids is to think of H^+ as combining with water to form a hydronium ion (H_3O^+) and to think of the hydronium ion as being the positive ion produced by an acid. Strong acids and bases are very caustic and can burn your hands if they spill. In the case of either being spilled on one's hands, the solutions should be flushed with water.

The **pH scale** was created to identify the strength of an acid or a base based on the concentration of hydrogen and hydroxide ions. The scale runs from 0 to 14, with a pH below 7 as acidic, a pH above 7 as basic, and a pH of 7 as neutral (neither acidic nor basic). A pH of 0 indicates an extremely strong acid, whereas a pH of 6 indicates that the acid is fairly weak. On the other hand, a pH of 14 indicates a very strong base, and a pH of 8 means the base is fairly weak. A substance that changes color in an acid or base is called an acid-base **indicator**, such as litmus, phenolphthalein, or bromthymol blue.

Decomposition Reactions

Decomposition reactions involve one reactant that is broken down into two or more simpler products. Often heat is used to drive this type of reaction.

$$H_2CO_3 \rightarrow H_2O + CO_2$$

Heated carbonic acid decomposes into water and carbon dioxide.

Basic Chemistry

201

SECTION A

SECTION B

SECTION C

COMPREHENSIVE PRACTICE Test 1

COMPREHENSIVE PRACTICE Test 2

COMPREHENSIVE PRACTICE Test 3

REACTION RATES AND CATALYSIS

Terms to Be Defined

activation energy   exothermic   equilibrium

catalyst   endothermic

A reaction depends on two things.

1. The two substances must come into contact.

2. Enough energy has to be available. If the appropriate amount of energy, the **activation energy**, is available, then the reaction can proceed.

Reaction rates are thus influenced by any factors that affect these two conditions. For instance, the reaction rate is increased by raising the temperature because an elevated temperature causes particles to move around in a quicker and more erratic manner. The increased movement heightens the probability that two particles will come into contact. Increasing the surface area of a substance also boosts reaction rate. Finally, a very important influence on rate is that of **catalysts**. These are substances that increase the rate of a reaction by lowering the activation energy needed. It is important to remember that catalysts only affect the rate of the reaction and are not used up in it. A reaction that releases energy is called **exothermic**; its products contain less energy than its reactants. A reaction that absorbs energy is called **endothermic**; its products contain more energy than its reactants.

Most chemical reactions do not go to completion but instead reach equilibrium. At **equilibrium**, the rate of the forward reaction is equal to the rate of the reverse reaction. The synthesis of ammonia is an example. The double arrows indicate that this is a reversible reaction.

$$N_2 + 3H_2 \rightleftharpoons 2NH_3$$

ORGANIC CHEMISTRY

Terms to Be Defined

organic compound   monosaccharide   glycerol

hydrocarbon   disaccharide   protein

alcohol   polysaccharide   amino acid

aldehyde   starch   dehydration synthesis

ketone   glycogen   hydrolysis

structural formula   lipid

carbohydrate   fatty acid

Organic chemistry is the study of **organic compounds**, which are compounds that contain carbon. Examples of organic compounds include **hydrocarbons**, such as methane or butane, **alcohols**, **aldehydes**, **ketones**, ethers, and esters. Organic compounds are often represented with **structural formulas**. These are similar to Lewis diagrams, but they use a dash in place of a colon (:) to represent a bond. Figure 25 shows several examples.

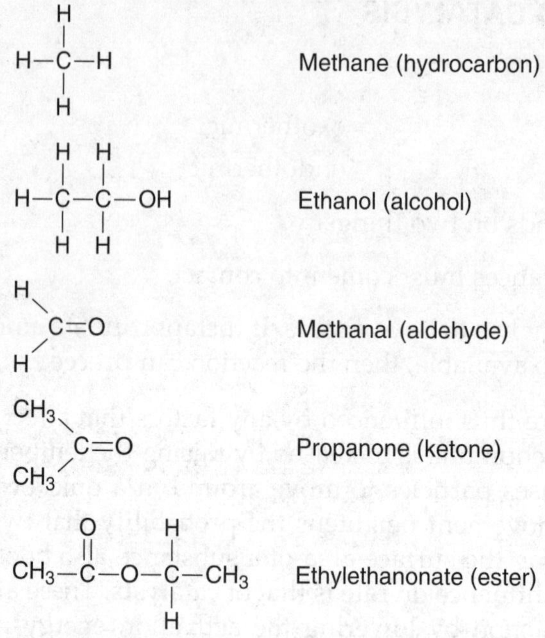

H—C—H   Methane (hydrocarbon)

H—C—C—OH   Ethanol (alcohol)

C=O   Methanal (aldehyde)

C=O   Propanone (ketone)

CH_3—C—O—C—CH_3 Ethylethanonate (ester)

Figure 25. Example Structural Formulas

Biochemistry is the chemistry of living things. Among the organic compounds that are important in biochemistry are nucleic acids, carbohydrates, lipids, and proteins. **Carbohydrates** contain carbon, hydrogen, and oxygen, and the ratio of hydrogen to oxygen is typically 2:1. Carbohydrates can be found in different sizes and are classified by size. **Monosaccharides** are the so-called simple sugars, whereas **disaccharides** are made from two monosaccharides and include table sugar, or sucrose. **Polysaccharides** are chains of monosaccharides and are commonly known as starch and glycogen. **Starch** is formed in plants, whereas **glycogen** is found in animals.

Lipids are fats and steroids. Fats are made of **fatty acids** and **glycerol**. Each fat molecule is made up of one glycerol molecule attached to three fatty acids. In saturated fats, the bonds between the carbons are single; in unsaturated fats, the bonds tend to be double or triple bonds.

Proteins are made up of **amino acids**, of which there are about 20 types. The amino acids are linked in chains, and the sequence determines the properties of the protein. Examples of proteins include enzymes, collagen (making up cartilage, tendons, bones), and keratin (hair and nails).

Two important types of reactions are dehydration synthesis and hydrolysis. **Dehydration synthesis** is a reaction in which small units, such as monosaccharides or amino acids, are joined to form larger molecules. In this reaction, one molecule gives up a hydrogen atom and the other an OH to form water, and the two molecules bond. **Hydrolysis** is the opposite; a large molecule is broken down into smaller molecules by adding water (H_2O) and putting the H and OH back.

Physics

The aim of physics is to understand the physical laws and principles that influence every aspect of daily life. Physicists examine the behavior and interaction of energy and matter in the universe to increase their understanding of everyday phenomena. An understanding of the principles of physics enables you to appreciate your physical world. This section provides an overview of the principles of physics.

MECHANICS

Terms to be Defined

displacement	newton	joule
motion	friction	power
speed	gravity	machine
velocity	weight	efficiency
acceleration	density	simple machine
vector	torque	inclined plane
deceleration	lever arm	wedge
momentum	centripetal force	screw
conservation of momentum	Newton's third law	lever
Newton's first law	energy	pulley
inertia	kinetic energy	wheel and axle
Newton's second law	potential energy	compound machine
force	work	

The **displacement** of an object is the distance that an object is from some starting point, and it is measured in units of length. When an object is in **motion**, its displacement is constantly changing. Motion is described by displacement, velocity (speed), and acceleration.

- **Speed** is the distance traveled by an object per unit of time.

$$\text{speed} = \frac{\text{distance traveled}}{\text{time}}$$

- **Velocity** is speed in a given direction; it therefore tells us two things about a moving object: its speed and its direction.

- Sometimes velocity, as well as displacement, can change with time. The rate of change in velocity is called **acceleration**. Acceleration refers to any change of velocity, either positive or negative. **Deceleration** is sometimes used to refer to negative acceleration or a decrease in velocity and can cause a change in direction.

$$\text{acceleration} = \frac{\text{final velocity} - \text{original velocity}}{\text{time}}$$

SECTION A

SECTION B

SECTION C

COMPREHENSIVE PRACTICE Test 1

COMPREHENSIVE PRACTICE Test 2

COMPREHENSIVE PRACTICE Test 3

An object traveling at a specific velocity has a quantity called momentum. Velocity and acceleration can both be described as **vectors** because they have both magnitude and direction. Speed is not a vector quantity because it does not specify direction. All moving objects have momentum. **Momentum** is equal to the mass of an object multiplied by its velocity. The mass of an object is the amount of matter in it.

$$momentum = mass \times velocity$$

One of the main laws of classical physics is the **conservation of momentum**, which states that the total momentum of an isolated system is always constant. During a collision between two bodies, the momentum of each body changes, but the total momentum is conserved. None of the momentum is lost. One object may lose momentum, but the momentum lost by the one object is gained by the other. When a moving object hits a stable object, such as a bullet hitting a wall, the bullet delivers an impulse to the wall. The impulse is said to be the change in the object's momentum.

Newton's Laws

Classical mechanics is based on the application of Newton's laws. **Newton's first law**, the law of inertia, states that objects in motion tend to stay in motion and that objects at rest tend to stay at rest. **Inertia** is the property of matter that resists any change in motion. **Newton's second law** describes the relationship between **force**, mass, and acceleration. It states that the force applied on an object equals the mass of the object times its acceleration:

$$force = mass \times acceleration \text{ or } F = ma$$

Newton's second law explains why a small car has better gas mileage than a big car. According to this law, the force required to accelerate the big car (with the greater mass) is greater than the force required to accelerate the small car. The big car therefore has to burn more gas in its engine to produce the additional force. The **newton** (N) is the unit that represents a force that accelerates a mass of 1 kilogram 1 meter per second.

You might think something is wrong with Newton's analysis. In the real world, when you slide a box along the floor, giving it a velocity, it does not continue at that speed forever but stops. This is due to the friction between the box and the floor. Whenever a force is exerted on an object along a surface or whenever an object has a velocity along the surface, and the two surfaces touch, there is a force called **friction**. In the case of the box being pushed along the floor, friction opposes the motion or the force being applied. Note that the force of friction is always in the direction to stop the object from moving.

A force we are all familiar with is gravitational force. **Gravity** is the force of attraction between all objects in the universe. The greater the mass of an object is, the greater its gravitational force will be. The earth's gravitational force is great because the earth has a large mass. If you drop an object, it falls to the earth because earth exerts a gravitational force on it. The force due to gravity is not the same on every object but depends on the object's mass. However, the acceleration toward earth is the same for all objects, independent of their mass.

The pull of gravity on an object determines its **weight**. A change in the force of gravity results in a change in an object's weight but not in its mass. For example, the earth has more mass than the moon. So the earth exerts a greater gravitational force than the moon. On the moon you would weigh about 1/7th of what you weigh on earth because the gravitational pull of the moon is about 1/7th of the gravitational pull of the earth. Yet your body mass would stay exactly the same as it is on earth. In addition, the force of gravity between two objects decreases as the distance between the objects increases. For example, the earth's gravitational pull on a rocket decreases as the rocket moves away from the earth. A way of comparing substances so that they are comparable is to use **density**, which is mass per unit volume: $\text{density} = \dfrac{\text{mass}}{\text{vol}}$. A pound of iron and a pound of feathers both weigh a pound. However, a pound of feathers takes up much more space than the iron.

The ability of a force that is applied perpendicularly to rotate an object around an axis, such as using a wrench to turn a bolt, is measured by a quantity called torque. **Torque** is the perpendicular force times the lever arm. The **lever arm** is the distance from the axis of rotation to the point where the force is exerted (e.g., the length of the wrench). The farther the force is from the axis of rotation, the easier it is to rotate the object and the more torque is produced.

To keep a ball at the end of a string moving in a circle, you must continually exert a force pulling the ball back toward the center of the circle. This force is called the **centripetal force**, and, in the case of the ball on a string, the string provides the force.

Newton's third law of motion states that for every action there is an equal and opposite reaction. A rocket works on this principle. The blast from the back of the rocket pushes the rocket forward.

In mechanics, objects are defined as having energy. **Energy** is the ability to do work. There are two types of energy.

1. **Kinetic energy** is energy associated with motion. Any moving body has this type energy because it is able to do work by moving other bodies. The kinetic energy of a body tells us how much work that body can do by moving other bodies until it is brought to rest. Kinetic energy is defined as one half of the product of mass and velocity squared:

$$\text{kinetic energy} = \frac{1}{2}(\text{mass} \times \text{velocity})^2$$

2. **Potential energy** is the energy stored in a body because of its position. When you lift an object up, you provide it with potential energy. An object has more potential energy at the top of a building than it does on the first floor.

When you do work on an object, you change its energy by giving it some of your energy. **Work** is defined as the product of the force applied to an object and the distance through which the force is applied:

$$\text{work} = \text{force} \times \text{distance}$$

A **joule** is the unit of energy equal to the work done by a force of 1 newton acting over a distance of 1 meter.

Power is the rate at which work is done. The power of a machine is the total work done divided by the time taken. Since work equals force times distance, the formula for power is:

$$\text{power} = \frac{\text{force} \times \text{distance}}{\text{time}} = \frac{\text{work}}{\text{time}}$$

A **machine** is a device that makes work easier by changing the force or the direction of an applied force. The **efficiency** of a machine is the work done divided by the energy used to power the machine, or the ratio of work input to work output. Because of friction, no machine can be 100% efficient.

There are six **simple machines**:

1. An **inclined plane** is a slanted surface used to raise an object.

2. A **wedge** is a moving inclined plane.

3. A **screw** is an inclined plane wrapped around a cylinder.

4. A **lever** is a simple machine that is free to move around a fulcrum when force is applied.

5. A **pulley** is a chain or rope wrapped around a wheel.

6. A **wheel and axle** act as a lever that rotates in a circle.

A **compound machine** is a combination of two or more simple machines.

THERMODYNAMICS

Terms to Be Defined

atom	Boyle's law	Celsius
kinetic theory of matter	Charles's law	Kelvin
solid	temperature	Fahrenheit
liquid	heat	ice point
gas	specific heat	steam point
molecules	phase change	triple point
pressure	latent heat	absolute zero

All matter is made up of **atoms**, which are the smallest particles of an element that retain all the chemical properties of the element. According to the **kinetic theory of matter**, the atoms in matter are in a constant state of motion. The motion and spacing of atoms determine the state of simple matter. The three ordinary states of matter are **solid**, **liquid**, and **gas**. When matter is in the gas or liquid state, **molecules**, which are groups of atoms, are free to move around.

Gases and liquids do not have definite shapes of their own. When a liquid or gas is placed in a container, the atoms or molecules move around freely in the container and take its shape. These molecules move in all possible directions and keep colliding with the walls of the container. Each time a molecule collides with the wall, it delivers an impulse to the wall. The greater the quantity of gas or liquid in a container, the more frequent the collisions are. **Pressure** is the result of the impulses from the collision of molecules with the walls of the container.

There are two important laws in thermodynamics:

1. **Boyle's law** states that the volume of a fixed amount of gas varies inversely with the pressure of the gas. If the volume of the gas is decreased, both the number of particle collisions and the pressure of the gas increase. If the volume of the gas is increased, the pressure of the gas decreases.

2. **Charles's law** defines the relationship between the temperature and volume of a gas. According to this law, the volume of a fixed amount of gas varies directly with its temperature. If the temperature of a gas increases, the volume increases.

Temperature is a very familiar concept, but what exactly is it? **Temperature** is a measure of the average kinetic energy of the particles in a substance. It tells how warm or cold a substance is with respect to other substances. Temperature determines whether a substance gains or gives up heat when put into contact with other bodies. A substance with a high temperature is said to be hot, or to contain heat. **Heat** is a form of energy that causes the particles of matter to move faster and farther apart. When a substance is heated, its temperature increases. The **specific heat** of a substance is the heat needed to raise the temperature of 1 gram by 1°.

When the temperature of a substance changes, its phase may change. **Phase change** refers to the physical change of a substance from one state to another. For example, when ice is heated, it eventually melts. The **latent heat** is the heat energy needed per unit mass to change the phase of a substance.

Temperature is measured with a thermometer using different scales. In science the most commonly used temperature scale is the **Celsius** scale. Two other scales are the **Fahrenheit** scale and the **Kelvin**, or absolute temperature, scale. The **ice point** is the temperature at which ice melts or water freezes. On the Fahrenheit scale, the ice point is 32°; on the Celsius scale the ice point is 0°. The **steam point** is the point at which water at standard pressure boils. On the Celsius scale the steam point is 100°; it is 212° on the Fahrenheit scale. The **triple point** (273.16 K) on the Kelvin scale is the temperature at which water exists simultaneously as a gas, a liquid, and a solid. On the Kelvin scale, the lowest possible temperature is known as **absolute zero**, or zero Kelvin (0 K).

The relationship of the Kelvin to the Celsius scale is:

$$\text{temperature}_{\text{Kelvin}} = \text{temperature}_{\text{Celsisus}} + 273$$

The relationship of the Fahrenheit to the Celsius scale is:

$$\text{temperature}°_{\text{Fahrenheit}} = \left(\frac{9}{5} \text{temperature}°_{\text{Celsisus}} \right) + 32$$

Therefore,

$$\text{A temperature change in } °\text{Fahrenheit} = \frac{9}{5} \text{ change in } °\text{Celsius}$$

WAVES

Terms to be Defined

motion	trough	pitch
wave	wavelength	loudness
longitudinal wave	wave speed	Doppler effect
transverse wave	diffraction	reflection
periodic motion	interference	refraction
periodic wave	resonance	dispersion
period	photon	lens

SECTION A

SECTION B

SECTION C

COMPREHENSIVE PRACTICE Test 1

COMPREHENSIVE PRACTICE Test 2

COMPREHENSIVE PRACTICE Test 3

frequency

hertz

amplitude

crest

electromagnetic waves

electromagnetic spectrum

visible light

convex lens

focal point

concave lens

Motion is a change in position relative to a frame of reference. A **wave** is a rhythmic disturbance that travels through matter or space, and wave motion is a means of transferring energy. The two basic types of waves are longitudinal and transverse waves. A **transverse wave** is a wave in which matter vibrates at right angles to the direction in which the wave travels. For example, water waves approximate a transverse wave, and light and heat appear to be transmitted by transverse waves. A **longitudinal wave** is a wave in which matter vibrates back and forth along the path that the wave travels. Sounds, for example, are transmitted by longitudinal waves.

Periodic motion is motion that repeats itself over and over again, such as the motion of a pendulum. A **periodic wave** is motion that repeats itself at regular intervals and that transfers energy but not mass. The time it takes for the motion to repeat itself is measured in seconds and is called the **period**. A cycle is equal to one complete repetition of a periodic event. The **frequency** (f) of a wave tells us how often a cycle repeats itself in a specific time unit. Frequency is often measured in **hertz** (Hz), which is equivalent to cycles per second.

Amplitude refers to the maximum distance a wave rises or falls as it travels, and it is related to the energy that the wave carries. For example, amplitude relates to brightness with light waves and to loudness with sound waves. The louder the sound or the brighter the light is, the higher the amplitude is. The **crest** of a transverse wave is the maximum upward displacement, and the **trough** is the maximum downward displacement. The **wavelength** of a transverse wave is the distance between two successive crests. **Wave speed** is the frequency of the wave times the wavelength.

The phenomena of **diffraction** is the bending of waves around an obstacle. When two waves meet, they combine to make a new wave. How the waves interact with each other when they go through the same portion of a medium at the same time is called **interference**. **Resonance** between two systems occurs when the vibration of one system results in the vibration of the other system at the same frequency.

Light waves are made up of streams of **photons**, or tiny packets of energy. The amount of energy in the photons determines the kind of light wave produced. Light waves are called **electromagnetic waves** because the moving photons generate electric and magnetic fields. The complete spectrum of light, arranged in order of their wavelengths, is called the **electromagnetic spectrum**. **Visible light**, only a small part of this spectrum, is the portion that is visible to the human eye. The electromagnetic spectrum consists of:

radio waves

infrared waves

visible light

ultraviolet light

x-rays

gamma rays

The photons of visible light contain a moderate amount of energy, while x-rays are made up of high-energy photons and radio waves, which contain low-energy photons. Gamma rays have the highest-energy photons and the shortest wavelengths of all the electromagnetic waves.

Sound waves are longitudinal waves; they vibrate in the direction of their motion. The **pitch** of a sound wave has to do with the frequency. High-frequency sound waves have a high pitch, and low-frequency waves have a low pitch. The **loudness** of a sound wave is determined by its amplitude. The **Doppler effect** occurs whenever there is relative motion between the source of waves and the observer. For example, the pitch of a siren gets higher as an ambulance approaches you and lower as it drives away. The siren has not changed its frequency, but the motion of the ambulance toward you increases the frequency of the sound waves you hear. As the siren moves away, the frequency you hear is less than the source frequency, and the pitch is lower.

When a light wave bounces off a surface that does not absorb its energy, it is reflected. The type of surface that light strikes determines the kind of **reflection**. Because a mirror has a smooth, flat surface, the reflected rays are not scattered and the image reflected is clearly defined. According to the law of reflection, the angle of incidence of a ray striking the mirror and the angle of reflection will be equal. **Refraction** is the bending of light rays as they pass obliquely from one medium to another because light moves at different speeds through different mediums. As light passes from one medium to another, it either speeds up or slows down. A prism is a piece of glass that separates light into its component colors. This phenomenon is called **dispersion**.

A **lens** is any transparent material that refracts light. When parallel rays of light pass through a lens, they are refracted so that they either come together or spread out. A lens that is thicker in the center than it is at the edges is a **convex lens**. When parallel rays of light pass through a convex lens, they converge, or bend toward the center. The **focal point** is the point at which the light rays meet. A **concave lens** is thicker at the edges than it is in the middle. When light rays pass through a concave lens, they diverge because they are bent toward the edges, or the thickest part, of the lens. Images of an object produced by concave lenses are smaller than the object.

ELECTRICITY AND MAGNETISM

Terms to Be Defined

neutron	generator	ampere
proton	electrical potential energy	ammeter
electron	potential difference	resistor
Coulomb's law	transformer	series circuit
magnetism	voltage	parallel circuit
magnetic fields	voltmeter	power
torque	current	watt

Two types of electric charge exist in our universe: positive and negative. Some particles have no charge (**neutrons**), some have a positive charge (**protons**), and some have a negative charge (**electrons**). Like charges repel each other, and unlike charges attract each other. **Coulomb's law** applies to this force of attraction and repulsion.

SECTION A

SECTION B

SECTION C

COMPREHENSIVE PRACTICE Test 1

COMPREHENSIVE PRACTICE Test 2

COMPREHENSIVE PRACTICE Test 3

Coulomb found that the electric force between two charges is proportional to the product of the two charges. Therefore, if one charge is doubled, the electric force is doubled. If both charges are doubled, the electric force increases four times. Coulomb also found that the electric force varied inversely as the square of the distance between the charges. Thus, when the distance between two forces doubles, the force between them decreases to $\frac{1}{4}$ of the original force. When the two forces are brought closer together, the force between them increases.

Electricity is closely related to **magnetism**, which is a force of attraction. All magnets have a north and a south pole, each of which attracts its opposite and repels its similar pole. **Magnetic fields** exist whenever electric charges are moving. When the moving charges are in a wire that loops, a **torque** results. This effect is the basis for electric motors. A **generator** is a device that converts mechanical energy, such as water coming down a waterfall, into electric energy.

Electrical potential energy can be compared to the gravitational force associated with an object's position; because of the force, the object has potential energy. Similarly, electrical potential energy is associated with the potential interaction of two objects' charges. **Potential difference** is the change in electrical potential energy. The device that changes the potential difference of electricity is called a **transformer**. **Voltage**, another term for potential difference, is a measure of the electrical energy available. A **voltmeter** is a device that measures the potential difference between two points in an electric circuit.

Electricity moving through a circuit is called a **current**. An **ampere** is the unit used to measure electrical current. An **ammeter** is a device that measures the current going through any specific point on the circuit. The way by which the ability to flow through a circuit is limited is a **resistor**. There are two different types of circuits:

1. A **series circuit** has all its resistors in a row so that all current must travel through all resistors.

2. In a **parallel circuit**, all the resistors are arranged side by side, so that they are all at the same voltage.

Electrical **power** is equal to the voltage times the current:

$$\text{power} = \text{voltage} \times \text{current}$$

Power is expressed as **watts**:

$$\text{watt} = \text{volts} \times \text{amperes}$$

MODERN PHYSICS

Terms to Be Defined

mass defect	nuclear reaction	photoelectric effect
radioactivity	fusion	ionization
radioactive decay	fission	theory of relativity
transmutation	quantum mechanics	

In the early twentieth century, scientists began to understand the structure of the atom. They discovered that the atom has a nucleus of positively charged protons and uncharged neutrons and that the nucleus is surrounded by negatively charged electrons. The mass of a nucleus is heavier then all the protons and neutrons that make it up. This mass difference is known as the **mass defect**. The mass defect represents the energy in the bonds holding the nucleus together.

It was also discovered that an atom's nucleus could spontaneously disintegrate while giving off energy in the form of alpha and beta particles and gamma rays. This phenomenon is known as **radioactivity**. The spontaneous change in the nucleus of an atom is known as **radioactive decay**. The conversion of one element into another element is referred to as **transmutation**. When a radioactive nucleus goes through a transmutation, it is called a **nuclear reaction**. There are two main processes of nuclear reactions.

1. In **fusion**, the nuclei of several light atoms combine to form a single heavy nucleus with a release of energy.

2. In **fission**, a heavy nucleus splits into two main pieces with the release of a huge amount of energy.

Another discovery attributable to modern physics is the nature of light. For years, scientists have been arguing over whether light consists of particles or acts like waves. As it turns out, the only theory that can accurately explain the behavior of light is **quantum mechanics**, which asserts that the behavior of light is actually an interesting combination of particles and waves. An example that illustrates this wave-particle duality is the **photoelectric effect**. When a light wave strikes certain metallic surfaces, electrons are emitted. This effect, called **ionization**, means that an atom loses an electron (or several electrons) and becomes an ion.

Albert Einstein's **theory of relativity**, devised in 1905, was one of the greatest accomplishments of modern physics. The main consequence of this theory is the identification of the existence of an upper limit on velocity. This upper limit (c, also known as the speed of light through a vacuum) is the fastest that any particle can travel. According to this theory, the speed of light is absolute, and material particles can never reach the speed of light.

SECTION A

SECTION B

SECTION C

COMPREHENSIVE PRACTICE Test 1

COMPREHENSIVE PRACTICE Test 2

COMPREHENSIVE PRACTICE Test 3

Health

NUTRITION, DIET, AND EXERCISE

Terms to Be Defined

caloric intake	nutrient	lipid
caloric need	protein	mineral
obesity	carbohydrate	vitamin
nutrient-dense food	saturated fat	cholesterol
balanced diet	trans-fat	atherosclerosis

When we consider diet, we must be conscious of the calories of energy contained in our food. Each of us has a specific number of calories that we need to run our bodies (**caloric need**). If we look at the caloric content of the food we eat, we can calculate our **caloric intake**. To maintain our current weight, our caloric intake should be equal to our caloric need. If the caloric intake is greater than the caloric need, we gain weight. If caloric intake is less than the caloric need, we lose weight. The caloric needs of individuals differ depending on factors such as age, gender, and amount of physical activity. **Obesity** (a condition of overweight in which a person has a body mass index in excess of 30) is a serious problem for many people, and diet and exercise are the principal means in managing body weight.

The substances in food that we need are called **nutrients**, such as **proteins**, **carbohydrates**, **lipids**, **minerals**, and **vitamins**. **Nutrient-dense foods** are foods that provide substantial amounts of minerals and vitamins with relatively few calories. To maintain a **balanced diet**, it is important to get appropriate amounts of the various nutrients. Lipids (fats and oils) should not comprise more than 10% of our diets. We should avoid **saturated fats** and **trans-fats**, which increase **cholesterol** concentrations in our blood vessels and lead to clogged arteries and coronary disease. Clogged arteries (**atherosclerosis**) can lead to heart attacks, strokes, and other health issues. Carbohydrates (starches and sugars) in our diets should include high-fiber forms and should not include large amounts of processed sugar. Sugar added to foods increases our caloric intake and adversely affects our teeth.

STERILIZATION, ANTISEPSIS, AND CLEANLINESS

Terms to Be Defined

pathogen	virus	antiseptics
bacteria	prion	disinfectants
fungus	antisepsis	pasteurization
protozoa	antibiotics	

Disease is caused by **pathogens**, which are infectious organisms (germs) and which include **bacteria**, **fungi**, **protozoa**, **viruses**, and **prions**. They cause disease and affect us in different ways, such as

- producing poisonous metabolic products (staphylococcus, diphtheria, botulism toxin, and many others),

- destroying vital organs and tissues (prions, polio, rabies viruses), or

- interfering with body chemistry (toxic fungi).

To prevent the spread of disease, it is important to prevent the spread of these organisms from one host to another. The easiest prevention method is washing our hands with soap. In a hospital, for example, the staff strives to maintain a sterile environment, in which they kill or eliminate all pathogens. **Antisepsis** is the prevention of infection by inhibiting the growth of pathogens. Among the means we use to achieve antisepsis are:

- **antibiotics** that kill pathogens in the body,

- **antiseptics** that kill pathogens on the body,

- **disinfectants** that kill pathogens on nonliving things, and

- **pasteurization**, heatings milk to a temperature that eliminates most pathogens.

SMOKING, ALCOHOL, AND DRUGS

Terms to Be Defined

emphysema	depressant	opioids
nicotine	hallucinogens	stimulant
cirrhosis	cannabinoids	

Smoking tobacco is hazardous to health. It is directly linked to lung cancer, heart disease, and **emphysema** (a disease of the lungs). Tobacco contains **nicotine**, which is addictive and makes it hard for smokers to stop smoking.

Alcohol used in moderation is not harmful. However, we should be aware that excess drinking over a long time can damage the liver, resulting in **cirrhosis** of the liver. Pregnant women should not drink alcohol because it can pass through the placental barrier and harm the fetus. Intoxication can affect one's judgment and ability to respond, which is why drunken driving results in so many accidents.

Drugs that are abused fall into specific categories and have different effects on the body. Commonly abused drugs include:

- **cannabinoids**, such as marijuana,

- **depressants**, such as barbiturates and tranquilizers,

- **hallucinogens**, such as LSD and mescaline,

- **opioids**, such as heroin and morphine, and

- **stimulants**, such as amphetamine, cocaine, and methamphetamine.

FOOD PREPARATION AND STORAGE

Terms to Be Defined

food-borne illness   *E. coli*   dangerous temperature zone
Salmonella

Food-borne illness is a disease that is caused by a pathogen in food, such as *Salmonella* or *E. coli*. It is what we commonly call food poisoning. The symptoms vary depending on the particular pathogen but often include nausea, vomiting, diarrhea, headache, tiredness, and fever.

Because pathogens need warm, moist conditions to survive, you can do several things to prevent the spread of these diseases:

• Wash your hands after handling raw meats.

• Cook food to a temperature that kills the bacteria (above 140°F).

• Keep food refrigerated (below 40°F) or frozen.

• Wash utensils, such as knives, between use on meat or poultry and other foods.

The **dangerous temperature zone**, in which bacteria can double in 20 to 30 minutes, is between 41° and 139°F. Freezing and refrigeration stop bacteria from increasing but do not kill them. A good way to reheat food is in a microwave oven, which kills pathogens.

DISEASE TRANSMISSION

Terms to Be Defined

disease transmission   airborne   immunity
direct contact   vector   vaccination
sexually transmitted disease (STD)   lymphocytes   noninfectious disease
indirect contact   antibodies

Disease transmission is the spread of an infectious disease from one person to another. Infectious diseases my be spread by **direct contact** with someone who is already infected. Person-to-person contact may take place through:

• kissing,

• touching,

• exchanging body fluids (as is the case for **sexually transmitted diseases [STD]**),

• blood transfusions, as is the case with AIDS,

• animal-to-person interaction, as in the case of Rabies,

• or mother-to-unborn-child interaction through the placenta (e.g., Rubella).

Indirect contact involves transmission through an inanimate object. For example, a person with a cold might use a telephone and leave cold viruses on its surface; the viruses are then transmitted to the next person using the phone. Transmission may also be **airborne**; that is, germs may spread through the air. For example, a sick individual may spread germs by sneezing or coughing in such a way that droplets with the germ are in the air; these droplets then are exposed to another person's eyes, nose, or mouth.

Another means of transmission is through **vectors**, organisms such as mosquitoes that spread the disease from one person to the next. Malaria, yellow fever, West Nile virus, and Lyme disease are examples of diseases spread by a vector. (We have already discussed food-borne illness.)

When bodies are invaded by pathogens, our immune system takes over, and our white blood cells go into action. One group of white blood cells, called **lymphocytes**, produces **antibodies**, which fight specific foreign proteins. Once we produce antibodies for a specific pathogen, we develop **immunity** to it. **Vaccination** is the injection of dead or weakened germs into the body to stimulate the production of antibodies and thus create immunity.

Some diseases are classified as **noninfectious**. These diseases are not spread from person to person; they are not communicable. Among these are vitamin deficiency diseases (such as pellagra and scurvy), glandular diseases (such as diabetes), and hereditary diseases (such as hemophilia and sickle cell anemia). Cancers are also generally noninfectious, although some are linked to specific carcinogens.

HEALTH BIBLIOGRAPHY

Crumpler, Kathy T., Prothrow-Smith, Deborah, and Pruitt, B. E. *Health: Skills for Wellness*. Boston: Pearson Prentice Hall, 2001.

SECTION A

SECTION B

SECTION C

COMPREHENSIVE PRACTICE Test 1

COMPREHENSIVE PRACTICE Test 2

COMPREHENSIVE PRACTICE Test 3

I. Science

45 minutes

DIRECTIONS

The science tests consist of questions on biology, chemistry, physics, human anatomy, physiology, and health. You should be able to answer all the questions in the test in 45 minutes.

Each test question consists of an incomplete sentence or a question, followed by four choices. Read each question carefully, and then decide which choice is the correct answer.

If you finish the science test before the 45 minutes are up, go back and check your work.

Your score will be the total number of correct answers. You may answer a question even if you are not completely sure of the correct response. Do not spend too much time on any one question. If you cannot answer a question, go on to the next one. Since it is important to be able to answer these questions in the allotted time, it is a good idea to use a timer while you complete the questions in each section.

Read each question carefully, and then select the correct answer. (The correct answers and their explanations are at the end of Section C.)

1. A person who has a high blood level of cholesterol is at risk for which of these conditions?
   a. heart disease
   b. lung disease
   c. hypoglycemia
   d. osteoporosis

2. A risk group for the disease AIDS (acquired immunodeficiency syndrome) is intravenous drug users. To prevent further spread of the disease, which of these measures would be most effective for this group to take?
   a. Undergo screening for the AIDS virus.
   b. Avoid sharing hypodermic needles with other drug users.
   c. Increase the fiber in their diets.
   d. Limit bodily contact with other drug users.

3. The nicotine in tobacco is classified as a
   a. food supplement.
   b. drug.
   c. preservative.
   d. food dye.

SECTION A

SECTION B

SECTION C

COMPREHENSIVE PRACTICE Test 1

COMPREHENSIVE PRACTICE Test 2

COMPREHENSIVE PRACTICE Test 3

The next question refers to the following diagram of a model of a thorax showing inspiration.

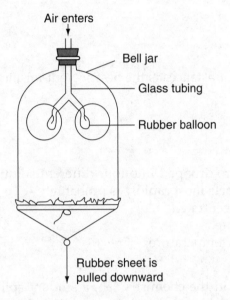

4. The rubber balloons in this diagram most likely represent the human
   a. lungs.
   b. rib cage.
   c. bronchi.
   d. trachea.

The next two questions refer to the following diagram of the human female reproductive system.

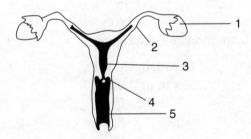

5. Which of the structures produces female sex hormones?
   a. 1
   b. 2
   c. 4
   d. 5

6. The oviduct (fallopian tube) is represented by number
   a. 2.
   b. 3.
   c. 4.
   d. 5.

7. A wooden box is dragged along the floor toward the east. The direction of the force of friction on the box is toward the
   a. north.
   b. south.
   c. east.
   d. west.

8. Which of these substances is the best solvent for most salts?
   a. alcohol
   b. water
   c. oil
   d. acetone

9. Pieces of zinc are dropped into four different solutions of hydrochloric acid. The solution that reacts most rapidly is probably
   a. the most concentrated.
   b. the most dilute.
   c. at the lowest temperature.
   d. the freshest.

10. While working in the chemistry lab, a student spills a strong acid on her hand. What is the first action the student should take?
    a. Pour a strong base on the spill to neutralize the acid.
    b. Flush the hand with water.
    c. Notify the instructor.
    d. Dry the hand with a towel.

11. In plants, the chemical that is used to convert light energy into food is
    a. sulfur dioxide.
    b. nitrogen.
    c. chlorophyll.
    d. iodine.

12. The following table indicates the ranges of wavelengths of different colors of light.

Color	Wavelength (m)
violet	less than 4.5×10^{-7}
blue	$4.5-5.0 \times 10^{-7}$
green	$5.0-5.7 \times 10^{-7}$
yellow	$5.7-5.9 \times 10^{-7}$
orange	$5.9-6.1 \times 10^{-7}$
red	greater than 6.1×10^{-7}

   What is the color of light having a wavelength of 5.6×10^{-7} m?
   a. blue
   b. green
   c. yellow
   d. orange

13. The process of killing pathogenic nonspore-forming bacteria in milk by heating is known as
    a. homogenization.
    b. sterilization.

c. pasteurization.

d. detoxification.

14. In the Bowman's capsule of the human nephron, materials diffuse from the blood into the kidney tubules. This process is known as

a. resorption.

b. active transport.

c. filtration.

d. urination.

15. The following diagram shows the paths taken by three rays of light from the flame of a candle as they pass through a lens.

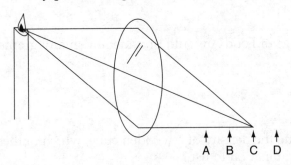

At which point should a screen be placed to get the sharpest image of the flame?

a. A

b. B

c. C

d. D

16. While some peony plants were being transplanted, the root hairs were destroyed, and the plants died in a few days. The most probable reason for the death of the plants is that

a. the auxin concentration of the plant was reduced.

b. the plant's anchorage was decreased.

c. the absorption area of the plant was reduced.

d. the pull for water from the plant was too great.

The following chart lists the nutritional content *per serving* of four foods. The next three questions refer to this chart.

	Food A	Food B	Food C	Food D
Nutritional Information				
Calories	150	141	100	110
Protein (g)	12	4	0	2
Carbohydrate (g)	17	27	0	22
Fat (g)	4	2	11	1
Sodium (mg)	0	320	80	570
% of U.S. Recommended Daily Allowance				
Protein	30	6	less than 2	4
Calcium	40	2	less than 2	4
Vitamin A	2	0	less than 2	0
Vitamin C	0	0	less than 2	0

SECTION A

SECTION B

SECTION C

COMPREHENSIVE PRACTICE Test 1

COMPREHENSIVE PRACTICE Test 2

COMPREHENSIVE PRACTICE Test 3

17. Which of these foods would be the most beneficial for a woman wishing to avoid developing osteoporosis?
    a. Food A
    b. Food B
    c. Food C
    d. Food D

18. Approximately how many servings of Food A would a person have to eat in a day to fulfill the U.S. Recommended Daily Allowance (RDA) for protein?
    a. 30–40
    b. 9–10
    c. 3–4
    d. 1–2

19. Two servings of Food A would provide how many grams of protein?
    a. 12
    b. 30
    c. 24
    d. 60

20. To determine the density of a wooden cube, which of these pairs of instruments is the best combination to use?
    a. a balance and a ruler
    b. a graduated cylinder and a ruler
    c. a balance and a thermometer
    d. a thermometer and a ruler

21. The stimulant drugs that are sometimes referred to as "pep pills" belong to which of these classes of drugs?
    a. barbiturates
    b. hallucinogens
    c. narcotics
    d. amphetamines

22. Which of these foods should be avoided by people who are intolerant of lactose?
    a. eggs
    b. honey
    c. fish
    d. milk

23. A cell with 10 chromosomes undergoes division, forming two daughter cells, each with 10 chromosomes. For this to happen, the DNA in the original cell had to first undergo
    a. translation.
    b. replication.
    c. transpiration.
    d. protein synthesis.

24. The following graph shows the electronegativities of the five halogens. Electronegativity is an indication of an atom's attraction for electrons from other atoms.

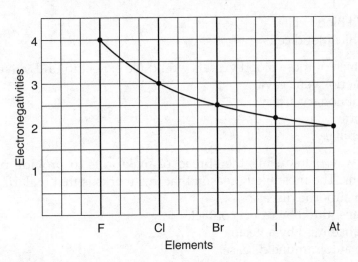

Which one has an electronegativity of 2.2?
a. Cl
b. Br
c. I
d. At

25. A device used to protect a circuit when the amount of current in it becomes too great is called a
   a. fuse.
   b. switch.
   c. capacitor.
   d. resistor.

26. If the stamens were removed from a complete flower, which of these processes could no longer occur?
   a. pollen formation
   b. seed formation
   c. meiosis
   d. pollen tube growth

27. Whole grains, raw fruits, and vegetables are important to the diet because they supply large amounts of
   a. protein.
   b. thiamin.
   c. fiber.
   d. amino acids.

28. *Panthera leo*, the scientific name of the lion, refers to the lion's
   a. kingdom and phylum.
   b. kingdom and genus.
   c. genus and species.
   d. class and order.

29. A boy had a bacterial infection in his toe. Which of these blood components would engulf the bacteria causing the infection?
   a. antibodies
   b. platelets

SECTION A

SECTION B

SECTION C

COMPREHENSIVE PRACTICE Test 1

COMPREHENSIVE PRACTICE Test 2

COMPREHENSIVE PRACTICE Test 3

    c. red blood cells
    d. white blood cells

30. In which of these blood vessels would we expect to find valves?
    a. inferior vena cava
    b. pulmonary artery
    c. aorta
    d. capillary

31. One way of reducing the spread of malaria is to provide people with window screens. The most likely reason that this works is that malaria is
    a. an airborne disease.
    b. transmitted by direct contact.
    c. transmitted by a vector.
    d. an autoimmune disease.

32. Which of the following molecules is not found in DNA?
    a. guanine
    b. uracil
    c. cytosine
    d. adenine

33. Which of these electromagnetic waves has the greatest energy?
    a. radio
    b. visible light
    c. ultraviolet
    d. x-rays

34. Which of these motors has the *most* power?
    a. a motor that can lift 10 kg to a height of 10 m in 10 sec
    b. a motor that can lift 20 kg to a height of 20 m in 10 sec
    c. a motor that can lift 10 kg to a height of 20 m in 20 sec
    d. a motor that can lift 10 kg to a height of 10 m in 20 sec

35. Which of these substances is an acid–base indicator?
    a. litmus paper
    b. Lugol's solution
    c. Benedict's solution
    d. indophenol

36. Which of these processes occurs in deciduous trees but not in coniferous trees?
    a. shedding of leaves
    b. bearing of cones
    c. photosynthesis
    d. root formation

37. Steel wool gains weight as it burns because
    a. hot iron is heavier than cold iron.
    b. the iron combines with oxygen from the air.
    c. the iron magnetizes the oxygen in the air.
    d. the iron releases hot gases when it burns.

The next three questions refer to the following diagrams.

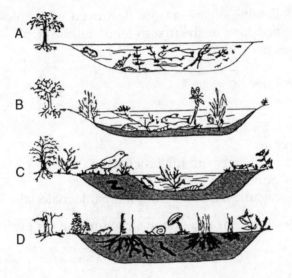

38. Which of these processes is most obviously represented by the diagrams?
    a. evolution
    b. ecological succession
    c. the formation of a marine biome
    d. spontaneous generation

39. Diagram D probably represents
    a. a climax community.
    b. pioneer organisms.
    c. predation.
    d. a blowout.

40. Diagram A can best be described as representing
    a. a population.
    b. a species.
    c. an ecosystem.
    d. a biosphere.

41. As part of a laboratory demonstration, some food was tested for the basic nutrients with Benedict's reagent. Three test tubes were used, each with a different food but with the same reagent. Upon heating, the following occurred: The solution in test tube A remained blue, the solution in test tube B turned green, and the solution in test tube C turned orange-red.

    The nutrient that most likely caused the reaction in test tube C is
    a. starch.
    b. glucose.
    c. protein.
    d. fat.

42. An automobile accident leaves a person with a damaged cerebellum. This damage will most likely cause the person to
    a. have difficulty remembering.
    b. be paralyzed in the arms and legs.
    c. have difficulty coordinating voluntary muscle movements.
    d. lose feeling in part of the body.

SECTION A

SECTION B

SECTION C

COMPREHENSIVE PRACTICE Test 1

COMPREHENSIVE PRACTICE Test 2

COMPREHENSIVE PRACTICE Test 3

43. All of the following organisms are destroyed by a volcanic eruption. Which one would be expected to be the first to reinhabit the area?
    a. deciduous trees
    b. lichens
    c. coniferous trees
    d. deer

44. An oak tree is an autotroph because it
    a. uses enzymes.
    b. needs water to carry out life functions.
    c. produces carbon dioxide.
    d. produces organic materials from inorganic materials.

45. A group of cells having a common structure and/or performing the same function is called
    a. a tissue.
    b. an organ.
    c. a system.
    d. a biome.

46. A tincture is a solution in which the solvent is
    a. alcohol.
    b. water.
    c. oil.
    d. hydrochloric acid.

47. In humans, most of the exchange of gases between the external air and blood occurs at the
    a. bronchi.
    b. trachea.
    c. alveoli.
    d. glomeruli.

48. Signals picked up by the eardrum of humans are transmitted to the inner ear by
    a. the vibration of bones in the middle ear.
    b. nerve fibers connecting the eardrum with the inner ear.
    c. the vibration of a fluid found between the eardrum and the inner ear.
    d. direct contact of the eardrum with the inner ear.

49. Which of these substances is a carbohydrate?
    a. C_6H_6
    b. $C_6H_{12}O_6$
    c. $C_6H_{11}OH$
    d. CH_2NH_2COOH

50. Diffusion is defined as
    a. the random movement of molecules from an area of high concentration to an area of low concentration.
    b. the random movement of molecules from an area of low concentration to an area of high concentration.

c. the engulfment of particles by the plasma membrane of a cell.

d. the breakdown of molecules within a cell.

51. Which of these parts of the human nervous system interprets the five senses?

    a. cerebrum

    b. cerebellum

    c. medulla

    d. spinal cord

52. Which of these equations shows the synthesis of a compound?

    a. $2Hg + O_2 \rightarrow 2HgO$

    b. $2Na + Hg(NO_3)_2 \rightarrow 2NaNO_3 + Hg$

    c. $HgBr_2 \rightarrow Hg + Br_2$

    d. $2NaCl + Hg(NO_3)_2 \rightarrow 2NaNO_3 + HgCl_2$

53. The following graph shows the effect of heat, added at a steady rate, on the temperature of a substance. The substance is a solid at 20°C. What is the melting point of the substance?

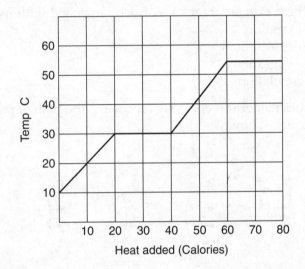

    a. 0°C

    b. 10°C

    c. 30°C

    d. 80°C

54. During protein synthesis, amino acids are brought to the ribosome by

    a. DNA.

    b. m-RNA.

    c. t-RNA.

    d. ATP.

The next question refers to the following diagram.

SECTION A

SECTION B

SECTION C

COMPREHENSIVE PRACTICE Test 1

COMPREHENSIVE PRACTICE Test 2

COMPREHENSIVE PRACTICE Test 3

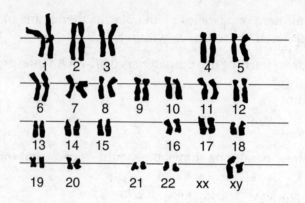

55. The diagram represents
    a. a blood type.
    b. a karyotype.
    c. an x-ray.
    d. an electron micrograph.

56. Which of these human organs is correctly matched with its function?
    a. colon—excretion
    b. kidney—respiration
    c. trachea—digestion
    d. heart—circulation

57. Which of these diagrams correctly represents the path of parallel light rays passing through the lens shown?

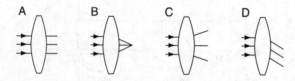

    a. A
    b. B
    c. C
    d. D

58. In which part of the human alimentary canal does protein digestion begin?
    a. mouth
    b. esophagus
    c. stomach
    d. small intestine

I. Science

227

SECTION A

SECTION B

SECTION C

COMPREHENSIVE PRACTICE Test 1

COMPREHENSIVE PRACTICE Test 2

COMPREHENSIVE PRACTICE Test 3

59. Which of these compounds is an isomer of

$$
\begin{array}{ccc}
 & H & H \\
 & | & | \\
H- & C- & C-O-H \;? \\
 & | & | \\
 & H & H
\end{array}
$$

a.

$$
\begin{array}{ccc}
 & H & H \\
 & | & | \\
H-O- & C- & C-H \\
 & | & | \\
 & H & H
\end{array}
$$

b.

$$
\begin{array}{ccc}
 H & & H \\
 | & & | \\
H-C- & O- & C-H \\
 | & & | \\
 H & & H
\end{array}
$$

c.

$$
\begin{array}{cccc}
 H & H & H \\
 | & | & | \\
H-C- & C- & C-O-H \\
 | & | & | \\
 H & H & H
\end{array}
$$

d.

$$
\begin{array}{ccc}
 H & & O \\
 | & & \| \\
H-C- & C- & O-H \\
 | & | \\
 H & H
\end{array}
$$

60. Light waves of different colors must differ in
   a. frequency.
   b. speed.
   c. amplitude.
   d. intensity.

II. Science

45 minutes

Read each question carefully, and then select the best answer. (The correct answers and explanations are at the end of Section C.)

1. A drug used by dentists to prevent pain while pulling a tooth is called
   a. a depressant.
   b. a stimulant.
   c. an anesthetic.
   d. a tranquilizer.

2. Which of the following animals is a mammal?
   a. worm
   b. robin
   c. whale
   d. alligator

3. Which of the following diseases is caused by a vitamin deficiency?
   a. tuberculosis
   b. pellagra
   c. malaria
   d. diabetes

4. Structures that tend to prevent blood loss after injury are called
   a. valves.
   b. clots.
   c. capillaries.
   d. sphincters.

5. Which of the following metals is a liquid at room temperature?
   a. mercury
   b. sodium
   c. magnesium
   d. cobalt

6. Most disease-producing organisms in food are killed by
   a. washing.
   b. freezing.
   c. refrigerating.
   d. cooking.

7. A group of organisms that are classified as fungi include
   a. mushrooms.
   b. cacti.
   c. crab grass.
   d. pine trees.

SECTION A

SECTION B

SECTION C

COMPREHENSIVE PRACTICE Test 1

COMPREHENSIVE PRACTICE Test 2

COMPREHENSIVE PRACTICE Test 3

8. When white light is passed through a prism, we observe
   a. the visible spectrum.
   b. ultraviolet light.
   c. infrared light.
   d. diffuse reflection.

9. A scientist surgically removed the pancreas of a rat. Which of the following conditions is most likely to develop in the rat?
   a. goiter
   b. anemia
   c. diabetes
   d. cretinism

10. Which of the following particles contains the other three?
    a. electron
    b. proton
    c. neutron
    d. atom

11. A pure black guinea pig is mated with a pure white guinea pig. All of the offspring are black. This means that white color in guinea pigs is
    a. recessive.
    b. not hereditary.
    c. dominant.
    d. hybrid.

12. Iodized salt is used by many people to ensure the proper functioning of the
    a. liver.
    b. thyroid gland.
    c. pancreas.
    d. kidneys.

13. Which organism can get its energy directly from sunlight?
    a. paramecium
    b. clam
    c. rabbit
    d. bean plant

14. Which of the following glands is part of the digestive system?
    a. adrenal
    b. thyroid
    c. salivary
    d. pituitary

15. A group of sedative drugs that may produce psychological dependency and severe withdrawal symptoms are the
    a. stimulants.
    b. barbiturates.
    c. amphetamines.
    d. hallucinogens.

16. Blood returns to the heart through the
    a. veins.
    b. capillaries.

c. arteries.
d. ducts.

17. Which two senses are stimulated by contact with molecules of specific chemical substances?
a. vision and hearing
b. taste and hearing
c. taste and smell
d. vision and smell

18. Which of the following is not necessary for burning?
a. a burnable substance
b. a supply of carbon dioxide
c. a temperature above the kindling point
d. a supply of oxygen

19. The organ that balances the amount of salt and water in the blood is the
a. small intestine.
b. liver.
c. esophagus.
d. kidney.

20. Which of the following diseases is an example of an STD?
a. syphilis
b. typhoid
c. tuberculosis
d. Rubella

21. Most of the exchange of materials between the blood cells and the other body cells occurs through the
a. arteries.
b. capillaries.
c. veins.
d. heart.

22. A vital inorganic substance in the body fluids is
a. sodium ion.
b. glucose.
c. amino acid.
d. protein.

23. Suppose a donor of blood type B were to give blood to a patient of blood type A. What would probably occur?
a. The two types of blood would combine, with no harmful effect to the patient.
b. Any children the patient might have in the future would have type AB blood.
c. The oxygen-carrying capacity of the patient's blood would increase.
d. The patient's blood cells would clump together.

24. Which of these phenomena is *not* an example of static electricity?
a. lightning
b. a shock from a toaster
c. a shock when touching a doorknob
d. hair clinging to a comb

SECTION A

SECTION B

SECTION C

COMPREHENSIVE PRACTICE Test 1

COMPREHENSIVE PRACTICE Test 2

COMPREHENSIVE PRACTICE Test 3

25. To test what the cotyledons of seeds contribute to the sprouting of seeds, 10 lima beans were planted with both of their cotyledons intact. Another 10 were planted after careful removal of one cotyledon from each seed. As a control in this experiment, one should
    a. use seeds from different plants.
    b. vary the amount of water provided to each group of seeds.
    c. keep the germinating seeds in partial light.
    d. provide each seed with the same amount of water.

26. The atoms in a hydrogen molecule are held together by
    a. ionic bonds.
    b. hydrogen bonds.
    c. non-polar covalent bonds.
    d. polar covalent bonds.

27. Opposite-sex (female–male) twins are conceived when
    a. one egg is fertilized by two sperm.
    b. one fertilized egg splits into two parts.
    c. two eggs are fertilized at the same time by two sperm.
    d. two eggs are fertilized at the same time by one sperm.

28. Quantities having both magnitude and direction are called
    a. line segments.
    b. scalars.
    c. vectors.
    d. directrixes.

The next three questions refer to the following pyramid.

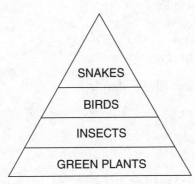

29. What first, if any, result would you expect if a disease decreases the population of snakes?
    a. No change will occur.
    b. The number of green plants will increase.
    c. The number of insects will increase.
    d. The number of birds will increase.

30. Which of these organisms represent herbivores?
    a. green plants
    b. insects
    c. birds
    d. snakes

31. According to this pyramid, to support 100 kg of birds, which of the following is needed?
    a. more than 100 kg of insects
    b. more than 100 kg of snakes
    c. less than 100 kg of green plants
    d. 100 kg of insects

32. Thirty grams is nearly the same as
    a. 1 m.
    b. 1 oz.
    c. 1 lb.
    d. 1 L.

33. Which of these organisms removes carbon dioxide from the earth's atmosphere?
    a. horses
    b. most bacteria
    c. trees
    d. yeasts

34. Which of the following phenomena is most likely to speed the evolutionary rate of a species?
    a. lack of environmental changes
    b. increase in mutations
    c. decrease in migration
    d. increase in death rate

35. Which structures are most closely involved in the body's responses to external stimuli?
    a. spleen and blood cells
    b. neurons and ganglia
    c. Isles of Langerhans
    d. alveoli and diaphragm

36. In the formula $F = ma$, the F stands for
    a. force.
    b. farads.
    c. Fahrenheit degrees.
    d. friction.

37. A heart–lung machine is used to
    a. exchange gases into and out of the blood.
    b. help a person breathe.
    c. regulate the heart rhythm.
    d. remove bacteria from the blood.

38. Which factor determines whether an object floats or sinks in water?
    a. volume of the object
    b. depth of the water
    c. weight of the object
    d. density of the object

39. With regard to higher animals, which of the following structures includes the other three?
    a. tissue
    b. organ
    c. system
    d. organism

40. The chromosomes of new cells in a growing tissue culture are exactly the same as a result of
    a. mitosis.
    b. segregation.
    c. fertilization.
    d. meiosis.

41. Which of the following terms is the metric unit for work?
    a. joule
    b. watt
    c. ampere
    d. meter

Questions 42 and 43 are based on the following information:

One reaction for preparing oxygen in the laboratory is:

$$2KClO_3 \rightarrow 2KCl + 3O_2$$

42. This reaction is an example of
    a. decomposition.
    b. chemical union.
    c. double replacement.
    d. single replacement.

43. MnO_2 is often added to the reactants in this reaction to speed up the reaction, without itself being changed. It is being used as a/an
    a. oxidizing agent.
    b. catalyst.
    c. enzyme
    d. reducing agent.

44. Which of the following statements best describes the functioning of the endocrine glands?
    a. They secrete directly into the bloodstream.
    b. Each of them acts independently.
    c. They regulate digestion.
    d. They act only in emergencies.

45. A fuse blows because electrical energy has been converted to
    a. light energy.
    b. heat energy.
    c. mechanical energy.
    d. potential energy.

SECTION A

SECTION B

SECTION C

COMPREHENSIVE PRACTICE Test 1

COMPREHENSIVE PRACTICE Test 2

COMPREHENSIVE PRACTICE Test 3

46. Which of these statements comparing cellular respiration to burning is true?
    a. Burning produces heat, and cellular respiration does not.
    b. Burning uses fuels that contain carbon and hydrogen, and cellular respiration does not.
    c. Cellular respiration uses oxygen, and burning does not.
    d. Burning and cellular respiration produce carbon dioxide and water.

47. In which of the following materials are the attractions between particles the strongest?
    a. iron
    b. ice
    c. milk
    d. air

Questions 48 and 49 refer to the following statement:

A green water plant is placed in a container in such a way that a test tube collects any gas the plant gives off.

48. The gas collected in the test tube is most probably
    a. hydrogen.
    b. carbon dioxide.
    c. nitrogen.
    d. oxygen.

49. The gas collected in the test tube was probably a result of
    a. osmosis.
    b. photosynthesis.
    c. respiration.
    d. oxidation.

50. Which of the following is a chemical compound?
    a. mercury
    b. water
    c. oxygen
    d. chlorine

51. Organisms that live in water possess certain structures that enable them to live there successfully. These structures are called
    a. vertebrae.
    b. protoplasm.
    c. cells.
    d. adaptations.

52. Which of these materials is attracted by an electromagnet?
    a. aluminum
    b. silver
    c. iron
    d. all of the above

53. A student focuses the low-power lens of a microscope and observes a dark object. When the slide is moved back and forth, the object remains in the same place.

When the student switches to the high-power lens, the object looks the same. The student should conclude that the

a. coverslip is dirty.
b. eyepiece is dirty.
c. diaphragm should be opened more.
d. high-power lens should be focused better.

54. A feather usually falls more slowly than a brick because the feather
a. is much lighter.
b. has a greater density.
c. has greater porosity.
d. is more affected by air resistance.

55. Which of these is a chemical change?
a. the electrolysis of water
b. the evaporation of alcohol
c. the dissolving of salt
d. the freezing of water

56. Which one of the following graphs shown represents an object at rest?

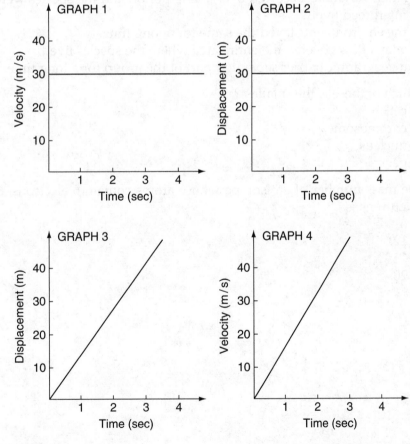

a. Graph 1
b. Graph 2
c. Graph 3
d. Graph 4

SECTION A

SECTION B

SECTION C

COMPREHENSIVE PRACTICE Test 1

COMPREHENSIVE PRACTICE Test 2

COMPREHENSIVE PRACTICE Test 3

57. The diameter of the field of a microscope under low power is 2 mm. The following diagram represents a long, narrow cell as seen under this microscope. What is the approximate length of this cell?

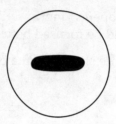

 a. 1 μm
 b. 500 μm
 c. 1000 μm
 d. 2000 μm

58. According to the theory of evolution, two species might have developed from a single one if
 a. small variations occurred over a long period and the species were able to interbreed freely.
 b. the environment stayed the same for a long time.
 c. a lava flow covered the entire area where the species lived.
 d. a geographic barrier separated part of the group for a long time.

59. Which of these is the smallest?
 a. cell
 b. chromosome
 c. nucleus
 d. gene

60. The mass number of an isotope whose atoms contain 6 electrons, 6 protons, and 8 neutrons is
 a. 6.
 b. 12.
 c. 14.
 d. 20.

SECTION A

SECTION B

SECTION C

COMPREHENSIVE PRACTICE Test 1

COMPREHENSIVE PRACTICE Test 2

COMPREHENSIVE PRACTICE Test 3

III. Science

45 minutes

Read each question carefully, and then select the best answer. (The correct answers and explanations are at the end of Section C.)

1. During vigorous exercise, the body loses a substantial amount of
   a. water only.
   b. salt only.
   c. water and salt.
   d. neither water nor salt.

2. The blocking of arteries can be caused by chemical deposits in the arterial walls. One of these chemicals is
   a. thiamine.
   b. urea.
   c. hemoglobin.
   d. cholesterol.

3. A person with athlete's foot should not share his clothing or towels with others. This is done to avoid spreading the
   a. fungus.
   b. bacteria.
   c. virus.
   d. worms.

4. The cell is the basic unit of structure and function
   a. in plants, but not in animals.
   b. in animals, but not in plants.
   c. in both animals and plants.
   d. in neither animals nor plants.

5. If 10 g of NaCl are mixed thoroughly with 1,000 mL of water, the resulting mixture is
   a. an emulsion.
   b. a colloid.
   c. a solution.
   d. a suspension.

6. Which of the following is *not* typically classified with the other three?
   a. rib
   b. skull
   c. vertebra
   d. tendon

7. Cooking pots should be placed with their handles pointing away from the front of the stove. This is done to prevent
   a. heat loss.
   b. burns.

    c. food waste.

    d. energy waste.

8. Which of the following structures includes the other three?

    a. cochlea

    b. hammer

    c. semicircular canals

    d. ear

9. Which is a base?

    a. HCl

    b. NaOH

    c. CH_3COOH

    d. C_2H_5OH

10. Which of the following is produced by the pancreas?

    a. insulin

    b. adrenalin

    c. thyroxin

    d. estrogen

The next question refers to the following diagram showing a ray of light as it strikes a mirror at an angle of 30°.

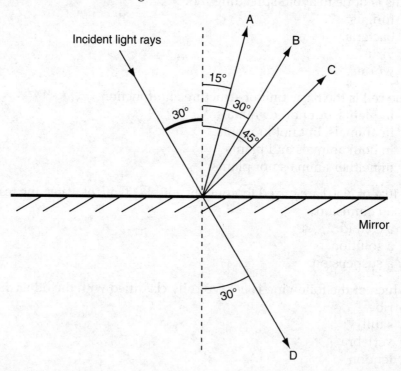

11. Which of the rays in this diagram best represents the reflected ray?

    a. A

    b. B

    c. C

    d. D

12. The structures that carry blood away from the heart are called
    a. arteries.
    b. capillaries.
    c. valves.
    d. veins.

Carbohydrates, proteins, and fats are chemically digested as food passes through the human alimentary canal. The following chart shows the percentage of undigested food in each organ of the canal. The next two questions relate to this chart.

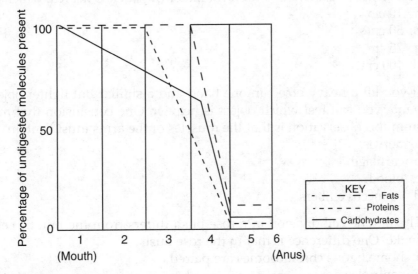

13. Proteins are digested in which of these organs as represented by numbers?
    a. 1 only
    b. 1, 2, and 3 only
    c. 3 and 4 only
    d. 4 only

14. Based on the net change in the percentage of undigested molecules present, the organ represented by 4 is most likely the
    a. stomach.
    b. small intestine.
    c. large intestine.
    d. esophagus.

15. Which group of chemicals does *not* normally occur in most living things?
    a. carbohydrates
    b. proteins
    c. silicates
    d. nucleic acids

16. If the force of gravity were to decrease, how would this affect a falling object?
    a. It would not fall.
    b. It would fall more slowly.
    c. It would fall at the same rate.
    d. It would fall more rapidly.

17. A group of organisms that once existed and are now extinct are the
    a. primates.
    b. reptiles.

c. buffalo.

d. dinosaurs.

18. Which of the following is *not* a usual property of most metals?
    a. They are good conductors of electricity.
    b. They become liquid at 100°F.
    c. They are capable of being hammered into thin sheets.
    d. They have a lustrous appearance.

19. The center of gravity of a uniform meter (m) stick is nearest which mark?
    a. 10 cm
    b. 50 cm
    c. 75 cm
    d. 100 cm

20. If you lift a heavy object in one hand and a similar but lighter object in the other hand, you can feel which object is heavier. One conclusion that might be drawn from this observation is that the muscles of the arms must contain
    a. nerves.
    b. cartilage.
    c. blood.
    d. connective fibers.

21. The mitotic cell division in a rose bush differs from the mitotic cell division in a snake. One difference is that in the rose bush
    a. homologous chromosomes are paired.
    b. centrioles are replicated.
    c. spindle fibers are produced.
    d. cell plates are synthesized.

22. Penicillin is a drug that is classified as a/an
    a. antiseptic.
    b. anesthetic.
    c. antibiotic.
    d. disinfectant.

23. The organs of the body are made up of different kinds of
    a. nuclei.
    b. tissue.
    c. systems.
    d. organisms.

24. Polluted water may be purified by boiling if the water is polluted by
    a. bacteria.
    b. organic chemicals.
    c. inorganic chemicals.
    d. industrial wastes.

Questions 25 and 26 refer to the following experiment:

A mixture of gelatin, sugar, salt, and water is placed in a cellophane bag and hung in a jar of water. Some of the sugar and salt pass through the cellophane into the jar of water, but none of the gelatin will.

25. The results show that
    a. molecules of sugar are larger than the pores in the cellophane.
    b. pores in the cellophane are smaller than the particles of salt.
    c. molecules of salt are larger than molecules of gelatin.
    d. molecules of gelatin are larger than the pores in the cellophane.

26. The term used for the movement of sugar and salt is
    a. diffusion.
    b. distillation.
    c. osmosis.
    d. precipitation.

27. Which of the following are most numerous in a drop of normal blood?
    a. clots
    b. platelets
    c. white blood cells
    d. red blood cells

28. The following diagram shows four sealed containers partially filled with water at various temperatures. In which of these containers is the vapor pressure the greatest?

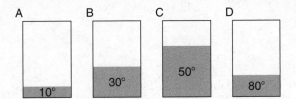

    a. A
    b. B
    c. C
    d. D

29. Which cell structure is adapted for cellular respiration?
    a. chloroplast
    b. vacuole
    c. nucleus
    d. mitochondrion

30. A reading on the Celsius scale is 255°. On the Kelvin scale, the reading would be closest to
    a. 528K
    b. 225K
    c. 48K
    d. 30K

31. Which of these is the proper order of organs through which liquid wastes leave the body?
    a. bladder, ureter, kidney, urethra
    b. kidneys, bladder, ureter, urethra
    c. kidneys, ureter, bladder, urethra
    d. ureter, kidneys, urethra, bladder

SECTION A

SECTION B

SECTION C

COMPREHENSIVE PRACTICE Test 1

COMPREHENSIVE PRACTICE Test 2

COMPREHENSIVE PRACTICE Test 3

32. The following chart shows the energy levels for a hydrogen atom.

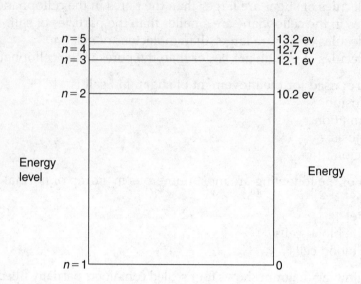

How much energy will an electron emit if it jumps from level $n = 4$ to level $n = 2$?
a. 12.7 ev
b. 12.1 ev
c. 10.2 ev
d. 2.5 ev

33. An example of a food-borne disease is
a. salmonella.
b. diabetes.
c. scurvy.
d. syphilis.

34. If a glowing splint is thrust into a full bottle of oxygen, the splint will
a. stop glowing.
b. cause the gas to explode.
c. cause the gas to burn.
d. burst into flames.

35. Which of the following organisms probably have bacteria that can digest cellulose in their digestive systems?
a. humans and dogs
b. cows and horses
c. lions and horses
d. tigers and lions

36. Which of these substances is the best conductor of heat?
a. air
b. water
c. wood
d. iron

37. Oxygen released during photosynthesis comes from the splitting of molecules of
a. chlorophyll.
b. carbon dioxide.

c. water.

d. glucose.

38. Which of the following gases are compounds?
    a. air and carbon dioxide
    b. chlorine and oxygen
    c. ammonia and hydrogen
    d. carbon monoxide and sulfur dioxide

39. Materials enter and leave a cell through which of the following cell structures?
    a. vacuoles
    b. mitochondria
    c. plasma membrane
    d. nucleus

40. When concentrated sulfuric acid is added to table sugar, the acid–sugar combination bubbles up into a black mass of carbon, and steam is released. This result is considered to be evidence that sugar is an
    a. inorganic compound.
    b. organic compound.
    c. ionic compound.
    d. inert compound.

Questions 41 and 42 refer to the following diagram, in which a viewer's eye is opposite point E on the mirror. A candle is opposite point A, and the space between A and E is divided into four equal parts by points B, C, and D.

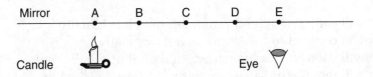

41. What reflection will the viewer see when looking at point E in the mirror?
    a. the area to the left of the candle
    b. the candle
    c. the area between the candle and the eye
    d. the eye

42. Where will the candle appear to be, as viewed in the mirror?
    a. at the reflective surface of the mirror
    b. at the same distance from the mirror as the candle is, and in front of the mirror
    c. at the same distance behind the mirror as the candle is in front of the mirror
    d. at the same distance to the right of the eye as the candle is to the left of the eye

43. Which of the following animals is *not* a vertebrate?
    a. monkey
    b. lobster
    c. elephant
    d. lizard

44. The "lub-dub, lub-dub" sounds of the heartbeat are made by
    a. the valves closing.
    b. the heart muscle contracting.

SECTION A

SECTION B

SECTION C

COMPREHENSIVE PRACTICE Test 1

COMPREHENSIVE PRACTICE Test 2

COMPREHENSIVE PRACTICE Test 3

   c. the blood moving.
   d. the chambers filling.

45. An element consists of
   a. atoms of only one kind.
   b. atoms of only a few kinds.
   c. substances that can vary in proportion.
   d. substances that can be separated by chemical reaction.

46. When a monoploid egg and a monoploid sperm combine to form a zygote, the zygote is
   a. polyploid.
   b. triploid.
   c. monoploid.
   d. diploid.

47. Increasingly heavier weights are hung from a spring. The length (cm) of stretch that occurs as each weight is added is listed in the following table. What will happen to the spring when all the weights are removed?

Weight in kilograms	Stretch in centimeters
1	1
3	3
4	4
5	7.5
6	9.5

   a. It will contract to a shorter length than it originally had.
   b. It will contract to the length that it originally had.
   c. It will contract to a longer length than it originally had.
   d. It will remain the same length that it was stretched to.

Questions 48 to 50 refer to an historic experiment:

In 1858, Gregor Mendel pollinated pea plants bearing yellow peas with pollen from pea plants bearing green peas.

48. The next year (1859), Mendel planted the resulting seeds. All the plants produced yellow peas. He decided that the trait of yellowness in peas was
   a. dominant.
   b. recessive.
   c. blended.
   d. universal.

49. The following year (1860), Mendel planted 8,023 of these yellow peas and allowed them to self-pollinate. From these plants grew 6,022 plants with yellow peas and 2,001 plants with green peas. Which values best represent these results?
   a. 80% yellow; 20% green
   b. 75% yellow; 25% green
   c. 67% yellow; 33% green
   d. 60% yellow; 40% green

SECTION A

SECTION B

SECTION C

COMPREHENSIVE PRACTICE Test 1

COMPREHENSIVE PRACTICE Test 2

COMPREHENSIVE PRACTICE Test 3

50. When he studied two traits such as tallness and color, he found that their inheritance had nothing to do with each other. This is explained by his law of
    a. independent assortment.
    b. dominance.
    c. segregation.
    d. natural selection.

51. The element capable of forming long chains of the same type of atom is
    a. chlorine.
    b. hydrogen.
    c. oxygen.
    d. carbon.

52. A balanced ecological community must contain
    a. producers, consumers, and predators.
    b. algae, trees, and animals.
    c. plants, animals, and parasites.
    d. producers, consumers, and decomposers.

53. A chlorine ion (Cl^-) contains 17 protons and 18 neutrons. How many electrons does it contain?
    a. 1
    b. 17
    c. 18
    d. 35

54. Proteins are synthesized from smaller molecules called
    a. amino acids.
    b. monosaccharides.
    c. lipids.
    d. nucleic acids.

55. The following graph shows the velocity of an object during a 10-sec period.

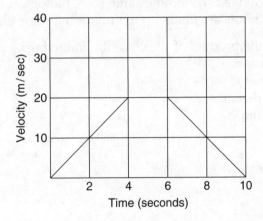

At which of these times does the object have no acceleration?
    a. 0 sec
    b. 2 sec
    c. 5 sec
    d. 8 sec

56. Four beakers containing different amounts of water at different temperatures are shown below.

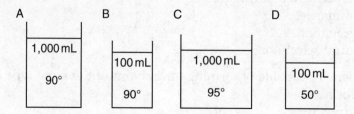

Which one requires the smallest amount of heat to come to a boil?
a. A
b. B
c. C
d. D

57. Which of these is an example of potential energy?
a. a hammer striking a nail
b. a climber starting up a mountain
c. a swing at the top of its arc
d. an electric switch in the off position

58. In the laboratory preparation of oxygen, the measured weight of the final products of the reaction
a. is less than the total weight of the starting materials.
b. is the same as the total weight of the starting materials.
c. is more than the total weight of the starting materials.
d. cannot be determined from the total weight of the starting materials.

59. Which of the following is *not* a true statement about living things?
a. There is a great variety of form in living things.
b. All living things are composed of many cells.
c. All living things carry on the same basic biological functions.
d. All living things are made up mainly of the same elements.

60. Work equals the product of which of the following?
a. force × distance
b. force × time
c. energy × distance
d. energy × time

Answers

I. Science

SECTION A

SECTION B

SECTION C

COMPREHENSIVE PRACTICE Test 1

COMPREHENSIVE PRACTICE Test 2

COMPREHENSIVE PRACTICE Test 3

1. **The answer is a.** A high concentration of cholesterol in the blood is correlated with arteriosclerosis, or the development of plaques on the inner walls of the arteries. The plaques develop from deposits of cholesterol and interfere with circulation. If arteriosclerosis, or hardening of the arteries, occurs in the coronary arteries of the heart, a heart attack can occur.

2. **The answer is b.** The human immunodeficiency virus (HIV), which causes acquired immunodeficiency syndrome (AIDS), is carried in the bloodstream. Thus intravenous drug users who share hypodermic needles are at a high risk for HIV. Using clean needles is a preventive measure taken against exposure to HIV. Limiting bodily or sexual contact is a preventive measure as well; however, this is not the most effective measure in an intravenous drug-using population.

3. **The answer is b.** Nicotine is an addictive drug found in tobacco. A substance does not have to be taken in pill form to be considered a drug.

4. **The answer is a.** The bell jar represents the rib cage, and the glass tubes represent the trachea and bronchi. The balloons, representing the lungs, inflate and deflate as the rubber sheet, representing the diaphragm, is pulled downward and released.

5. **The answer is a.** The ovaries produce estrogen and progesterone. Number 2 is pointing at the fallopian tubes, along which the egg travels and is fertilized. Number 3 is pointing at the uterus, where the fertilized egg implants. Number 4 is pointing at the cervix, which is the opening to the uterus. Number 5 is pointing at the vaginal canal, or birthing canal.

6. **The answer is a.** An egg is released each month and travels through the fallopian tubes, where it may be fertilized. If fertilization occurs, the fertilized egg travels to the uterus, where it implants in the uterine lining, or endometrium.

7. **The answer is d.** The force of friction always acts to oppose the motion. In this case the box is moving east, so the force of friction is to the west.

8. **The answer is b.** Most salts, or ionic compounds, dissociate into their component ions in water, which is a polar solvent.

9. **The answer is a.** The most concentrated hydrochloric acid (HCl) provides the most ^+H ions to react with the zinc to form zinc chloride $(ZnCl_2)$ and hydrogen (H_2) gas.

10. **The answer is b.** Immediately flush toxic substances that come in contact with a body part. The student should call for help while flushing her hand with water.

11. **The answer is c.** Light energy is absorbed by chlorophyll, a green pigment contained in chloroplasts. This energy is used to fuel photosynthesis.

12. **The answer is b.** According to the table, green light has a wavelength range of $5.0 - 5.7 \times 10^{-7}\,m$. The wavelength of $5.6 \times 10^{-7}\,m$ fits into that range.

13. **The answer is c.** Pasteurization is the process of applying heat to milk to kill or retard the growth of pathogenic bacteria. Sterilization would kill all pathogens, but would change the nature of the milk.

14. **The answer is c.** The pressure of the blood causes materials (urea, salts, and water) to flow into the capsule from the bloodstream. Bowman's capsule is porous and thus acts as a filter to prevent large molecules from entering the tubules. The filtrate then continues through the nephron.

15. **The answer is c.** The screen should be placed at point c on the diagram. Point c is at the focal point, where the light rays converge. This point would provide the sharpest image on the screen.

16. **The answer is c.** Root hairs increase the surface area of roots and thus aid in mineral and water absorption.

17. **The answer is a.** Food A contains the most calcium, which aids in the prevention of osteoporosis by strengthening bones.

18. **The answer is c.** 12 grams is less than one-third of the US RDA (30%). Thus 3–4 servings would satisfy the requirement.

19. **The answer is c.** $2 \times 12 \text{ g} = 24 \text{ g}$

20. **The answer is a.** Density is equal to the mass of an object divided by the volume of the object. To determine the mass of an object, a triple-beam balance is necessary. Volume is equal to the product of the length times the width times the height. A ruler would enable you to determine the volume of the cube and a balance would help in determining its mass.

21. **The answer is d.** Amphetamines are central nervous system stimulants; they cause wakefulness and euphoria.

22. **The answer is d.** Milk contains lactose that requires a specific enzyme, lactase, to break it down. People who are lactose intolerant do not have enough lactase.

23. **The answer is b.** This example describes mitosis, which produces two identical daughter cells, each with a full complement of DNA. For each cell to have a full complement of DNA, the doubling or replication of the chromosomes must take place before division occurs.

24. **The answer is c.** The graph indicates that iodine (I) has an electronegativity of 2.2.

25. **The answer is a.** A fuse acts to protect a circuit when the current becomes too great for it.

26. **The answer is a.** The stamen is responsible for producing pollen grains.

27. **The answer is c.** All of these nutrients supply dietary fiber.

28. **The answer is c.** The scientific names of organisms are always made up of the organism's genus and species.

29. **The answer is d.** One of the most important functions of white blood cells is to engulf and destroy bacteria.

30. **The answer is a.** Veins contain valves to prevent backflow. Choice a, inferior vena cava, is the only vein among the choices.

31. **The answer is c.** Malaria is spread from one person to another by a mosquito that acts as a vector.

32. **The answer is b.** Uracil is found in RNA, but not DNA.

33. **The answer is d.** X-rays have the greatest energy of this selection. X-ray photons are high-energy photons. On the electromagnetic spectrum, only gamma rays have higher energy than x-rays.

34. **The answer is b.** Power is defined as work divided by time. Work is force times distance. The motor that lifts 20 kg to a height of 20 m in 10 sec has the most power because it does the most work in the least time.

35. **The answer is a.** Litmus paper is an acid–base indicator; Lugol's solution tests for starch, Benedict's solution for glucose, and indophenol for vitamin c.

36. **The answer is a.** Deciduous trees lose their leaves. Cones are characteristic of conifers.

37. **The answer is b.** When a substance burns, it is reacting with oxygen. When steel wool, which contains iron, burns, it gains atomic oxygen and increases in mass.

38. **The answer is b.** The diagrams represent ecological succession because each stage shows a change in the community.

39. **The answer is a.** Of the choices presented, diagram D most likely represents a climax forest because it seems to be the last phase of the succession.

40. **The answer is c.** Diagram A represents an ecosystem—the sum of living and nonliving things that support a chain of life events within a particular area.

41. **The answer is b.** Benedict's solution is used to indicate the presence of monosaccharides, i.e., glucose.

42. **The answer is c.** The cerebellum is responsible for muscle coordination.

43. **The answer is b.** After such a severe destruction, the first thing to reoccupy the area would be a simple organism that can grow in minimal conditions. A lichen has much fewer requirements than trees and deer and is a pioneer organism.

44. **The answer is d.** An autotroph uses photosynthesis to make its own food out of carbon dioxide and water.

45. **The answer is a.** Tissue is made up of a group of cells. An organ is often made up of many types of tissues. An organ system contains a number of different organs that work together.

46. **The answer is a.** Alcohol is the solvent in a tincture.

47. **The answer is c.** The functional units of the lungs are alveoli. At the level of the alveolus, oxygen is delivered to the blood to be transported, and carbon dioxide is delivered to the alveolus to be exhaled.

48. **The answer is a.** Sound waves reach the inner ear via vibrations of the eardrum and ossicles.

49. **The answer is b.** Carbohydrates are made up of carbon, hydrogen, and oxygen, and they can be characterized by the 2:1 ratio of hydrogen to oxygen.

SECTION A

SECTION B

SECTION C

COMPREHENSIVE PRACTICE Test 1

COMPREHENSIVE PRACTICE Test 2

COMPREHENSIVE PRACTICE Test 3

50. **The answer is a.** Diffusion is the movement of particles from a higher to a lower concentration until the concentration of both solutions reaches equilibrium.

51. **The answer is a.** The cerebrum contains a number of lobes that are responsible for responding to the five senses.

52. **The answer is a.** A synthesis reaction is the formation of one product from two or more reactants. Reaction b is a single replacement, c is a decomposition, and d is a double replacement reaction.

53. **The answer is c.** When a substance changes phase, the temperature remains constant, even though the number of Calories increases. This is due to the fact that all of the energy that is input during a phase change is used to break bonds to change a solid to a liquid or a liquid to a gas. Thus, at 20 Calories and 30° Celsius, the substance is still a solid, but at 40 Calories and 30° Celsius, the substance becomes a liquid.

54. **The answer is c.** Transfer RNA (t-RNA) transfers amino acids to the ribosome. Messenger RNA (m-RNA) carries information from the nucleus to the ribosome, and DNA in the nucleus is the template. ATP is not part of protein synthesis.

55. **The answer is b.** A karyotype is a printed array of a person's chromosomal makeup. As seen in the diagram, 23 pairs of chromosomes are present (46 chromosomes). Often, karyotyping is done to check for chromosomal abnormalities such as Down's syndrome, which is characterized by an extra copy of chromosome 21.

56. **The answer is d.** The heart is an organ that pumps blood, that is, circulation. None of the other pairings is correct.

57. **The answer is b.** Parallel light waves passing through a convex lens bend toward the center and converge at the focal point, as represented in diagram B.

58. **The answer is c.** Salivary amylase in the mouth begins the digestion of starches. The esophagus is a passageway between the pharynx and the stomach. The small intestine is the location where most food digestion occurs; however, some digestion is initiated in the stomach. For instance, enzymes in the stomach catalyze proteins, which is completed by enzymes found in the small intestine.

59. **The answer is b.** Isomers are compounds with the same mass and composition of elements but different structures.

60. **The answer is a.** Wavelength determines color, and wavelength is inversely proportional to frequency. So frequency also determines color. The visible spectrum consists of light waves with frequencies between 430 trillion hertz and 760 trillion hertz. Each color has a certain frequency. Moving along the spectrum, from red to violet, the frequency of the waves increases, and the wavelength decreases.

II. Science

1. **The answer is c.** An anesthetic interferes with normal sensation, especially pain. A dentist would use a local anesthetic to prevent the patient from feeling pain when the tooth is pulled.

2. **The answer is c.** Mammals are warm-blooded, usually have hair or fur, suckle their young with milk, and usually bear live young. (Monotremes, such as the spiny anteater and the platypus, are exceptions.) Reptiles (alligator) and worms are cold-blooded; birds, though warm-blooded, lay eggs and have feathers instead of hair. None of the other three produce milk.

3. **The answer is b.** Pellagra is a disease that is caused by a vitamin deficiency. Tuberculosis is caused by a bacterium and malaria by a protozoan. Diabetes is a glandular problem.

4. **The answer is b.** Blood clots form at the site of an injury due to the action of several clotting proteins. Hemophilia is a disorder in which the blood clotting function is absent.

5. **The answer is a.** Remember your mercury thermometer!

6. **The answer is d.** The high temperatures used by cooking can kill most bacteria. Freezing and refrigeration tend to prevent the growth of the organisms; however, left at room temperature, these organisms proliferate.

7. **The answer is a.** Mushrooms are examples of fungi, which have plant-like cells but are heterotrophic and thus do not photosynthesize. Cacti, crab grass, and pine trees are all autotrophs and contain chlorophyll, the green pigment necessary for capturing light energy to fuel photosynthesis.

8. **The answer is a.** A glass prism can be used to separate light into its component colors, which make up the visible spectrum. Ultraviolet light and infrared light are not visible to humans. An irregular surface produces diffuse reflection.

9. **The answer is c.** The pancreas contains cells called the Islets of Langerhans, which produce insulin and glucagon. These two hormones control glucose levels in the bloodstream. When the glucose levels are not controlled, diabetes results.

10. **The answer is d.** An atom contains three types of subatomic particles: protons, neutrons, and electrons. Though protons and neutrons are contained in the nucleus of an atom, the electrons reside outside the nucleus.

11. **The answer is a.** Since the offspring are 100% black, the allele for black must be dominant to the allele for white. The data indicates that each of the parents was homozygous because this is the only way in which all of the offspring would have the same phenotype. Thus, the following cross occurred:

$$BB \times bb = 100\%Bb$$

B = dominant allele

b = recessive allele

BB = black

SECTION A

SECTION B

SECTION C

COMPREHENSIVE PRACTICE Test 1

COMPREHENSIVE PRACTICE Test 2

COMPREHENSIVE PRACTICE Test 3

Bb = black

bb = white

12. **The answer is b.** The thyroid gland produces thyroid hormones that are responsible for regulating our metabolism. A necessary component of thyroid hormone is iodine. In a diet lacking iodine, the thyroid gland produces a nonfunctional thyroid hormone and thus continues to receive messages from the body to produce this hormone. As a result, the thyroid gland swells in size due to the great demand, and the swelling is called a goiter. Iodized salt is a preventive measure taken to ensure that people receive iodine in their diet.

13. **The answer is d.** A bean plant contains chlorophyll, which can absorb light energy from the sunlight and use this energy to fuel photosynthesis. The other three are heterotrophs.

14. **The answer is c.** Salivary glands produce salivary amylase, which is a digestive enzyme that begins the process of breaking down starch. The other three are endocrine glands.

15. **The answer is b.** Barbiturates are medications that produce sedation and can lead to dependency.

16. **The answer is a.** Blood leaves the heart via the pulmonary arteries and the aorta (an artery) and returns to the heart via the pulmonary veins and vena cavae. Arteries transport blood away form the heart, while veins transport blood to the heart. Capillaries connect arteries and veins. Ducts transport secretions from glands and are not part of the circulatory system.

17. **The answer is c.** Vision is sparked by light stimulus, and hearing involves sound wave stimulus. Taste and smell result from the stimulus of receptors by molecules of chemical substances.

18. **The answer is b.** Burning involves the reaction of oxygen with a burnable substance at an appropriate temperature. Carbon dioxide is a product of combustion, not a reactant in it.

19. **The answer is d.** The nephrons, which are the functional units of the kidney, are responsible for altering the composition of water and ions in the blood by producing urine of the appropriate concentration to meet the needs of an individual. For instance, a person who is running a marathon produces urine that is more concentrated (the body retains more water) than a sedentary person's urine.

20. **The answer is a.** Syphilis is a sexually transmitted disease; the others are not.

21. **The answer is b.** The exchange between blood and body cells occurs at the level of the capillaries, which are thin enough to allow diffusion to occur.

22. **The answer is a.** Of the four choices, only sodium is inorganic (it contains no carbon).

23. **The answer is d.** A person of blood type A carries antibodies against the antigen in blood that is type B. When the antibodies are placed in contact with blood type B, agglutination (or clumping) occurs. This is called a transfusion reaction.

SECTION A

SECTION B

SECTION C

COMPREHENSIVE PRACTICE Test 1

COMPREHENSIVE PRACTICE Test 2

COMPREHENSIVE PRACTICE Test 3

24. **The answer is b.** Static electricity results from charges that build up on objects, as opposed to current running through a circuit. The toaster is the only example of an electric circuit; the other three phenomena are due to static electricity.

25. **The answer is d.** In a controlled experiment, we want to keep the number of variables to just the one that we are studying. Since we are investigating the function of the cotyledon, keeping the water provided to each specimen constant eliminates water concentration as a variable. Choices a and b would increase the number of variables, and light should not affect seed germination.

26. **The answer is c.** Atoms of the same element are held together in molecules by nonpolar covalent bonds. To form polar bonds or ionic bonds, the atoms must be different (different attractions for electrons). Hydrogen bonding occurs between polar molecules.

27. **The answer is c.** Identical twins result from a fertilized egg splitting into two parts, and fraternal twins result from two eggs being fertilized by two sperm. Since the twins are of different gender, we know that they are fraternal.

28. **The answer is c.** By definition, vectors are quantities with magnitude and direction.

29. **The answer is d.** The diagram shows a food chain in which snakes feed on birds. If the number of snakes declines, then the number of birds will increase.

30. **The answer is b.** Herbivores are animals that feed on plants. Thus, insects are herbivores because they consume green plants.

31. **The answer is a.** The diagram increases in size in the direction of birds to insects, indicating that more insects are required to support a certain amount of birds. Thus, 100 kg of birds will consume an amount of insects exceeding 100 kg.

32. **The answer is b.** Approximately 454 g are equal to 1 lb, and there are 16 oz in a pound. Thus, each ounce is approximately 30 g. Also recognize that a gram is a measurement of mass or weight, as is a pound. A meter is a unit of length, and a liter is a volume measurement.

33. **The answer is c.** Trees photosynthesize and thus remove carbon dioxide from the atmosphere.

34. **The answer is b.** Mutations of DNA are the original source of variation and alter the gene pool in a population. An increase in the number of mutations would increase the variation in the gene pool and thus speed up the evolutionary rate of a species.

35. **The answer is b.** The nervous system is mostly involved with the body's response to external stimuli and is made up of neurons and ganglia.

36. **The answer is a.** The equation $F = ma$ stands for force equals mass times acceleration.

37. **The answer is a.** A heart–lung machine is used during heart surgery to bypass the heart and lungs and to exchange gases in the blood.

38. **The answer is d.** If an object is denser than water, it sinks. If it is less dense, it floats. The density of an object relates its mass to its volume. This relationship determines

whether an object floats or sinks in water, which has a density of 1 g/mL. If an object has a density that is greater than lg/mL, it sinks. Otherwise, it floats.

39. **The answer is d.** An organism is made up of organ systems, which are made up of organs, which are made up of tissues.

40. **The answer is a.** Mitosis is a type of cell division that results in the formation of two identical cells from one cell. They are identical due to the fact that the chromosomes double before division occurs, and thus each contains the identical genetic information.

41. **The answer is a.** The joule is the unit of energy equal to the work done by a force of 1 newton acting over a distance of 1 m.

42. **The answer is a.** A reaction in which one reactant produces two or more products is called a decomposition reaction and usually requires heat to occur.

43. **The answer is b.** A catalyst speeds up a reaction by lowering activation energy and is not used up during the reaction. Enzymes are protein catalysts. Oxidizing agents and reducing agents undergo change.

44. **The answer is a.** Endocrine glands release their products directly into the bloodstream. Usually, one hormone that is released from an endocrine gland stimulates the production and release of other hormones.

45. **The answer is b.** When a fuse blows, it is because of a short circuit. A short circuit has little or no resistance, and all the electricity is converted quickly into heat.

46. **The answer is d.** When a hydrocarbon reacts with oxygen, carbon dioxide and water are produced, along with a great deal of energy. Likewise, cellular respiration involves the reaction of a hydrocarbon (glucose) with oxygen to produce carbon dioxide, water, and energy.

47. **The answer is a.** In a solid, the molecules or atoms are held much more closely together and with greater strength than in a liquid or a gas. Comparing ice and iron, look at some of the properties of these two substances. The fact that ice melts much more easily than iron indicates that the particles are more strongly attracted to each other in iron than in ice.

48. **The answer is d.** Green plants photosynthesize and produce oxygen and glucose as a result.

49. **The answer is b.** Photosynthesis is the process by which plants synthesize substances for energy and give off oxygen.

50. **The answer is b.** Water is made up of two atoms of hydrogen and one atom of oxygen bonded together. Mercury, oxygen, and chlorine are elements.

51. **The answer is d.** Structures that increase an organism's ability to survive in its environment are adaptations.

52. **The answer is c.** Not all metals are attracted to an electromagnet. Only ferromagnetic metals, such as iron, are attracted—not aluminum or silver.

53. **The answer is b.** If the slide moves back and forth and the dark object does not move, the object must be dirt on the microscope. Since changing to the high-power objective does not change the magnification, the dirt must be on the eyepiece.

54. **The answer is d.** Air resistance provides a small amount of force on a falling object. Since a feather is so much lighter than a brick, it is affected much more by the air resistance.

55. **The answer is a.** When water undergoes electrolysis, it is separated into hydrogen and oxygen gases. These two substances no longer retain the properties of water. In the other three cases, it is possible to retrieve the initial substance via condensation, evaporation, or melting.

56. **The answer is b.** Displacement is the distance that an object is from some starting point. Graph 2 shows an object with constant displacement. It is not moving.

57. **The answer is c.** The field is 2 mm, which equals 2000 μm. The cell takes up half of the field; therefore the approximate length of the cell is 1 mm, or 1000 μm.

58. **The answer is d.** If a geographic barrier was present, the two groups may evolve differently from each other over time. If the groups were able to interbreed freely, the traits would be spread evenly throughout the population and two distinct groups would not be able to form. If the environment did not change, there would be no selective pressure for new traits. Finally, a lava flow would wipe out the whole species!

59. **The answer is d.** Genes are found on chromosomes, which are contained in the nucleus of a cell.

60. **The answer is c.** The mass number is the sum of the number of protons and the number of neutrons.

SECTION A

SECTION B

SECTION C

COMPREHENSIVE PRACTICE Test 1

COMPREHENSIVE PRACTICE Test 2

COMPREHENSIVE PRACTICE Test 3

III. Science

1. **The answer is c.** During exercise, sweating occurs, which serves to maintain body temperature. Cooling occurs as water evaporates from the skin, taking heat from the body as it evaporates. Salt is also lost with water from the sweat glands.

2. **The answer is d.** Cholesterol buildup in the arteries can lead to heart disease.

3. **The answer is a.** Athlete's foot is a fungus, which can be spread on clothing or towels.

4. **The answer is c.** The cell is the basic structural and functional unit in all living things.

5. **The answer is c.** Since salt dissolves in water, the result of this mixture is a solution. A solution is a homogeneous mixture, meaning the composition is the same throughout.

6. **The answer is d.** The skeletal system can be divided into two parts: the appendicular and the axial skeletons. The appendicular skeleton is mostly comprised of the limbs and the pelvis, and the axial skeleton includes the ribs, skull, and vertebral column. Tendons connect muscles to bones.

7. **The answer is b.** Cooking pots should be placed with the handles turned in to prevent burns. The pots can tip over on a child who pulls on the handle or when anyone accidentally hits the handle.

8. **The answer is d.** The hammer is a small bone in the middle ear, and the semicircular canals and cochlea are both found in the inner ear.

9. **The answer is b.** Bases are compounds that release OH^- into solution. NaOH is a base, HCl and CH_3COOH are acids, and C_2H_5OH is an alcohol.

10. **The answer is a.** Insulin is a hormone that is released from the pancreas in response to the presence of glucose in the blood. Insulin binds to cells and allows glucose to be taken up by the liver and stored as glycogen.

11. **The answer is b.** Reflection is the bouncing back of a wave after it strikes a surface that does not absorb its energy. According to the law of reflection, the angle of incidence equals the angle of reflection. This ray struck a mirror at a $30°$ angle; therefore, the reflected ray will be $30°$.

12. **The answer is a.** Arteries carry blood away from the heart; veins carry blood to the heart. Valves ensure the proper direction of blood flow between the atria and the ventricles, and between the ventricles and the arteries. As arteries carry blood away from the heart, they branch until they form capillaries, which are thin enough to allow for gas exchange.

13. **The answer is c.** Numbers 3 and 4 represent the activity of the stomach and small intestine, where protein is digested.

14. **The answer is b.** The greatest portion of digestion occurs in the small intestine.

15. **The answer is c.** Carbohydrates are energy sources, proteins are necessary for structural purposes, and nucleic acids (RNA and DNA) contain our genetic information. Silicates, such as sand, are generally not found in living organisms.

16. **The answer is b.** If gravity were to decrease, the downward force pulling objects down would be weaker. The standard acceleration down of 9.8 m/s would also be decreased, and objects would fall at a slower rate.

17. **The answer is d.** Dinosaurs no longer exist.

18. **The answer is b.** Metals usually do not have low melting points; rather, it is more common that they have high ones. The melting point of 100°F, which is less than the boiling temperature of water, is too low.

19. **The answer is b.** The center of gravity of a uniform stick is in the middle of the stick. This is clearly nearest to the 50-cm mark on a meter (or 100-cm) stick.

20. **The answer is a.** Nerve fibers would communicate this information to the brain.

21. **The answer is d.** During cytokinesis (the division of the cytoplasm) in plant cells, a cell plate divides the two new cells in half. In animal cells, the cytoplasm is pinched in half to form the two daughter cells.

22. **The answer is c.** Penicillin is an antibiotic, which is taken internally to kill bacteria. Antiseptics are used externally and disinfectants are used on inanimate objects. Anesthetics are used to treat pain.

23. **The answer is b.** Similar cells make up tissues, which make up organs.

24. **The answer is a.** Bacteria are destroyed at high temperatures, such as boiling.

25. **The answer is d.** The molecules of salt and sugar pass through the pores in the cellophane bag by diffusion. Diffusion is the process by which particles move from areas of high particle concentration to areas of low particle concentration. Gelatin cannot fit through the pores and thus remains in the bag.

26. **The answer is a.** Diffusion is the movement of solutes from higher concentration to lower concentration through a semipermeable membrane.

27. **The answer is d.** Red blood cells make up approximately 45% of blood, and white blood cells make up less than 1%.

28. **The answer is d.** Water molecules naturally alternate between vapor and liquid form until the boiling temperature is reached. At this point, more liquid molecules enter the gas phase as boiling continues. The vapor pressure is the highest in the container with the highest temperature.

29. **The answer is d.** Mitochondria are the sites of cellular respiration.

30. **The answer is a.** K = °C + 273

    255 + 273 = 528K.

31. **The answer is c.** Blood is filtered in the kidney forming urine, which leaves the kidneys through the ureters and enters the bladder. Here it is stored until released through the urethra.

SECTION A

SECTION B

SECTION C

COMPREHENSIVE PRACTICE Test 1

COMPREHENSIVE PRACTICE Test 2

COMPREHENSIVE PRACTICE Test 3

32. **The answer is d.** The energy emitted as an electron moves between two levels is the difference in the energy of the two energy levels: 12.7 ev − 10.2 ev = 2.5 ev.

33. **The answer is a.** Salmonella is a food-borne pathogen. Diabetes and scurvy are noninfectious diseases, and syphilis is an STD.

34. **The answer is d.** Oxygen itself does not burn, but it is needed for the burning of other substances.

35. **The answer is b.** Plant cells contain cellulose. Thus, cows and horses, which are both herbivores, require bacteria in their gut to help them digest cellulose.

36. **The answer is d.** Of the choices, iron is the best conductor of heat.

37. The answer is c. The release of oxygen (O_2) during photosynthesis occurs during the light reactions from splitting water (H_2O) molecules.

38. **The answer is d.** Air and the substances listed are gases. Compounds are made up of atoms of more than one type bonded together. Air is a mixture of different molecules. Chlorine, oxygen, and hydrogen are elements. Carbon dioxide, sulfur dioxide, and ammonia are all compounds.

39. **The answer is c.** The plasma membrane is semipermeable (selectively permeable), meaning it controls the entry and exit of particles.

40. **The answer is b.** The black mass that formed is charcoal, or carbon. Thus, sugar must contain carbon, which means that it is an organic compound.

41. **The answer is d.** The angle of incidence is always equal to the angle of reflection. In this case, both angles are 90°, so the light from the eye reflects right back to the eye.

42. **The answer is c.** It appears that the light is coming from behind the mirror at a distance equal to the distance of the candle in front of the mirror.

43. **The answer is b.** A lobster is an invertebrate. It contains an external skeleton rather than an internal one. Vertebrates include fish, amphibians, reptiles, birds, and mammals.

44. **The answer is a.** The first sound is made as the atrioventricular valves close, and the second sound occurs as the valves leading to the aorta and pulmonary arteries close.

45. **The answer is a.** An element is made up of isotopes of the same atoms. For example, sodium, an element, is made up solely of sodium atoms.

46. **The answer is d.** The zygote is diploid, receiving one set of chromosomes from each parent. Only gametes are monoploid. Triploid and polyploid zygotes would result from meiosis failing to occur and are abnormal.

47. **The answer is b.** The stretch of a spring is proportional to the force exerted divided by the spring constant (k). $F = -kx$. Since the force is zero when no weight is hanging, it will not stretch but return to the length it originally had.

48. **The answer is a.** Since the yellow trait showed up in plants that originally bore green peas, the trait for the yellow color is dominant.

49. **The answer is b.** The yellow pea plants (6,022) are approximately 75% of all the plants (8,023). When heterozygotes are crossed, 25% of the offspring have the recessive phenotype.

50. **The answer is a.** Independent assortment tells us that traits carried on different chromosomes are sorted independently of each other.

51. **The answer is d.** Carbon is capable of forming long chains of the same type of atom. This is because of the structure of carbon atoms, with four valence electrons.

52. **The answer is d.** Decomposers are necessary to recycle inorganic substances and make them available for plants. Plants photosynthesize and produce glucose, becoming excellent sources of nutrients for consumers.

53. **The answer is c.** In a chloride ion, there is one more electron than protons.

54. **The answer is a.** Monosaccharides make up polysaccharides, fatty acids make up lipids, and nucleic acids such as DNA and RNA are made up of nucleotides.

55. **The answer is c.** At $t = 5$ sec, the velocity is constant at 20 m/sec. The acceleration is zero whenever velocity is constant.

56. **The answer is b.** The specific heat of a substance is the energy required to change the temperature of 1 kg of that substance by $1°C$: The boiling point of water is $100°C$. For the water in container A to boil, the temperature of 1,000 mL of water must be raised $10°C$. For the water in container B to boil, the temperature of 100 mL of water must be raised $10°C$. For the water in container C to boil, the temperature of 1,000 mL of water must be raised $5°C$. For the water in container D to boil, the temperature of 100 mL of water must be raised $50°C$. Container B requires the least amount of heat for the water to reach a boil.

57. **The answer is c.** A swing is a perfect example of an object changing back and forth between potential and kinetic energy. When the swing is at the top of its arc, it has all potential energy.

58. **The answer is b.** According to the law of conservation of mass, in a reaction mass can neither be created nor destroyed.

59. **The answer is b.** Some living things are unicellular.

60. **The answer is a.** Work is defined as the product of force and distance.

SECTION A

SECTION B

SECTION C

COMPREHENSIVE PRACTICE Test 1

COMPREHENSIVE PRACTICE Test 2

COMPREHENSIVE PRACTICE Test 3

BIBLIOGRAPHY

Avila, Vernon. *Investigation Life on Earth*. Jamul, CA: Bookmark Publishers, 1995.

Cambell, Neil A. *Biology*. San Francisco: Benjamin/Cummings Publishing Company, Inc., 1996.

Marieb, Elaine. *Essentials of Anatomy and Physiology*. San Francisco: Benjamin/Cummings Publishing Company, Inc., 1991.

Olmsead, J., and G. M. Williams. *Chemistry: The Molecular Science*. Dubuque, IA: William C. Brown Publishers, 1997.

Serway, R., and Jerry Faughn. *Physics*. New York: Holt, Rinehart & Winston, 1999.

Comprehensive Practice Tests

Comprehensive Practice Test 1

Verbal Ability

Word Knowledge and Reading Comprehension

60 Minutes

WORD KNOWLEDGE: Read each sentence carefully. Then, on the basis of what is stated in the sentence, select the answer to the incomplete statement. (The correct answers are found at the end of this test).

1. The lens was thinner at the center. It was
   a. concise.
   b. concordant.
   c. concave.
   d. convex.

2. Field glasses and opera glasses are both examples of
   a. microscopes.
   b. telescopes.
   c. monoculars.
   d. binoculars.

3. The apartment was in good enough condition to be lived in. The apartment was
   a. decorous.
   b. rearranged.
   c. habitable.
   d. convenient.

4. When he spoke of his past, he spoke with animation.
   Animation means
   a. indifference.
   b. liveliness.
   c. longing.
   d. bitterness.

5. Sonia doubted his explanation. She was
   a. reassured.
   b. naive.
   c. skeptical.
   d. preoccupied.

6. Researchers have found that the harmful effects of smoking increase progressively over the years. The effects are
   a. incidental.
   b. multifaceted.
   c. cumulative.
   d. substantive.

7. Her position seemed dangerously uncertain. It seemed
   a. precarious.
   b. unassailable.
   c. recalcitrant.
   d. intractable.

8. Some medications alleviate pain.
   Alleviate means
   a. increase.
   b. prevent.
   c. hide.
   d. lessen.

9. The happy couple wandered aimlessly across the meadow. The couple was
   a. foraging.
   b. interloping.
   c. meandering.
   d. trespassing.

10. It is essential for a nurse to understand the jargon of the profession.
    Jargon is
    a. repartee.
    b. minutia.
    c. technical vocabulary.
    d. underlying philosophy.

11. The rules of behavior that people are expected to follow in a particular social setting are called
    a. etiquette.
    b. initiation.
    c. socialism.
    d. elitism.

12. The class learned how to type a letter with a postscript.
    A **postscript** is
    a. a salutation.
    b. an attention line.
    c. an added note.
    d. an inside address.

13. The teacher reported Helen's bizarre behavior to her counselor.
    Bizarre means
    a. wild.
    b. very strange.
    c. undisciplined.
    d. somewhat dangerous.

14. A horse that can be easily managed is considered
    a. doleful.
    b. docile.
    c. fulsome.
    d. flippant.

15. When they approached the courthouse, they experienced a sense of foreboding.
    Foreboding means
    a. wonder.
    b. dread.
    c. joy.
    d. relief.

16. The manual typewriter has become almost obsolete.
    Obsolete means
    a. outmoded.
    b. unusual.
    c. useless.
    d. antique.

READING COMPREHENSION: There are five reading passages in this section. Read each passage carefully. Then, on the basis of what you have read in the passage, select the correct answer for each question.

I

Fat people must lie. What else would explain all the studies—at least 30 of them at last count—that conclude overweight people don't eat more than others? Obese people must sneak candy bars when the researchers aren't looking, then fib about it. Right?

"To be honest," says Robert Klesges, a clinical psychologist and authority on obesity . . . , "we assumed what everyone else assumes, and set out to find support for the notion that the obese lie about their gluttony."

To that end, Klesges gathered 42 families, evenly divided between those in which the parents were obese and those in which their weight was normal. . . . He told them all they were part of a study of family factors and health, which happened to be a lie. Midway through a day of psychological tests, Klesges excused the families for lunch. He suggested they eat at the university cafeteria.

In a second experiment he told 40 adults—evenly divided between obese and normal weight—that they were part of a study on the effects of caffeine and personality. Again, midway through the tests, the subjects were excused for lunch with the suggestion that they dine at the university cafeteria. The real test was about to begin.

"Of course," says Klesges, "everyone at the cafeteria worked for us—the counter help, the people busing tables, even some of the customers."

All the portions were precisely measured, as were the leftovers. The subjects were closely watched to see if they were sneaking seconds on pie or whatever it is that overweight people must eat and then lie about to confound researchers. The families were particularly tricky. "They like to play 'Let's Make a Deal' with their food," Klesges recalls.

The next day the subjects were told that what they had eaten might have skewed the tests, and were asked to recall what and how much they ate. The parents were asked to report not only their own meals, but those of their children.

"We put our data through every analysis we could think of," Klesges says, "and we came up with the same conclusion every time: The fat people in our study were just as accurate in reporting their dietary intake as the other people. In fact, both groups tended very slightly to overreport." Not only that, but the obese subjects in Klesges' studies didn't, on the whole, eat more than the others.

Klesges' work adds more weight, as it were, to the growing evidence that obesity is due to a lack of physical activity and a metabolism that slows down when the person tries to diet. "People are more likely to be cured of most forms of cancer," Klesges suggests, "than they are of obesity."

(By Eric Olsen, "Fat People Don't Lie." Excerpted from *Hippocrates—The Magazine of Health & Medicine.* Copyright © 1987, Hippocrates, Inc.)

17. According to this article, the statement, "Fat people must lie," represents
    a. a lie nobody believes.
    b. the conclusion of the researcher.
    c. an incorrect assumption.
    d. the result of scientific studies.

18. At the end of the sixth paragraph, the comments about the eating behavior of family groups imply that
    a. some family members take more than their share of food.
    b. families tend to trade the food items on their plates.
    c. family members encourage each other to overeat.
    d. the family meal is a stressful situation that leads to overeating.

19. Based on the information in this passage, we may infer that the number of persons observed by the researchers was
    a. fewer than 50.
    b. exactly 84.
    c. probably 150 or more.
    d. at least 400.

20. Which of these statements is true about the subjects' reporting of their eating habits?
    a. Overweight people tend to report as accurately as people of normal weight.
    b. All people tend to report less than they actually eat.
    c. People of normal weight are more truthful in reporting their eating habits than obese people.
    d. Neither normal weight nor overweight people report their eating habits accurately.

21. The structure and results of the first study involving 42 families might lead Klesges to conduct further obesity experiments concerning the
    a. nutritional content of restaurant food.
    b. importance of heredity and physical activity.
    c. effect of gluttony on short-term memory.
    d. relationship between body image and overeating.

22. If the results of Klesges' study are substantiated, the advice that doctors could give to most obese people would be to
    a. take metabolism-slowing drugs.
    b. cut out fats.
    c. exercise more vigorously.
    d. discontinue dieting.

II

In the early years of California history, those who traveled across the desert found it barren, lifeless, and downright hostile. Surviving the trip was considered enough of a reward; nobody expected to enjoy it.

But things are different today. We don't have to go straight through the desert. We can stop and observe the treasures it offers us. Wildflower lovers, birdwatchers, rock climbers, hikers, campers, and hunters all can and do find things to intrigue, enchant, and challenge them.

For me, one of the most remarkable aspects of the desert is how little it has changed. If we could bring back Death Valley Scotty or any of the other hardy prospectors of the late 1800s and early 1900s, I think they'd feel right at home in many places. The highways would amaze them, no doubt, but they could still wander where the overall look and feel of the desert—the vastness, the majesty, the solitude—would remain unchanged.

Covering more than a fourth of the state's land surface, the California Desert spreads south from Death Valley National Monument to the Mexican border, and east from the San Jacinto and San Bernardino mountains to the Colorado River. At 25 million acres, the California Desert is larger than 13 of the nation's states.

While its immensity has helped shield it from change, the desert is hardly impervious to the impacts of civilization. Just the opposite is true:

Because of its dryness and extremes of heat and cold, the desert heals slowly. What may take decades or even hundreds or thousands of years to grow can be wiped out literally overnight.

Consider Devil's Garden. Located north of Palm Springs, it once contained thousands of acres of yuccas and cacti—perhaps the most concentrated and varied collection in the entire California Desert. Then, in the 1920s, city people began to appreciate the beauty of desert plants. They came from Los Angeles in their Model Ts and uprooted what they thought would look best on their front porches and patios. Sixty years later, Devil's Garden has yet to recover. Today the casual visitor would never know the area was once a wonderland of desert life.

The human population boom that now threatens the desert is a recent phenomenon: It began in earnest after World War II, with the arrival of air conditioning and the modern off-road vehicle. As California's population continues to grow and tourism increases, more and more demands will be made on this fragile environment. What we lose today because of carelessness or poor management could remain lost for untold generations.

(From Senator Alan Cranston, "In Defense of the Desert," *Sierra*, November/December 1986. Copyright © 1986, Sierra Club.)

23. Which of these titles is the most appropriate for this passage?
    a. "Desert Memories"
    b. "Dangers of Desert Travel"
    c. "Plea for the Desert"
    d. "Little Known Desert Life"

24. According to the writer, the desert should be valued for its
    a. tourist attractions.
    b. historical interest.
    c. agricultural potential.
    d. intrinsic majesty.

25. One may infer that better management of the desert as a natural resource would result in
    a. an increase in tourist activities in the desert.
    b. a gradual return to the former condition of the desert.
    c. the identification of new desert plants.
    d. the decline of desert wildlife.

26. It can be inferred that a prospector from the 1800s would find today's Devil's Garden in the California Desert
    a. destroyed.
    b. threatening.
    c. vast and beautiful.
    d. exactly as it was.

27. According to the passage, one of the factors that helped to increase the tourist's use of the desert was
    a. the availability of air conditioning.
    b. the baby boom.
    c. the ending of World War II.
    d. the growth of motel chains.

28. The author of this passage would probably support regulations to forbid which of these activities in the California Desert?
    a. smoking
    b. camping
    c. digging up plants
    d. hunting native wildlife

III

Ah, autumn in the country. The sky a deep blue, the leaves a bright gold, the grass a rich purple.

Purple? Well, not in the world as we know it. But if things had evolved just a bit differently, the lavender lawn may have been perfectly commonplace.

SECTION A

SECTION B

SECTION C

COMPREHENSIVE PRACTICE Test 1

COMPREHENSIVE PRACTICE Test 2

COMPREHENSIVE PRACTICE Test 3

Andrew Goldsworthy, a biologist at the Imperial College in London, recently began investigating why the chlorophyll that gives plants their color evolved in green and not some other shade. The answer, he already knew, wasn't in some life-giving property of greenness. Chlorophyll absorbs red and blue light and uses it to produce energy; the green is reflected away, giving plants their color. What stumped him was why plants would choose red and blue—colors from the edges of the visible spectrum—while ignoring the easier-to-target green in the middle.

The biologist thinks he has found a clue in the obscure bacterium *Halobacterium halobium*. What makes the organism unusual is that although, like a plant, it makes energy from light, it contains no chlorophyll. Rather, *H. halobium* uses a chemical called bacteriorhodopsin that feeds on green light and reflects away blues and reds. This phenomenon gives the bacterium a distinct purple complexion.

Goldsworthy hypothesizes that long before green plants evolved, organisms like *H. halobium* may have ruled the world. When plants as we know them did arrive on the primitive, watery Earth, they had to get their start with the red and blue light that filtered through the life floating above them. Since bacteriorhodopsin couldn't absorb these colors, the new life-forms needed a new chemical. It was then that they evolved chlorophyll. Over time, Goldsworthy believes, green plants developed the ability to live without the steady supply of organic food their purple predecessors depended on; eventually the green upstarts became dominant.

Goldsworthy thinks his findings can lead to a whole raft of new evolutionary ideas. Since purple organisms evolved so early, their legacy could extend to countless forms of present-day life. It's already known that many green plants contain chemicals similar to bacteriorhodopsin called carotenoids, which give carrots and tomatoes their color. And even we may be evolutionary heirs of *H. halobium*: We can see because our eyes use a chemical very similar to bacteriorhodopsin to detect light.

(Tom Waters, © *Discover*, 1987, Family Media, Inc.)

29. The main purpose of this article is to
    a. describe the origin of chlorophyll.
    b. explain why plants should really be purple.
    c. describe the hypothesis of a biologist.
    d. explain the importance of bacteriorhodopsin.

30. The third paragraph states that a characteristic of green light is that it is
    a. the easiest to target.
    b. necessary for plant life.
    c. at the end of the visible spectrum.
    d. necessary for chlorophyll to produce energy.

31. From the information given in the next-to-last paragraph, we can most safely conclude that
    a. plants first evolved in water.
    b. chlorophyll existed invisibly in *H. halobium*.
    c. in the future, purple life forms will again become dominant.
    d. light was nonexistent on the primitive, watery earth.

32. Also in the next-to-last paragraph, green plants are compared to "their purple predecessors."
    Predecessors means
    a. forerunners.
    b. competitors.
    c. cousins.
    d. neighbors.

33. According to Dr. Goldsworthy's hypothesis, green plants as we know them evolved
    because
    a. atmospheric changes reduced the amount of green light available.
    b. they made use of the light sources rejected by purple organisms.
    c. they made more efficient use of the organic food supply.
    d. bacteriorhodopsin began to absorb red and blue light.

34. If an organism were to absorb light from the red end of the spectrum only, it would most
    likely appear to our eyes to be
    a. blue-green.
    b. yellow.
    c. red.
    d. red and blue.

IV

The skyscraper, the architectural form of the 20th century, is a product of modern economics as much as of modern technology. Its status and worth are judged mainly by its height and its exterior form. From the tall office buildings of Chicago built around the turn of the century, to the curtain-walled glass boxes of Ludwig Mies van der Rohe and his many imitators, to today's slick corporate monoliths sporting the latest haphazardly historic postmodern divots and curves, the search for a skyscraper form has been reduced to a variation of surface, a question of superficial image-making.

The steel frame construction methods developed at the turn of the century have not changed, nor have the basic layout and function of the office building. Indeed, the basic conception of the skyscraper has remained unchanged since Louis Sullivan, one of the first great skyscraper archi-tects, spelled out the form's essential elements in his article "The Tall Office Building Artistically Considered," published in 1896. Sullivan connected this new and audacious architectural type with the dignified and acceptable form of the Greek column. The division of the column into its base, shaft, and capital translated into the organizational division of the skyscraper into its entrance, office spaces, and top. Despite the enormous increase in height and size of these structures, despite much superficial innovation, this simple design has not been altered. What has changed is the attention—or lack of it—to the detail and craft of the building. . . .

The romance of the skyscraper, the art and the craft of the tall office building, began with Adler and Sullivan's Wainwright Building. Built in downtown St. Louis in 1891, the nine-story Wainwright Building solved the problem of the tall office form. The massive stone-clad base planted the building firmly on the block, defining the street; yet the clearly defined vertical members carried the form upward as one sculptural gesture. The detailing of the structure, its delicate Celtic-inspired ornamentation, gave the building a grace and elegance that have seldom been seen since.

This blending of structural expressionism and romantic ornamentation culminated in the great Art Deco skyscrapers of the 1930s. The Chrysler Building by William van Allen and the Empire State Building by Shreve, Lamb, and Harmon marked not only the end of economic prosperity, but of architectural extravagance. In their towering forms, these two skyscrapers capture the myth of the skyscraper, appearing mountainous at their bases, yet launching into the sky, glamorously punctuated at their peaks by spires as delicately designed as jewelry.

(Excerpted by permission from Maya Lin, "Beauty and the Bank," *The New Republic*, December 23, 1985. Copyright © 1985, The New Republic, Inc.)

35. Which of these titles is appropriate for this passage?
    a. "The Flexible Skyscraper"
    b. "Monoliths of the Future"
    c. "The Skyscraper's Form"
    d. "Extravagant Grace"

36. According to the passage, Sullivan drew an analogy between the skyscraper and the
    a. booming economy.
    b. Greek column.
    c. office building.
    d. Wainwright Building.

37. An architect wishing to design a skyscraper must still divide the column into its
    a. commercial and residential uses of space.
    b. base, shaft, and capital.
    c. angular and circular geometric forms.
    d. skeletal frame, protective covering, and finish.

38. In the second paragraph, the skyscraper is referred to as a "new and audacious architectural type."
    Audacious means
    a. expensive.
    b. elegant.
    c. improved.
    d. daring.

39. The author's protest regarding the architecture of skyscrapers is that today's skyscrapers are
    a. slick and haphazard in design.
    b. unsound in their basic structure.
    c. restrictive in the use of space.
    d. ornate on the exterior.

40. The highlighting of the Art Deco skyscrapers of the 1930s is intended by the author to promote
    a. the construction of ever-taller skyscrapers.
    b. the craft of sculpturing skyscrapers.
    c. the expansion of shopping malls at the base of the skyscrapers.
    d. the use of air rights by building skyscrapers.

SECTION A

SECTION B

SECTION C

COMPREHENSIVE PRACTICE Test 1

COMPREHENSIVE PRACTICE Test 2

COMPREHENSIVE PRACTICE Test 3

V

Even ordinary sleepiness can cause mistakes, according to a study conducted by Dr. Torbjorn Akerstedt of the Karolinska Institute in Stockholm. He instrumented 11 locomotive engineers on runs between Malmo and Stockholm with electrodes measuring their brain waves and eye movements.

The engineers, he found, divided into an "alert" group of five engineers and a "sleepy" group of six. Exhibiting drooping eyelids and brain waves associated with nodding off, all of the sleepies dozed during the trip, but only four admitted it. Two of them careened through warning signals, for all practical purposes asleep. Akerstedt's research shows that when body clock and work schedule clash, people can drift in and out of so-called microsleeps without being aware of them.

Such assaults on body rhythms afflict an estimated 60 million shift workers, says Dr. Martin C. Moore-Ede, associate professor of physiology at Harvard and a circadian rhythms specialist. Moore-Ede has worked with 50 companies worldwide, including utilities that operate nuclear power plants, helping to revamp schedules and train personnel to stay awake. "Most managers are not aware that as many as 80 percent of their workers are nodding off on the night shift," he says.

"The typical shift worker rotates from the day shift to the night and then to the evening shift. This routine is like working a week in Denver, a week in Paris, and a week in Tokyo. Put a lone operator in a dimly lit, automated computer control room with nothing important to do, and you almost guarantee the worker will fall asleep," he says.

Though airlines continue to provide one of the safest forms of transportation, pilot sleepiness is a real—if seldom discussed—issue. Moore-Ede describes the wear and tear to the circadian rhythms of crews who fly day and night across multiple time zones: "They sleep about two hours less than usual on trips, so they're sleep deprived, and they operate at all hours in the cramped, monotonous, dark environment of the cockpit."

He told me of a jetliner on final approach to Chicago's O'Hare Airport that veered toward the American Airlines terminal building instead of the runway: "Despite being warned by the other crew members, the copilot was in a zombie state—'No problem,' he said. The captain took control."

The management of another airline later approached Moore-Ede, intent on addressing pilot fatigue. Moore-Ede's first priority is to revise crew scheduling, which he says is "totally random and erratic. Billions of dollars are spent optimizing equipment," he says, "but we have an underinvestment in the most complex piece of machinery in the airplane, the brain of the pilot."

(From Michael Long, "What Is This Thing Called Sleep?" *National Geographic*, December 1987. Copyright © National Geographic Society.)

41. Which of these phrases taken from the passage best states the main idea of the entire passage?
    a. "Even ordinary sleepiness can cause mistakes . . ."
    b. " . . . people can drift in and out of so-called microsleeps without being aware of this."
    c. " . . . you almost guarantee the workers will fall asleep."
    d. " . . . we have an underinvestment in . . . the brain of the pilot."

42. From the information given in the passage, we may infer that a factor that can contribute to a worker's tendency to doze off is
   a. the use of drugs or alcohol.
   b. an unstable private life.
   c. neurological abnormalities.
   d. a dark work environment.

43. After reading this passage, business travelers who frequently cross time zones might wish to
   a. ask flight attendants to awaken them periodically.
   b. seek the help of a circadian-rhythm expert to help them prevent fatigue.
   c. switch from plane to train or bus transportation.
   d. reexamine their everyday working environment.

44. From the description of Dr. Akerstedt's research on the engineers, we can conclude that
   a. most of the "sleepers" were aware of their dozing.
   b. the subjects were attached to monitoring equipment.
   c. only two of the subjects actually fell asleep.
   d. most of the engineers on this train line are not alert.

45. The first two paragraphs of this passage indicate that sleepiness among shift workers is caused by
   a. the monotony of repetitive duties.
   b. drooping eyelids and reduced brain activity.
   c. the mistakes of managers and researchers.
   d. a discrepancy between the body's rhythm and the work schedule.

46. Which of these administrators would probably be most interested in the information presented in this passage?
   a. a dentist's office manager
   b. a high school principal
   c. a hospital administrator
   d. the supervisor of a secretarial pool

WORD KNOWLEDGE: Read each sentence carefully. Then, on the basis of what is stated in the sentence, select the correct word or phrase to complete the statement.

47. Before making a decision, the director thought over the situation thoroughly. The director
   a. became embroiled.
   b. procrastinated.
   c. was confounded.
   d. cogitated.

48. A word that is no longer in common use is considered to be
   a. colloquial.
   b. archaic.
   c. loquacious.
   d. connotative.

SECTION A

SECTION B

SECTION C

COMPREHENSIVE PRACTICE Test 1

COMPREHENSIVE PRACTICE Test 2

COMPREHENSIVE PRACTICE Test 3

49. Facing the dying patient, the doctor felt impotent.
    Impotent means
    a. guilty.
    b. powerless.
    c. frustrated.
    d. useless.

50. The property of a rolling ball that allows it to keep rolling for a time before it comes to a stop is known as
    a. force.
    b. fulcrum.
    c. velocity.
    d. momentum.

51. When it comes to cooking, Sharon is a neophyte.
    Neophyte means
    a. failure.
    b. beginner.
    c. expert.
    d. gourmet.

52. The reporter thought that the senator's actions were incongruous.
    Incongruous means
    a. unpatriotic.
    b. in poor taste.
    c. out of place.
    d. illegal.

53. The newly promoted manager is unsure of her position in the company's administrative structure. She is unsure of her
    a. status.
    b. social standing.
    c. employee benefits.
    d. deposition.

54. After his trek through the desert, the explorer's face looked gaunt and tired. His face looked
    a. dissipated.
    b. mottled.
    c. bruised.
    d. haggard.

55. He thought that the teacher's comment was ambiguous. He thought that the comment
    a. was ridiculous in nature.
    b. was offensive.
    c. had more than one meaning.
    d. made no sense.

56. The Senate did not consider a tax cut to be feasible.
Feasible means
a. worthwhile.
b. possible.
c. appropriate.
d. necessary.

57. The lithe ballerina performed in *Swan Lake*.
Lithe means
a. foreign.
b. talented.
c. limber.
d. slender.

58. The article describing the deceased person's life and accomplishments was
a. an autobiography.
b. an obituary.
c. a retrospective.
d. a resume.

59. My uncle has a swarthy complexion.
Swarthy means
a. fair.
b. mottled.
c. livid.
d. dark.

60. Barbara's popularity proved to be ephemeral.
Ephemeral means
a. inexplicable.
b. temporary.
c. exaggerated.
d. widespread.

SECTION A

SECTION B

SECTION C

COMPREHENSIVE PRACTICE Test 1

COMPREHENSIVE PRACTICE Test 2

COMPREHENSIVE PRACTICE Test 3

Mathematics

45 Minutes

Work each problem carefully. Use scrap paper to do your calculations. (The correct answers and explanations are at the end of this test.)

1. What should the gas pump meter read to indicate that the equivalent of 8 gal has been pumped? (1 gal = 3.79 L)
   a. 8 L
   b. 25 L
   c. 30.32 L
   d. 33.45 L

2. Add 2.5, 18.07, 0.607, 26, 30.97, 86.
   a. 164.147
   b. 164.107
   c. 154.047
   d. 153.204

3. An insecticide label specifies a dilution ratio of $1\frac{1}{2}$ t per gallon of water. How much insecticide (in teaspoons) should be added to $\frac{1}{2}$ gal of water?

   a. $\frac{1}{8}$ t

   b. $\frac{1}{2}$ t

   c. $\frac{3}{4}$ t

   d. 3 t

4. A kilometer is 0.62 mi. In Europe, a road sign indicates that the next town is 85 km away. How far is this in miles?
   a. 137.10 mi
   b. 112.40 mi
   c. 96.71 mi
   d. 52.70 mi

5. Arrange the following numbers in order from smallest to largest: 0.37, 0.309, 1.4, 0.094, 0.319, 1.13.
   a. 0.309, 0.37, 0.094, 1.4, 1.13, 0.319
   b. 1.13, 0.319, 0.094, 1.4, 0.309, 0.37
   c. 0.094, 0.309, 0.319, 0.37, 1.13, 1.4
   d. 1.4, 1.13, 0.37, 0.319, 0.309, 0.094

6. What percentage is equivalent to $2\frac{1}{4}$?

   a. 25%
   b. 125%
   c. 200%
   d. 225%

7. If 80% of the 130 students enrolled in a class earned passing grades, how many did not?
   a. 26
   b. 30
   c. 45
   d. 130

8. Arrange in order from smallest to largest: $\frac{4}{13}, \frac{7}{15}, \frac{9}{64}, \frac{2}{3}$.

   a. $\frac{9}{64}, \frac{4}{13}, \frac{7}{15}, \frac{2}{3}$

   b. $\frac{7}{15}, \frac{4}{13}, \frac{2}{3}, \frac{9}{64}$

   c. $\frac{4}{13}, \frac{9}{64}, \frac{7}{15}, \frac{2}{3}$

   d. $\frac{2}{3}, \frac{9}{64}, \frac{7}{15}, \frac{4}{13}$

9. Arrange these integers from smallest to largest: 4, −1, 12, −4, −10, 1, −24, −36, 6, 9.
   a. −1, −4, −10, −24, −36, 1, 4, 6, 9, 12
   b. 12, 9, 6, 4, −36, −24, −10, −4, −1, 1
   c. −36, −24, −10, −4, −1, 12, 9, 6, 4, 1
   d. −36, −24, −10, −4, −1, 1, 4, 6, 9, 12

10. 70% is equal to what fraction in simplest form?

    a. $\frac{70}{100}$

    b. $\frac{7}{10}$

    c. $\frac{4}{7}$

    d. $\frac{4}{5}$

11. If $3x < 4$, then x could be
    a. 1

    b. $1\frac{1}{3}$

    c. 2
    d. 12

SECTION A
SECTION B
SECTION C
COMPREHENSIVE PRACTICE Test 1
COMPREHENSIVE PRACTICE Test 2
COMPREHENSIVE PRACTICE Test 3

12. Find the missing number: $\dfrac{2}{5} = \dfrac{x}{45}$.

    a. $x = 20$
    b. $x = 18$
    c. $x = 17$
    d. $x = 9$

13. A table top is $2\dfrac{3}{4}$ ft long. What is the length in feet and inches?

    a. 2 ft 3 in
    b. 2 ft 6 in
    c. 2 ft 7 in
    d. 2 ft 9 in

14. Name the fraction with 56 for a denominator that is equal to $\dfrac{3}{7}$.

    a. $\dfrac{25}{56}$

    b. $\dfrac{24}{56}$

    c. $\dfrac{18}{56}$

    d. $\dfrac{9}{56}$

15. The volume of a rectangular solid is obtained by multiplying the area of the base times the height. What is the volume of the solid in the diagram?

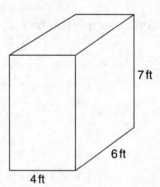

    a. 24 ft³
    b. 28 ft³
    c. 42 ft³
    d. 168 ft³

Mathematics   279

SECTION A

SECTION B

SECTION C

COMPREHENSIVE PRACTICE Test 1

COMPREHENSIVE PRACTICE Test 2

COMPREHENSIVE PRACTICE Test 3

16. To find the surface area (A) of a rectangular solid:

$$A = 2lw + 2wh + 2lh$$

where l = length, w = width, and h = height. Using the figure in problem 15, find the surface area.
   a. 188 ft²
   b. 140 ft²
   c. 132 ft²
   d. 104 ft²

17. One gram is 1,000 mg. A patient needs 500 mg each day. For a 30-day supply of drugs administered at this rate, how many grams are needed?
   a. 1,500 g
   b. 35 g
   c. 30 g
   d. 15 g

18. The ratio of substance A to substance B in a mixture is 2:3. If the mixture contains 12 mg of substance A, how much is there of substance B?
   a. 18 mg
   b. 16 mg
   c. 9 mg
   d. 8 mg

19. If 60 is decreased by 25%, the result equals
   a. 10
   b. 15
   c. 20
   d. 45

20. Which of these sets shows a one-to-one correspondence?
   a. The set of nurses and the set of patients.
   b. The set of real numbers and the set of integers.
   c. The set of positive integers and the set of negative integers.
   d. The set of real numbers and the set of fractions.

21. What percentage of 1,280 is 1,600?
   a. 25%
   b. 75%
   c. 125%
   d. 320%

22. A man runs a 12-km race (13,123 yd). Given that 1 mi = 1,760 yd, how many miles are in a 12-km race? (Solve to the nearest tenth of a mile.)
   a. 0.13
   b. 7.5
   c. 8.0
   d. 10.2

23. Solve this problem in its simplest form: $3\frac{9}{16} + 7\frac{1}{2} + 1\frac{3}{4} = ?$

    a. $12\frac{13}{16}$

    b. $12\frac{3}{4}$

    c. $11\frac{29}{16}$

    d. $11\frac{13}{16}$

24. How many inches would be in 15% of a yard?
    a. 540
    b. 15
    c. 6.2
    d. 5.4

25. A two-day automobile trip of 880 mi is planned. Traveling at a speed of 55 mph, half this distance is to be covered each day. How many hours will be driven each day? (Use distance = rate × time.)
    a. 16 hr
    b. 12 hr
    c. 10 hr
    d. 8 hr

26. This large cube is made up of smaller cubic units. How many cubic units does the cube contain?

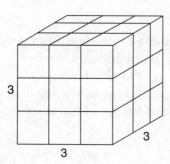

    a. 9
    b. 18
    c. 27
    d. 30

27. If the outside surface of the figure shown in the previous problem were painted red, how many of the smaller cubes contained in the large cube would have only one red surface?
    a. 4
    b. 6
    c. 8
    d. 12

28. Two out of five males in the United States between the ages of 18 and 29 live with their parents. If there are 60 million males between those ages in the country, how many of them live with their parents?
    a. 15,000,000
    b. 23,000,000
    c. 24,000,000
    d. 35,000,000

29. 48 is what percentage more than 40?
    a. 20%
    b. 23%
    c. 83.3%
    d. 120%

30. If two-thirds of the 132,000 lawyers in the country belong to the American Bar Association, how many do not belong?
    a. 33,000
    b. 44,000
    c. 66,000
    d. 88,000

31. In reference to the data in question 30, what percentage of the lawyers are not members of the American Bar Association?

    a. $66\frac{2}{3}\%$

    b. 66%

    c. $33\frac{1}{3}\%$

    d. 33%

32. The following temperatures were recorded each morning at 6 a.m. over a 7-day period: $-3\degree F$, $13\degree F$, $31\degree F$, $-1\degree F$, $21\degree F$, $11\degree F$, and $5\degree F$. What is the average of these temperatures?
    a. $81\degree F$
    b. $12\degree F$
    c. $11\degree F$
    d. $10\degree F$

33. From a 12-ft board, cut as many equal pieces as possible, each 1.75 ft long. How much of the 12-ft board will be left?
    a. 2 ft
    b. 1.5 ft
    c. 1.25 ft
    d. none

34. In a recent election, 260 registered voters in a community cast ballots. This was 40% of the registered voters. How many registered voters were there?
    a. 104
    b. 560
    c. 650
    d. 1,215

SECTION A

SECTION B

SECTION C

COMPREHENSIVE PRACTICE Test 1

COMPREHENSIVE PRACTICE Test 2

COMPREHENSIVE PRACTICE Test 3

35. Simplify: $\dfrac{[6n + 7n - (-n)]}{2}$

    a. $14n$
    b. $7n$
    c. $6n$
    d. $2n$

36. Find the perimeter of this figure.

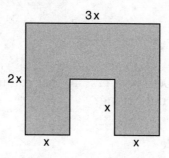

    a. $8x$
    b. $9x$
    c. $10x$
    d. $12x$

37. Find the area of the shaded part of the figure in the previous question.
    a. x^2
    b. $4x^2$
    c. $5x^2$
    d. $6x^2$

38. One number is two-thirds of another number. The average of the numbers is 30. Find the two numbers.
    a. 36 and 24
    b. 24 and 8
    c. 18 and 12
    d. 12 and 8

39. If the product of $(-\dfrac{3}{4})$ and another number is 1, what is the other number?

    a. $\dfrac{3}{4}$

    b. 0

    c. $-\dfrac{3}{4}$

    d. $-\dfrac{4}{3}$

SECTION A

SECTION B

SECTION C

COMPREHENSIVE PRACTICE Test 1

COMPREHENSIVE PRACTICE Test 2

COMPREHENSIVE PRACTICE Test 3

40. A rectangle is three times as long as it is wide and has an area of 48 square units. What is the length of the rectangle?
   a. 4
   b. 16
   c. 12
   d. $4x$

Science

45 Minutes

Read each question carefully, and then select the best answer. (The correct answers and explanations are at the end of this test.)

1. A substance that you might use to kill germs on your telephone is called
   a. a disinfectant.
   b. an anesthetic.
   c. an antibiotic.
   d. an antiseptic.

2. A woman driving under the influence of alcohol collides with a parked car. Which of these statements describes the effect of alcohol on her central nervous system?
   a. It slowed her judgment and muscle coordination.
   b. It anesthetized the sensations in her hands.
   c. It distorted the image of the oncoming car and roadway.
   d. It flooded her thinking with more thoughts than she could manage.

3. The following diagram shows a eudiometer tube in a water bath. The water levels inside and outside the tube are equal. If the atmospheric pressure is 750 torr, what is the pressure inside the tube?

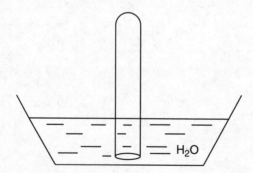

   a. 740 torr
   b. 750 torr
   c. 760 torr
   d. 800 torr

4. Which of these phenomena demonstrates a reflex arc in action?
   a. riding a bicycle
   b. a heart beating
   c. a smell triggering a memory of a past incident
   d. a knee-jerk response when a knee is tapped

5. A newly discovered fossil was described as having three pairs of jointed walking legs, two pairs of wings, and a body clearly demarcated into head, thorax, and abdomen. Which of the following organisms would most closely correspond anatomically to the fossil described?
   a. earthworm
   b. hydra
   c. grasshopper
   d. lobster

6. A diagnostic test that assesses the body's ability to produce a normal amount of insulin is called
   a. a glaucoma test.
   b. a vital capacity test.
   c. a glucose-tolerance test.
   d. an electroencephalogram.

7. When a pathogen penetrates the human body and comes into contact with the white blood cells in the bloodstream, the white blood cells produce antibodies that destroy the pathogen. This process provides
   a. desensitization.
   b. self-defense.
   c. allergy.
   d. immunity.

8. After 8 days, 100 g of a radioactive substance disintegrates to 25 g. What is the half-life of the substance?
   a. 2 days
   b. 4 days
   c. 8 days
   d. 25 days

Questions 9 and 10 refer to the following diagram of a cell:

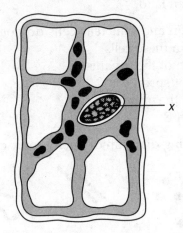

9. What is the name of the deeply chromatinic structure labeled *x*?
   a. nucleus
   b. cell wall
   c. vacuole
   d. chloroplast

SECTION A

SECTION B

SECTION C

COMPREHENSIVE PRACTICE Test 1

COMPREHENSIVE PRACTICE Test 2

COMPREHENSIVE PRACTICE Test 3

10. From what kind of organism does this cell come?
    a. animal
    b. blue-green algae
    c. bacterium
    d. plant

11. Which organelles are most likely to be observed using a compound microscope under low power?
    a. ribosomes and endoplasmic reticulum
    b. cell walls and chloroplasts
    c. lysosome and genes
    d. mitochondria and Golgi bodies

12. During respiration, when the rib cage moves upward and outward and the diaphragm flattens out,
    a. air is expelled from the lungs.
    b. air is drawn into the lungs.
    c. air pressure in the lungs rises.
    d. the abdominal muscles contract.

13. The energy associated with an object's motion is called its
    a. potential energy.
    b. nuclear energy.
    c. kinetic energy.
    d. thermal energy.

14. Photographs in an old family album reveal that an area now covered with shrubs and small trees, which occasionally gets swampy in the spring, once was a pond. This is an example of
    a. a food chain.
    b. an ecological succession.
    c. an ecosystem.
    d. the colonization of barren land.

15. Mutations that occur in skin and pancreas cells do not affect the evolution of a species. This is because mutations in these cells
    a. usually lead to the death of the organism.
    b. cannot be inherited by offspring.
    c. are usually beneficial to the organism.
    d. cannot be linked to cancer.

Question 16 refers to the following diagram of microscopic organisms.

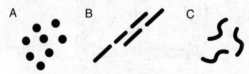

16. In the diagram, A, B, and C illustrate the three types of
    a. bacteria.
    b. viruses.
    c. protozoa.
    d. fungi.

Questions 17 and 18 refer to the following diagrams, representing different human cells.

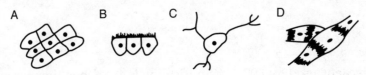

17. Which of these cells are most likely to be found in the trachea and bronchus?
    a. A
    b. B
    c. C
    d. D

18. Which of these cells are used in throwing a ball?
    a. A
    b. B
    c. C
    d. D

19. Sedative drugs that may produce psychological dependency and severe withdrawal symptoms, including depression, are found in which of these drug categories?
    a. stimulants
    b. barbiturates
    c. amphetamines
    d. hallucinogens

20. Skim milk and low-fat cheeses are included in a person's diet in an effort to reduce the intake of
    a. lipids.
    b. calcium.
    c. proteins.
    d. carbohydrates.

21. The following diagram represents a portion of a triple-beam balance that measures in grams. If the beams are in balance with the riders in the position shown, what is the total mass in grams of the object on the balance?

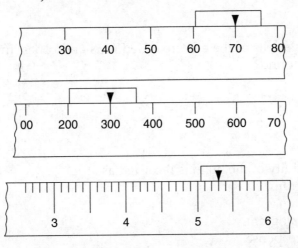

SECTION A

SECTION B

SECTION C

COMPREHENSIVE PRACTICE Test 1

COMPREHENSIVE PRACTICE Test 2

COMPREHENSIVE PRACTICE Test 3

a. 375.72
b. 375.30
c. 370.53
d. 370.20

22. If the objective lens used for 400× magnification is 40×, then the magnification of the eye-piece of the microscope must be
    a. 10×.
    b. 40×.
    c. 360×.
    d. 440×.

23. If the human body has an infection, such as rheumatic fever, the white blood cell (WBC) count shows
    a. a lower-than-normal count of white blood cells.
    b. a greater-than-normal count of white blood cells.
    c. a white blood cell count that is equal to the platelet count.
    d. a white blood cell count that is equal to the red blood cell count.

24. The following diagram represents a portion of a buret. Which of these readings is the correct reading of the meniscus?

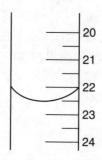

    a. 22.0
    b. 22.2
    c. 22.5
    d. 23.5

25. The light-sensitive cells of the eye are called rods and cones. In which of these layers of the eye are they found?
    a. cornea
    b. choroid
    c. sclera
    d. retina

26. The electrical activity of the brain is recorded as an
    a. electrocardiogram.
    b. angiogram.
    c. electroencephalogram.
    d. electromotor response.

27. Human body temperature is the result of a body process in which
    a. foods are broken down into nutrients.
    b. water is used to produce body fluids such as sweat, blood, and urine.
    c. oxygen and nutrients react to produce energy.
    d. blood is formed in the bones.

28. As a force acts on an object, there must be a change in the object's
    a. momentum.
    b. inertia.
    c. mass.
    d. weight.

Questions 29 and 30 refer to the following diagram.

	RY	Ry	rY	ry
RY	RRYY 1	RRYy 2	RrYY 3	RrYy 4
Ry	RRYy 5	RRyy 6	RrYy 7	Rryy 8
rY	RrYY 9	RrYy 10	rrYY 11	rrYy 12
ry	RrYy 13	Rryy 14	rrYy 15	rryy 16

Symbols

R   round seed
Y   yellow seed
r   wrinkled seed
y   green seed

Punnett square analysis of
cross between F pea plants

29. What proportion of the possible offspring of this cross would be homozygous for both traits?
    a. none
    b. $\dfrac{1}{8}$
    c. $\dfrac{1}{4}$
    d. $\dfrac{1}{2}$

30. What will be the phenotype of the seeds of the offspring indicated in box 10?
    a. round and yellow
    b. round and green
    c. wrinkled and yellow
    d. wrinkled and green

SECTION A

SECTION B

SECTION C

COMPREHENSIVE PRACTICE Test 1

COMPREHENSIVE PRACTICE Test 2

COMPREHENSIVE PRACTICE Test 3

31. The following graph shows the relationship between voltage and current (in amperes [A]) for a fixed resistor.

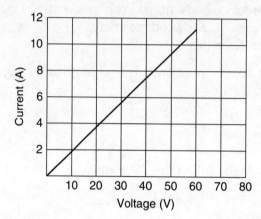

What is the current when the voltage applied across the resistor is 40 V?

a. 6.0 A
b. 6.5 A
c. 7.5 A
d. 8.0 A

32. A small foil disk was attached to a leaf of a plant that was placed in a well-lighted spot. After two days, the leaf was removed from the plant and chlorophyll extracted from it. How would the leaf appear after it was stained with Lugol's solution (iodine)?
a. uniformly black
b. uniformly white
c. mostly black, except for a white area corresponding to the presence of the disk
d. mostly white, except for a black area corresponding to the presence of the disk

33. Which of the following properties is associated with the cell membrane?
a. It is thick and impermeable.
b. It can be seen clearly.
c. It is selectively permeable.
d. It can manufacture protein.

34. If attempts to decompose a substance prove unsuccessful, this substance is probably
a. an element.
b. a compound.
c. a mixture.
d. a liquid.

35. In the reaction

$$2H_2O_2 \xrightarrow{MnO_2} 2H_2O + O_2$$

the catalyst is
a. H_2O_2.
b. MnO_2.
c. H_2O.
d. O_2.

SECTION A

SECTION B

SECTION C

COMPREHENSIVE PRACTICE Test 1

COMPREHENSIVE PRACTICE Test 2

COMPREHENSIVE PRACTICE Test 3

36. The results of a urine analysis can often indicate the presence of disease in a patient. Which of these findings suggests a serious illness?
    a. No glucose or protein was found.
    b. Urea and mineral salts were present.
    c. Glucose and protein were present.
    d. Urea was present, and glucose was absent.

The following diagram represents a group of unidentified cells observed through a compound microscope. The total magnification is 400×. The next question refers to this diagram.

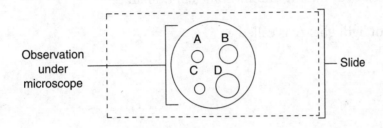

37. If the diameter of the field is 400 micrometers (μm), the diameter of the cell at D can be estimated to be approximately
    a. 100 μm.
    b. 200 μm.
    c. 300 μm.
    d. 400 μm.

38. A ray of light strikes a plane mirror at an angle of 30°. Which of the rays in the following diagram best represents the reflected ray?

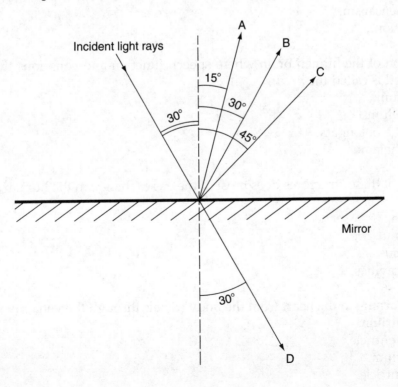

a. A
b. B
c. C
d. D

39. In the field of genetics, the initials "RNA" refer to a
    a. shorthand reference for heredity.
    b. nucleic acid.
    c. research geneticist.
    d. pair of sex-determining chromosomes in human cells.

40. A particle of light energy is called a
    a. positron.
    b. neutron.
    c. betatron.
    d. photon.

41. The blood vessels that carry out most of the exchange of nutrients, metabolic wastes, and respiratory gases with the interstitial fluid are called
    a. arteries.
    b. capillaries.
    c. veins.
    d. arterioles.

42. Bacteria in the intestines of cows break down cellulose. This is an example of
    a. mutualism.
    b. parasitism.
    c. commensalism.
    d. predation.

43. The region of the human brain where speech function and conscious thought processes are located is called the
    a. cerebrum.
    b. cerebellum.
    c. medulla oblongata.
    d. hypothalamus.

44. In which of these structures does most of the gas exchange in the human respiratory tract occur?
    a. trachea
    b. alveoli
    c. bronchus
    d. nasal cavities

45. Blood returning to the heart from the body travels through the vena cavae and enters the
    a. right atrium.
    b. right ventricle.
    c. left atrium.
    d. left ventricle.

46. One possible reason that animals, such as mice, moles, and rabbits, have such rapid rates of reproduction is that they
    a. are herbivorous.
    b. live together in burrows.
    c. are predators.
    d. serve as prey for many other animals.

47. A cross between a plant with red flowers and one bearing white flowers produces off-spring, all of which have pink flowers. This is an example of
    a. codominance.
    b. Mendel's law of independent assortment.
    c. Mendel's law of segregation.
    d. sex linkage.

48. When a human red blood cell is placed in distilled water, it will
    a. swell up and eventually burst.
    b. shrink in size.
    c. stay the same size.
    d. actively pump water out of the cell.

The following diagram represents a portion of a periodic wave.

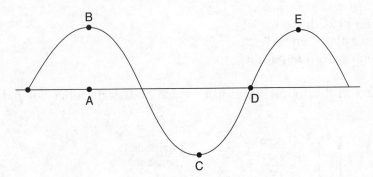

49. The amplitude of this wave is defined as the
    a. vertical distance between A and B.
    b. vertical distance between B and C.
    c. horizontal distance between C and E.
    d. horizontal distance between D and E.

50. The pH of a solution is 3. This solution is
    a. acidic.
    b. basic.
    c. neutral.
    d. amphiprotic.

51. A chemical change always involves the formation of a
    a. compound.
    b. gas.
    c. new element.
    d. new substance.

SECTION A

SECTION B

SECTION C

COMPREHENSIVE PRACTICE Test 1

COMPREHENSIVE PRACTICE Test 2

COMPREHENSIVE PRACTICE Test 3

52. The temperature at which the vapor pressure of a liquid is equal to the pressure on the liquid is called the liquid's
    a. freezing point.
    b. melting point.
    c. boiling point.
    d. triple point.

53. A structure associated with osmosis in the amoeba and paramecium is the
    a. nucleus.
    b. mitochondria.
    c. contractile vacuole.
    d. ribosome.

54. The interaction of bone and muscle that results in a specific musculoskeletal movement can best be characterized by the physical principle of a
    a. pulley.
    b. spring.
    c. wave.
    d. lever.

55. In an electric circuit, the current is measured with a
    a. voltmeter placed in series.
    b. a voltmeter placed in parallel.
    c. an ammeter placed in series.
    d. an ammeter placed in parallel.

Question 56 refers to the following graph, which shows the effect of pH on two digestive enzymes.

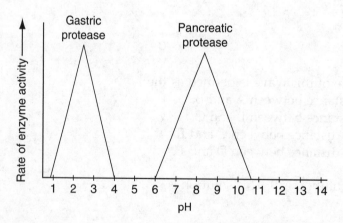

56. At what pH does protein digestion in the small intestine most probably occur?
    a. 2
    b. 4
    c. 6
    d. 8

57. Which of these types or combinations of types of muscles are involved in peristalsis?
    a. smooth and striated
    b. cardiac and smooth
    c. smooth only
    d. striated only

58. Which of these statements accurately describes what happens to an object as it falls freely (neglecting air resistance) near the surface of the earth?
    a. Its kinetic and potential energies decrease.
    b. Its kinetic energy decreases, and its potential energy increases.
    c. Its kinetic energy increases, and its potential energy decreases.
    d. Its kinetic and potential energies increase.

59. On the periodic table, the most metallic elements are found in the
    a. lower left.
    b. upper right.
    c. center of the table.
    d. lower right.

60. A sodium atom (Na) can become a sodium ion (Na^{+1}) by
    a. gaining a proton.
    b. losing a proton.
    c. gaining an electron.
    d. losing an electron.

SECTION A

SECTION B

SECTION C

COMPREHENSIVE PRACTICE Test 1

COMPREHENSIVE PRACTICE Test 2

COMPREHENSIVE PRACTICE Test 3

Answers to Comprehensive Practice Test 1

ANSWERS TO COMPREHENSIVE PRACTICE TEST 1: VERBAL ABILITY

1.	c	21.	b	41.	a
2.	d	22.	c	42.	d
3.	c	23.	c	43.	b
4.	b	24.	d	44.	b
5.	c	25.	b	45.	d
6.	c	26.	a	46.	c
7.	a	27.	a	47.	d
8.	d	28.	c	48.	b
9.	c	29.	c	49.	b
10.	c	30.	a	50.	d
11.	a	31.	a	51.	b
12.	c	32.	a	52.	c
13.	b	33.	b	53.	b
14.	b	34.	a	54.	d
15.	b	35.	c	55.	c
16.	a	36.	b	56.	b
17.	c	37.	b	57.	c
18.	b	38.	d	58.	b
19.	c	39.	a	59.	d
20.	a	40.	b	60.	b

ANSWERS TO COMPREHENSIVE PRACTICE TEST 1: MATHEMATICS

1. **The answer is c.** Set up the proportion, and cross-multiply.

$$\frac{L}{gal} = \frac{L}{gal}$$

$$\frac{3.79\ L}{1\ gal} = \frac{x\ L}{8\ gal}$$

SECTION A

SECTION B

SECTION C

COMPREHENSIVE PRACTICE Test 1

COMPREHENSIVE PRACTICE Test 2

COMPREHENSIVE PRACTICE Test 3

$x = 3.79 \times 8$
$x = 30.32$
You can also solve this problem by multiplying 8 gal by 3.79 L/gal.

2. **The answer is a.** Make sure to line up the decimal points. You can add zeros after the last digit to the right of the decimal point.

$$
\begin{array}{r}
2.500 \\
18.070 \\
0.607 \\
26.000 \\
30.970 \\
+\ 86.000 \\
\hline
164.147
\end{array}
$$

3. **The answer is c.** Set up the proportion. Cross-multiply, changing $1\frac{1}{2}$ to $\frac{3}{2}$.

$$\frac{t}{gal} = \frac{t}{gal}$$

$$\frac{1\frac{1}{2}t}{1\ gal} = \frac{x}{\frac{1}{2}\ gal}$$

$$x = \frac{3}{2} \times \frac{1}{2} = \frac{3}{4}t$$

You can also solve this problem by multiplying $1\frac{1}{2}$ tsp/gal by $\frac{1}{2}$ gal.

4. **The answer is d.** Set up a proportion, and cross-multiply.

$$\frac{km}{mi} = \frac{km}{mi}$$

$$\frac{1\ km}{0.62\ mi} = \frac{85\ km}{x\ mi}$$

$x = 0.62\ mi \times 85\ km$
$x = 5\ 2.7\ mi$
You can also solve this problem by multiplying 0.62 mi/km $\times$ 85 km = 52.7 mi.

5. **The answer is c.** The smallest number given is 0.094 and is listed first only in answer c.

6. **The answer is d.** Change $2\frac{1}{4}$ into a decimal.

$1 \div 4 = 0.25$
So
$$2\frac{1}{4} = 2.25\ (2 + 0.25)$$

To change a decimal into a percentage, move the decimal point two places to the right: $2.25 = 225\%$.

7. **The answer is a.** The question asks how many did not pass. If 80% passed, then 20% failed, and 20% of 130 is the number that failed. Change 20% to a decimal (20% = 0.20), and multiply by 130.
$0.20 \times 130 = 26$ students who failed

8. **The answer is a.** Change each fraction into a decimal.

$$\frac{4}{13} = 0.30$$

$$\frac{7}{15} = 0.46$$

$$\frac{9}{64} = 0.14$$

$$\frac{2}{3} = 0.66$$

Arrange the decimals from least to greatest: 0.14, 0.30, 0.46, 0.66.
$$\frac{9}{64}, \frac{4}{13}, \frac{7}{15}, \frac{2}{3}$$

9. **The answer is d.** The smallest number listed is -36, and it appears first in answers c and d. Comparing both answers item by item, we see they are the same until we get to 12 in c, compared to 1 in d. Since 1 is smaller than 12, d is the correct answer.

10. **The answer is b.** Seventy percent (70%) means $\frac{70}{100}$ reduced to $\frac{7}{10}$.

11. **The answer is a.** Given $3x < 4$, divide 4 by 3.

$$x < \frac{4}{3}$$

So any number less than $\frac{4}{3}$ ($1\frac{1}{3}$) is a solution. Choice a, 1, is the only number less than $1\frac{1}{3}$. You can also solve this problem by substituting each choice into the inequality.

12. **The answer is b.** Cross-multiply, and divide by 5.
$$\frac{2}{5} = \frac{x}{45}$$
$5x = 90$
$x = 18$

SECTION A

SECTION B

SECTION C

COMPREHENSIVE PRACTICE Test 1

COMPREHENSIVE PRACTICE Test 2

COMPREHENSIVE PRACTICE Test 3

13. **The answer is d.**

$$2 \text{ ft} + \left(\frac{3}{4} \times 12 \text{ in} \right) = 2 \text{ ft } 9 \text{ in}$$

14. **The answer is b.** Set up the proportion, cross-multiply, and divide by 7.

$$\frac{3}{7} = \frac{x}{56}$$

$7x = 168$

$x = 24$

If you are looking for x in $\frac{x}{56}$, then the answer is $\frac{24}{56}$.

15. **The answer is d.** To find the volume (V), use the formula

$V = lwh$

where l = length, w = width, and h = height.

$V = 4 \times 6 \times 7$

$V = 24 \times 7$

$V = 168 \text{ ft}^3$

16. **The answer is a.** Use $A = 2lw + 2wh + 2lh$.

$A = (2 \times 4 \times 6) + (2 \times 6 \times 7) + (2 \times 4 \times 7)$

$A = 48 + 84 + 56$

$A = 188 \text{ ft}^2$

17. **The answer is d.** For 30 days, at 500 mg/day, the total 500 mg $\times$ 30 days = 15,000 mg. To change milligrams into grams, divide by 1,000: 15,000 mg $\div$ 1,000 mg/g = 15 g. It may be easier to first change 500 mg to .5 g and then proceed.

$500 \text{ mg} = .5 \text{ g}$

$.5 \text{ g} \times 30 \text{ days} = 15 \text{ g/day}$

18. **The answer is a.** Use the following proportion, cross-multiply, and divide by 2.

$$\frac{12}{B} = \frac{2}{3}$$

$2B = 36$

$B = 18 \text{ mg}$

19. **The answer is d.** If 60 is decreased by 25%, 75% remains. Change 75% to a decimal: 75% $\div$ 100 = 0.75. Multiply 0.75 by 60: 0.75 $\times$ 60 = 45.

You can also solve for 25% of 60, which is 15, and subtract 15 from 60.

20. **The answer is c.** To have a one-to-one correspondence, each set must have the same number of elements (things). There are as many positive integers as there are negative integers.

21. **The answer is c.**

$$\frac{1,600}{1,280} = 1.25$$

$1.25 \times 100 = 125\%$

You can also set up a proportion to solve this problem:

$$\frac{x}{100} = \frac{1,600}{1,280}$$

22. **The answer is b.** If 1,760 yd = 1 mi, to change 13,123 yd into miles, divide 13,123 yd by 1,760 yd/mi.

$$13,123 \div 1,760 = 7.45 \approx 7.5 \text{ mi}$$

23. **The answer is a.** Find a common denominator for the fractions, which is 16.

$$3\frac{9}{16} = 3\frac{9}{16}$$

$$7\frac{1}{2} = 7\frac{8}{16}$$

$$1\frac{3}{4} = 1\frac{12}{16}$$

$$3\frac{9}{16} + 7\frac{8}{16} + 1\frac{12}{16} = 11\frac{29}{16} = 12\frac{13}{16}$$

24. **The answer is d.** Since there are 36 in/yd, we need to find 15% of 36. Use the proportion:

$$\frac{\%}{100} = \frac{is}{of}$$

$$\frac{15}{100} = \frac{x}{36}$$

Cross-multiply, and divide by 100.

$$100x = 540$$
$$x = 5.40$$

You can also solve this problem changing 15% to 0.15 and finding 0.15 × 36 in = 5.4 in.

25. **The answer is d.** In one day they cover half the distance of 880 mi, which is 880 ÷ 2, or 440 mi. Use the given formula (distance = rate × time), and divide by rate.

time = distance ÷ rate
time = 440 mi ÷ 55 mph = 8 hr

26. **The answer is c.** There are 27 cubic units in the large cube

$$3 \times 3 \times 3 = 27 \text{ units}^3$$

27. **The answer is b.** The middle square on each face of the large cube has only one side painted. There are six faces on the large cube, so there are six cubes with only one side painted.

28. **The answer is c.** Solve the proportion by cross-multiplying and dividing by 5.

$$\frac{2}{5} = \frac{x}{60,000,000}$$

$$5x = 120,000,000$$

$x = 24,000,000$ males living with their parents

You can also solve this problem by multiplying $\frac{2}{5}$ by 60,000,000 = 24,000,000.

29. **The answer is a.** The problem is to find the percentage of increase. Use the formula:

$$\% \text{ increase} = \frac{\text{change in value}}{\text{original value}}$$

$$\% \text{ increase} = \frac{48 - 40}{40} = \frac{8}{40} = \frac{1}{5}$$

Change $\frac{1}{5}$ into a decimal, and change the result to a percentage.

$1 \div 5 = 0.20 \times 100 = 20\%$

30. **The answer is b.** The question is how many do *not* belong. If $\frac{2}{3}$ belong, then $\frac{1}{3}$ do not belong.

$$\frac{1}{3} \times \frac{132,000}{1} = \frac{132,000}{3} = 44,000 \text{ lawyers who do not belong}$$

31. **The answer is c.** The problem is to change $\frac{1}{3}$ into a percentage. First change $\frac{1}{3}$ into a decimal: $1 \div 3 = 0.33$ (repeating). Second, change 0.33 (repeating) into a percentage. Move the decimal point two places to the right: 33.3 (repeating)%, or $33\frac{1}{3}\%$.

32. **The answer is c.** To find the average of seven numbers, find the sum, and then divide by 7.
$-3 + 13 + 31 + (-1) + 21 + 11 + 5 = 77$

$$\frac{77}{7} = 11°F$$

33. **The answer is b.** First find out how many 1.75-ft lengths are in the 12-ft board.
12 ft ÷ 1.75 ft = 6.9 units, 6 units used and .9 units not used

6 units × 1.75 ft/unit = 10.5 ft

Then subtract 10.5 ft from 12 ft to get 1.5 ft left over.

34. **The answer is c.** The problem is this: 260 is 40% of what number?
Use the proportion:

$$\frac{\%}{100} = \frac{\text{is}}{\text{of}}$$

$$\frac{40}{100} = \frac{260}{x}$$

Cross-multiply, and divide by 40.
$40x = 26,000$
$x = 650$

SECTION A

SECTION B

SECTION C

COMPREHENSIVE PRACTICE Test 1

COMPREHENSIVE PRACTICE Test 2

COMPREHENSIVE PRACTICE Test 3

You can also solve this problem by saying 40% of $x = 260$, changing 40% to 0.40, and dividing both sides by 0.40.

$$0.40x = 260$$

$$x = \frac{260}{0.40} = 650$$

35. **The answer is b.**

$$\frac{[6n + 7n - (-n)]}{2} =$$

$$\frac{6n + 7n + n}{2} =$$

$$\frac{14n}{2} = 7n$$

36. **The answer is d.** Add up all the sides: $2x + 3x + 2x + x + x + x + x + x = 12x$

37. **The answer is c.** To find the area of the shaded region, subtract the area of the open square from the area of the large rectangle.

area of rectangle − area of square = area of shaded region
$(3x \times 2x) - (x \times x)$ = area of shaded region
$6x^2 - x^2$ = area of shaded region
$5x^2$ = area of shaded region

38. **The answer is a.** One number = x; the other number = $\frac{2}{3}x$. Calculate the average.

$$\text{average} = \frac{x + \frac{2}{3}x}{2} = 30$$

Change both numbers to fractions, and multiply both sides by 2.

$$\left(\frac{3/3x + 2/3x}{2}\right) \times 2 = 30 \times 2$$

$$\frac{5}{3}x = 60$$

Multiply both sides by $\frac{3}{5}$.

$$x = \frac{3}{5} \times \frac{60}{1} = 36$$

$$\frac{2}{3} \times 36 = 24$$

The two numbers are 36 and 24.

39. **The answer is d.** You are given

$$-\frac{3}{4} \times x = 1$$

Remember that a fraction multiplied by its reciprocal is 1. The reciprocal of $-\dfrac{3}{4}$ is $-\dfrac{4}{3}$. Multiply both sides by $-\dfrac{4}{3}$.

$$-\frac{4}{3} \times \frac{3}{4}x = 1 \times -\frac{4}{3}$$

$$x = -\frac{4}{3}$$

40. **The answer is c.** Use the formula for area: area = length $\times$ width. Let width = w and length = $3w$.

$$3w \times w = 48$$
$$3w^2 = 48$$

Divide both sides by 3.

$$\frac{3w^2}{3} = \frac{48}{3}$$
$$w^2 = 16$$
$$w = \sqrt{16} = 4 \text{ units}$$

length $= 3w = 3 \times 4 = 12$ units

SECTION A

SECTION B

SECTION C

COMPREHENSIVE PRACTICE Test 1

COMPREHENSIVE PRACTICE Test 2

COMPREHENSIVE PRACTICE Test 3

ANSWERS TO COMPREHENSIVE PRACTICE TEST 1: SCIENCE

1. **The answer is a.** Disinfectants are used on inanimate surfaces, antibiotics are taken internally, antiseptics are used on the skin, and anesthetics are used to reduce pain.

2. **The answer is a.** Although the other choices may occur, they are related to choice a.

3. **The answer is b.** The system is in equilibrium; therefore the pressures are equal.

4. **The answer is d.** A reflex arc is the simplest response to an external stimulus. The other choices do not fit that criterion.

5. **The answer is c.** The grasshopper is a member of the phylum Arthropoda, class insecta. While all arthropods have an exoskeleton and jointed appendages, only insects have six legs and wings. The lobster is an arthropod, but not an insect. The other organisms are not arthropods.

6. **The answer is c.** A glaucoma test is done on the eyes, a vital capacity test on the lungs and an electroencephalogram measures electrical activity in the brain.

7. **The answer is d.** By definition, immunity is provided by the production of specific antibodies.

8. **The answer is b.** The half-life of a radioactive substance is defined as the amount of time required for half the original material to decay into other elements. Twenty-five grams is $\frac{1}{4}$ of the original mass; therefore, two half-lives have passed.

9. **The answer is a.** Eukaryotic cells have nuclei, and chromatin is found in the nucleus.

10. **The answer is d.** The cell has a cell wall, large vacuoles, and chloropasts, all characteristics of a plant cell.

11. **The answer is b.** Cell walls and chloroplasts can be seen with a compound microscope. Endoplasmic reticulum, ribosomes, lysosomes, Golgi bodies, and mitochondria all require an electron microscope.

12. **The answer is b.** These actions result in an increase in the volume of the chest cavity and a reduction in the pressure. The pressure gradient results in the movement of air into the lungs.

13. **The answer is c.** This is the definition of kinetic energy.

14. **The answer is b.** Ecological succession describes the gradual changes in ecosystems over time.

15. **The answer is b.** Mutations can affect evolution only if they can be inherited by the offspring (i.e., occur in the gametes). Mutations of skin and pancreas cells are not inherited by offspring.

SECTION A

SECTION B

SECTION C

COMPREHENSIVE PRACTICE Test 1

COMPREHENSIVE PRACTICE Test 2

COMPREHENSIVE PRACTICE Test 3

16. **The answer is a.** The diagrams represent the three basic morphologies of bacteria: cocci (A), bacilli (B), and spirilla (C).

17. **The answer is b.** The trachea and bronchi are lined with ciliated epithelial cells. Choice b clearly shows the cilia.

18. **The answer is d.** This choice shows striated, or voluntary, muscle tissue.

19. **The answer is b.** These symptoms are indicative of barbiturate withdrawal.

20. **The answer is a.** Skim milk and low-fat cheese contain reduced amounts of fat, which is a lipid.

21. **The answer is b.** The total mass is obtained by adding the masses of the riders on each of the three beams. The smallest markings represent tenths of grams.

22. **The answer is a.** The total magnification is the product of the eyepiece magnification and the objective magnification: $40\times \times 10\times = 400\times$.

23. **The answer is b.** The immune response to infection results in an increase in WBCs in the blood.

24. **The answer is c.** Liquids, such as water, commonly form a curve, known as the meniscus, in cylindrical vessels. The volume of the liquid is read at the bottom of the meniscus.

25. **The answer is d.** The retina contains the rods and cones, and it is connected to the brain by the optic nerve.

26. **The answer is c.** An electroencephalogram (EEG) measures the electrical activity in the brain.

27. **The answer is c.** The process of aerobic respiration yields energy. Some of this energy is used to maintain a constant body temperature.

28. **The answer is a.** An impulse is a type of force, which can change the momentum of an object.

29. **The answer is c.** To be homozygous for both traits, the offspring must have consistent alleles for both traits (either both dominant or both recessive). Boxes 1, 6, 11, and 16 satisfy this condition.

30. **The answer is a.** The phenotype is the expressed or observed condition. Capital letters conventionally represent the dominant trait.

31. **The answer is c.** Find the point on the line directly above the 40-V value on the horizontal axis; then find the corresponding value on the vertical axis.

32. **The answer is c.** Iodine turns black in the presence of starch, a secondary product of photosynthesis. The covered portion would not have undergone photosynthesis during the previous two days.

33. **The answer is c.** By definition, the cell membrane is selectively permeable.

34. **The answer is a.** Decomposition reactions result in simpler substances; the simplest substance is an element.

35. **The answer is b.** Catalysts in reactions are normally expressed above the arrow.

36. **The answer is c.** Glucose and protein in the urine may be an indication of a problem in the kidneys. The other choices reflect normal conditions in the urine.

37. **The answer is a.** Cell D is less than half the diameter of the field of view; therefore choice a is the only possible correct choice.

38. **The answer is b.** In a plane mirror, the angle of reflection is equal to the angle of incidence.

39. **The answer is b.** The initials "RNA" represent ribonucleic acid.

40. **The answer is d.** Light energy can be thought of as having both wavelike and particulate properties. As particles, they are called photons.

41. **The answer is b.** Capillaries are the smallest blood vessels and have thin walls that permit the exchange of materials.

42. **The answer is a.** Choice a represents the win–win (++) symbiotic relationship, b the win–lose (+−) symbiotic relationship, and c the win–neutral (+0) one. Predation is not a symbiotic relationship.

43. **The answer is a.** The cerebrum is responsible for higher-order thinking processes.

44. **The answer is b.** The alveoli are found in the lungs and are surrounded by blood vessels. The large total surface area of the alveoli permits efficient gas exchange.

45. **The answer is a.** The right atrium is the entryway to the heart.

46. **The answer is d.** Prey species need to produce large numbers of offspring if they are to survive as a species.

47. **The answer is a.** Most traits are expressed in two phenotypes, or observed traits. When a third trait is expressed, this is called codominance or incomplete dominance.

48. **The answer is a.** The plasma surrounding red blood cells normally has dissolved salts, and the red blood cell is isotonic to that. If the cell is put in pure water (which is hypotonic), it will absorb water by means of osmosis until it bursts.

49. **The answer is a.** Amplitude is defined as the total displacement of a wave in the vertical dimension above or below the normal.

50. **The answer is a.** A pH below 7 is acidic, a pH above 7 is basic, and a pH of 7 is neutral.

51. **The answer is d.** By definition, a chemical change results in the formation of a new substance, which may be either a compound or an element.

52. **The answer is c.** By definition, the boiling point of a substance is the temperature at which the vapor pressure equals the pressure on the liquid.

53. **The answer is c.** The contractile vacuole pumps excess water out of freshwater protozoa.

54. **The answer is d.** Levers transfer forces across a distance.

55. **The answer is c.** To measure current (amperes), the ammeter is placed in series in the circuit. Voltmeters measure voltage and are placed in parallel.

56. **The answer is d.** Pancreatic protease is released into the small intestine. According to the graph, the greatest rate of activity for this enzyme occurs at a pH of approximately 8.

57. **The answer is c.** Smooth muscles are responsible for involuntary action such as peristalsis. Striated muscles are involved in voluntary behavior, and cardiac muscle is the muscle tissue of the heart.

58. **The answer is c.** Total energy is conserved; as an object falls, some of its potential energy converts to kinetic energy.

59. **The answer is a.** On the periodic table, metals are on the left and nonmetals on the right. Metallic properties increase going down a group.

60. **The answer is d.** The loss of electrons (e^-) results in the formation of a positive ion.

Comprehensive Practice Test 2

Verbal Ability:
Word Knowledge and Reading Comprehension

45 minutes

WORD KNOWLEDGE: Read each sentence carefully. Then, on the basis of what is stated in the sentence, select the correct answer to the incomplete statement. (The correct answers are at the end of this test.)

1. Martin's presentation was smooth but seemed superficial. It was
    a. rehearsed.
    b. graphic.
    c. substantive.
    d. glib.

2. The ancient Romans looked to several deities for support.
    Deities means
    a. plants.
    b. gods.
    c. neighbors.
    d. groups.

3. The bookkeeper noted that the figures on the sales slips did not equal the amount in the cash box. He noted
    a. an omission.
    b. a dilemma.
    c. an embellishment.
    d. a discrepancy.

4. The time of embarkation will be announced long before the rest of the plans are completed.
    Embarkation means
    a. beginning.
    b. liquidation.
    c. surrender.
    d. automation.

5. After watching the sun set over the lake, the couple felt very serene.
   Serene means
   a. comfortable.
   b. calm.
   c. happy.
   d. sleepy.

6. The landlord had to contact all owners of contiguous property.
   Contiguous means
   a. adjoining.
   b. vacant.
   c. destroyed.
   d. mortgaged.

7. The seal on the certificate was stamped with a raised design. It was
   a. embossed.
   b. incised.
   c. embraced.
   d. engraved.

8. Even at a young age, the teenager manages a successful child care business; that teenager is a real
   a. entrepreneur.
   b. altruist.
   c. bigot.
   d. charlatan.

9. The buyers were unable to close the deal on the property because of the presence of a
   a. designation.
   b. tenant.
   c. lien.
   d. misdemeanor.

10. The candidate certainly talked for a long time; the newspaper was right to call him
    a. degenerate.
    b. munificent.
    c. notorious.
    d. loquacious.

11. As soon as the ship touched the mine, the mine
    a. dissipated.
    b. depleted.
    c. digressed.
    d. detonated.

12. When the child fell from the bicycle, she received several cuts and abrasions.
    Abrasions means
    a. bruises.
    b. scrapes.
    c. wounds.
    d. marks.

13. Sarah and I had a tacit agreement not to discuss anything that might lead to an argument. **Tacit** means
    a. unrealistic.
    b. unsworn.
    c. unsure.
    d. unspoken.

14. The person who states that he cannot know of the existence of a supreme being is
    a. an acolyte.
    b. a deist.
    c. an agnostic.
    d. a theologian.

15. An economy that is based on farm production is described as
    a. agrarian.
    b. cooperative.
    c. utopian.
    d. utilitarian.

16. Most people feel that in a political race the advantage is held by the candidate already in office. This person is the
    a. resident.
    b. opponent.
    c. candidate.
    d. incumbent.

READING COMPREHENSION: There are five reading passages in this section. Read each passage carefully. Then, on the basis of what you have read in the passage, select the best answer for each question.

I

An adult pelican looks as if it were a bird designed more to float than to fly. In profile, its wings seem bulky, and the standing bird looks top-heavy, its large, strange head and sword bill pulling it down. When the pelican turns, however, and you see those long, tapered wings and watch their lazy flap and see the bird rise in the air, turning, then spiraling with the wind currents as skillfully as a sailplane, you know that it is a master of flight. Those powerful wings, which normally stretch from six to ten feet, can carry a pelican through the air at 35 to 40 miles an hour and keep it soaring for hours.

A flock of brown pelicans flying to an early-morning or pre-dusk fishing engagement is an enchanting sight. Following a leader, the birds move with military precision in a long, slanting line. As the squadron leader flaps its wings, each bird behind it also flaps, almost in unison.

Spotting fish from 25 to 50 feet above the sea, the leader suddenly peels off, its long beak aimed like a spear at its victim. Wings half folded, it plummets in a spin, hitting the water and actually somersaulting under the surface. One by one, as they see fish, the other birds follow, always entering the water downwind and emerging facing the wind, ready for take-off.

SECTION A
SECTION B
SECTION C
COMPREHENSIVE PRACTICE Test 1
COMPREHENSIVE PRACTICE Test 2
COMPREHENSIVE PRACTICE Test 3

Sometimes they dive from lesser heights, swooping down sharply, leveling off, and smashing into the water with carefully calculated force—just hard enough to send their beaks, but not their bodies, beneath the surface.

How does the bird strike the water so hard without harming itself? Another of its wonders: the pelican is armored with inflatable air sacs under its skin. Not only do the air sacs provide protection when the brown pelican crash-dives into the hard wall of water, they also supply buoyancy and bring the bird quickly to the surface.

(Excerpt from "A Wonderful Bird Is the Pelican" by Jack Denton Scott, *Reader's Digest*, November, 1981. Reprinted by permission of the Putnam Publishing Group from *That Wonderful Pelican*, text copyright © 1975 by Jack Denton Scott.)

17. The main topic of the passage is the pelican's
    a. size.
    b. diet.
    c. offspring.
    d. flight.

18. The pelican's profile makes it look
    a. handsome.
    b. large.
    c. disproportionate.
    d. distorted.

19. According to the passage, the bill of the pelican is
    a. thick and bulky.
    b. long and thin.
    c. heavy and curved.
    d. wide and flat.

20. According to the passage, the pelican's wing span is, on the average
    a. 20 feet.
    b. 12 feet.
    c. 8 feet.
    d. 6 feet.

21. The air sacs provide protection by helping the pelican to
    a. dive straight from the air.
    b. fly in strong winds.
    c. return to the surface.
    d. float for long periods of time.

22. It can be inferred from the passage that a good time to see the pelican in flight is when the sun is
    a. directly overhead.
    b. just above the horizon.
    c. at a 45° angle to the horizon.
    d. completely set.

Verbal Ability

313

SECTION A

SECTION B

SECTION C

COMPREHENSIVE PRACTICE Test 1

COMPREHENSIVE PRACTICE Test 2

COMPREHENSIVE PRACTICE Test 3

II

In 1876 Edison set up a laboratory in Menlo Park, New Jersey. It was to be an "invention factory." He hoped to be able to produce a new invention every ten days. The "Wizard of Menlo Park" (as he came to be called) patented well over a thousand inventions before he died, a record no other inventor has ever approached.

In Menlo Park, Edison improved the telephone and made it workable. There he invented what proved to be his own favorite accomplishment: the phonograph. He put tinfoil on a cylinder, set a free-floating needle skimming over it, and connected a receiver to carry sound waves to and from the needle. This machine, he announced, will talk.

His own associates laughed at him, including the mechanic who had built the machine to Edison's specifications. But Edison won. He talked into the receiver while the foil-covered cylinder revolved under the needle. Then he placed the needle at the beginning of the cylinder and his own words came out at him: "Mary had a little lamb, its fleece was white as snow—"

"*Gott im Himmel,*" cried the mechanic who had built the machine.

A machine that talked! The whole world was astonished. Edison was a wizard indeed. So when he next announced he would invent an electric light, everyone believed him.

This time, however, Edison had bitten off almost more than he could chew. For a while it looked as though he would fail. It took him a year and $50,000 to find that platinum wires would not work.

After hundreds of experiments, Edison found what he wanted: a wire that would warm to white heat without melting or breaking. No metal was needed after all—only a scorched cotton thread; a fragile carbon filament.

On October 21, 1879, Edison set up a bulb with such a filament. It burned for forty continuous hours. The electric light was a reality! On the next New Year's Eve, the main street of Menlo Park was illuminated by electricity in a public demonstration. Newspaper reporters from all the world came to cover the event, and to marvel at history's greatest inventor.

That was the climax of Edison's life. He never again reached this peak, although he worked on for more than half a century. He patented crucial inventions that made motion pictures and the whole electronics industry possible. A stream of inventions issued out of Edison's workshop until he died on October 18, 1931, at the age of 84.

(Reprinted by permission. Copyright © 1959, by Scholastic Magazine, Inc., from *Breakthroughs in Science* by Isaac Asimov.)

23. The best title for this passage is
    a. "Thomas Edison: The Wizard of Menlo Park."
    b. "Edison at His Prime."
    c. "A Machine That Talked."
    d. "The Effects of Edison's Inventions on Our Life Today."

24. The part of the later phonograph that corresponds to the foil-covered cylinder is the
    a. arm.
    b. cartridge.
    c. tape.
    d. record.

25. Among his inventions, Edison thought most highly of the
    a. telephone.
    b. phonograph.
    c. incandescent bulb.
    d. motion picture.

26. At the time of the invention of the incandescent bulb, Edison was in his
    a. thirties.
    b. forties.
    c. fifties.
    d. sixties.

27. According to the passage, which of these statements about Edison is true?
    a. He produced more inventions than any other inventor.
    b. He invented the incandescent bulb accidentally.
    c. He finally found the metal needed to make the incandescent bulb possible.
    d. He reached the height of his creative efforts in the early twentieth century.

28. According to the passage, at times Edison had to face
    a. money problems.
    b. public opinion.
    c. doubting colleagues.
    d. lack of self-confidence.

III

Erosion of America's farmland by wind and water has been a problem since settlers first broke the virgin prairies in the 19th century. But it wasn't until after the Dust Bowl days of the 1930s when wind and water savaged 282 million acres of American farmland that erosion forced itself into the national consciousness.

In 1935, a shocked nation enacted new laws to protect the soil, as President Franklin D. Roosevelt created the U.S. Soil Conservation Service. Government agents instructed farmers in how to hold on to their soil, and billions of dollars were eventually spent building terraces, planting trees as windbreaks, and trying new methods of strip-cropping, plowing, and crop rotation.

The experiment worked. Erosion slowed down, and ravaged farmlands became lush and productive once more. Soon government began paying farmers to keep land idle as a way of preventing surpluses.

But by the early 1970s, with a huge new market for grain in Russia and a growing world demand, the United States stopped these subsidies. To boost harvest volumes and meet escalating production costs, land never before touched by the plow—much of it previously thought too fragile or not fertile enough—was hastily planted or dug out to accommodate giant irrigation systems. The old terraces and tree rows, in the way of gigantic modern farm machinery, were ripped out and the land seeded. As a result, after 40 years of conservation efforts, soil erosion is worse today than in Dust Bowl days.

Although few dust storms are now sweeping across the Plains states, some experts see signs of their return. In 1980, 5.1 million acres of Great Plains land were damaged by routine wind erosion, almost double that of the previous year. Nationally, water erosion is taking an even greater toll. Because marginal, hilly land has been

Verbal Ability

315

SECTION **A**

SECTION **B**

SECTION **C**

COMPREHENSIVE PRACTICE **Test 1**

COMPREHENSIVE PRACTICE **Test 2**

COMPREHENSIVE PRACTICE **Test 3**

planted, and because farmers no longer alternate grain crops with soil-conserving grasses, rain and melting snow annually strip billions of tons of soil from the land.

(Excerpt from "Where Has All Our Soil Gone?" by James Risser, *Reader's Digest*, July 1981, a condensation of an article published in *Smithsonian Magazine*, March 1981. Copyright by James Risser.)

29. Which of the following titles is most appropriate for this passage?
    a. "The Problem of Soil Erosion"
    b. "The Dust Bowl"
    c. "America's Farmlands"
    d. "The U.S. Soil Conservation Service"

30. One of the causes of soil erosion is
    a. windbreaks.
    b. strip-cropping.
    c. farm subsidies.
    d. the use of marginal land.

31. All of the following factors contribute to soil erosion **except**
    a. wind.
    b. tree rows.
    c. irrigation systems.
    d. water.

32. The word "subsidies," as used in the fourth paragraph, refers to
    a. payments to farmers for not planting crops.
    b. instructions to farmers in modern agricultural methods.
    c. the demonstration of soil conservation by government agencies.
    d. investments in model farms by government agencies.

33. The passage implies that
    a. subsidies will be resumed.
    b. conservation will be accelerated.
    c. not enough grain will be produced.
    d. erosion by water will increase.

34. It can be concluded from the passage that soil erosion
    a. is unavoidable.
    b. is on the decline.
    c. could be slowed.
    d. has developed only in recent years.

IV

Psychologists who write about laughter usually make the subject about as cheery as patricide, with ponderous treatises on "covariation of variables in the humor stimulus." In short order humor lies on the dissecting table like a dead frog, its innards "discouraging to any but the pure scientific mind," as E. B. White put it. Now a few scientists are leaving the nature of humor well enough alone and are asking instead what happens when people laugh. They have already shown that laughter is good medicine, primarily for relieving stress; they also suspect that it can cure headaches, fight infections, and alleviate hypertension.

Medieval physicians told their patients jokes, but mirth was not widely welcome in the modern examining room until editor Norman Cousins wrote in 1976 that he had laughed his way to recovery from a degenerative spinal condition. While many doctors disparaged Cousins's claim, pointing out that the disease sometimes goes into spontaneous remission, others began taking a serious look at the biology of laughter. Dozens of scientists presented papers at a symposium on humor last month in Washington, and a two-volume "Handbook of Humor Research" is due next year. Most of the research is heavy on theory and light on data, but there are some encouraging anecdotes. Patients at a gerontology center at the University of Southern California, for instance, became more sociable and more active when volunteers reawakened their sense of humor.

A hearty laugh produces well-documented physical effects, many of them akin to moderate exercise. Muscles in the abdomen, chest, shoulders, and elsewhere contract; heart rate and blood pressure increase. In a paroxysm of laughter, the pulse can double from 60 to 120, and systolic blood pressure can shoot from a norm of 120 to a very excited 200. Dr. William Fry of Stanford University describes laughter as a kind of "stationary jogging." Like other exercise, it may produce lasting benefits. Once the laughing stops, muscles are more relaxed than before it started, which could relieve some kinds of headaches. Heartbeat and blood pressure also dip below normal, a sign of reduced stress. "It is not too far-fetched," wrote psychologist Jeffrey Goldstein of Temple University in The Sciences, that "laughter is related in several ways to longevity"—mainly through the reduction of stress and hypertension.

The chemical effects of laughter are more elusive, mainly because people hooked to intravenous tubes that monitor chemicals in the blood have trouble laughing on command. Nevertheless, Fry reports that adrenaline in the blood increases, and other researchers suspect that similar chemicals flood the brain. Jogging increases the brain's supply of beta-endorphins, natural opiates that probably account for the "runner's high." Although there is no similar evidence for the effects of laughter, Goldstein believes that a rush of endorphins may make people feel better after laughing.

(From *Newsweek*, Copyright © 1982 by Newsweek, Inc. All rights reserved. Reprinted by permission).

35. Which of the following titles is best for this passage?
    a. "The Evolution of Laughter"
    b. "Laughter Ensures Longevity"
    c. "The Analysis of Laughter"
    d. "Laughter Is Good Medicine"

36. Which of the following individuals has claimed that laughter cured his degenerative disease?
    a. Norman Cousins
    b. E. B. White
    c. William Fry
    d. Jeffrey Goldstein

37. The term "spontaneous remission" in the second paragraph means that
    a. the illness was caused by a psychological factor that no longer is present.
    b. a remedy has been discovered for the illness.
    c. symptoms of the illness have subsided without specific treatment.
    d. the cause of the illness was unknown.

SECTION A

SECTION B

SECTION C

COMPREHENSIVE PRACTICE Test 1

COMPREHENSIVE PRACTICE Test 2

COMPREHENSIVE PRACTICE Test 3

38. The passage cites a study in which older people were encouraged to laugh more often. The older people were found to
   a. live longer.
   b. be more sociable.
   c. have fewer headaches.
   d. be more withdrawn.

39. Which of the following inferences might be drawn about psychologists who write about laughter?
   a. They treat humor as if it were a laboratory specimen.
   b. They report their findings in an interesting manner.
   c. They describe the real meaning of humor.
   d. They don't laugh very often.

40. Which of the following statements can be inferred from the passage?
   a. Laughter should be used as part of the treatment of chronic illnesses.
   b. Scientists have discovered the chemicals that the brain produces during laughter.
   c. Scientists are taking a fresh look at laughter as a potential form of medical treatment.
   d. Physicians have been using humor to treat human ills since medieval times.

V

Science has long known that the earth's orbit around the sun is but one of a hierarchy of motions. What has not been known until recently is the velocity of the earth and whether our world, the solar system, and our galaxy—the Milky Way—are moving somewhere independently of their standard orbits.

In a recent interview, Dr. David T. Wilkinson, a Princeton University astrophysicist, reported the results of 15 years of research on these questions.

His measurements show that the earth is moving at 380 miles a second. This was confirmed in simultaneous studies—"friendly, useful competition," Dr. Wilkinson called them—by Dr. George F. Smoot of the University of California at Berkeley.

Dr. Wilkinson also found that the earth and its galaxy were hurtling, at the same speed, toward a possible collision in the Virgo cluster of galaxies in a relatively "nearby" part of the universe—200 million trillion miles away.

As sometimes happens in science, Dr. Wilkinson and his associates set out to find the answer to one key question and came up with another discovery. Their original goal was to determine the shape of the universe and learn whether it was rotating or revolving on "some sort of axis."

It is not rotating or revolving, they say, and is not football-shaped, as some scientists theorize, but is "remarkably spherical," as Einstein stated in one of the fundamental assumptions in his General Theory of Relativity.

It was a dramatic discovery by radio astronomers in the mid-1960's that gave Dr. Wilkinson a long-sought opportunity to learn how fast the earth was moving through space. They found that the universe was blanketed by radio waves, which were "bathing" the earth from all directions.

Even more remarkable, Dr. Wilkinson noted, was the origin of this cosmic microwave radiation. It was a remnant of the Big Bang that is believed to have created the universe about 15 billion years ago.

(© 1982, by The New York Times Company. Reprinted by permission.)

41. Which of the following titles would be best for this passage?
    a. "Competition in Science"
    b. "Dr. David T. Wilkinson, Astrophysicist"
    c. "Where the Earth Is Going—and How Quickly"
    d. "Einstein's Theory of Relativity"

42. According to the passage, the results of Dr. Wilkinson's research on the earth's velocity are reasonable because
    a. Dr. Smoot wrote a critical review of the work.
    b. Dr. Smoot's research produced similar results.
    c. Dr. Smoot's work depended on Wilkinson's results.
    d. Dr. Smoot discovered the means for Wilkinson to measure the earth's velocity.

43. According to the passage, the radio waves around the earth appear to be
    a. frequently exploding.
    b. continually disappearing.
    c. periodically expanding.
    d. constantly moving.

44. According to the passage, the earth's galaxy is moving toward the Virgo cluster at a speed of
    a. 100 trillion miles per year.
    b. 15 miles per year.
    c. 380 miles per second.
    d. 200 million miles per second.

45. According to the passage, the universe has the shape of a
    a. basketball.
    b. football.
    c. pyramid.
    d. cone.

46. It can be inferred from the passage that the results of Wilkinson's work had what kind of relationship to Einstein's theory?
    a. They provided support for Einstein's theory.
    b. They depended on Einstein's theory.
    c. They disagreed radically with Einstein's theory.
    d. They added a new facet to Einstein's theory.

WORD KNOWLEDGE: Read each sentence carefully. Then, on the basis of what is stated in the sentence, select the correct completion of the statement.

47. After several additions were made to the building, its corridors formed a labyrinth.
    Labyrinth means
    a. tunnel.
    b. rectangle.

Verbal Ability

319

SECTION A

SECTION B

SECTION C

COMPREHENSIVE PRACTICE Test 1

COMPREHENSIVE PRACTICE Test 2

COMPREHENSIVE PRACTICE Test 3

c. maze.
d. pattern.

48. The farmer did not plant one of his fields this year; he left it
    a. organic.
    b. fallow.
    c. rejuvenated.
    d. passive.

49. When asked about his domicile, Peter claimed that he did not have one.
    Domicile means
    a. opinion.
    b. spouse.
    c. income.
    d. residence.

50. Animals that eat both plants and meat are
    a. carnivorous.
    b. omnivorous.
    c. herbivorous.
    d. obsequious.

51. The state representative recommended building a residence for indigent people.
    Indigent means
    a. impoverished.
    b. elderly.
    c. handicapped.
    d. illiterate.

52. East Indian society was divided into distinct social classes known as
    a. peers.
    b. degrees.
    c. aristocracies.
    d. castes.

53. The speaker's remarks made light of a serious topic. The remarks were
    a. sarcastic.
    b. flippant.
    c. intellectual.
    d. optimistic.

54. A chart that shows how a company is organized shows its
    a. posture.
    b. policy.
    c. hierarchy.
    d. finances.

55. The father apologized for his son's inexplicable behavior.
    Inexplicable means
    a. unalterable.
    b. undependable.

c. unaccountable.

d. unsurpassable.

56. The students practicing in the music building produce a cacophonous sound.
    Cacophonous means
    a. melodic.
    b. harsh.
    c. harmonious.
    d. rhythmic.

57. Susan's vitriolic comments were meant to hurt her opponent.
    Vitriolic means
    a. improbable.
    b. adamant.
    c. chaste.
    d. caustic.

58. The president of the company was so aggravated that he was almost impossible to placate.
    Placate means
    a. appease.
    b. inform.
    c. convince.
    d. console.

59. The movement failed to progress even though the zealots pushed with all their might.
    Zealot means
    a. practitioner.
    b. fanatic.
    c. character.
    d. rebel.

60. Paul refuses to soften his position; he's being very
    a. flaccid.
    b. pernicious.
    c. intemperate.
    d. obdurate.

Mathematics

45 minutes

Work each problem carefully. Use scrap paper to do your calculations. (The correct answers and explanations are at the end of this test.)

1. $0.206 \times 6.3 =$
   a. 1.2978
   b. 1.3608
   c. 1.5768
   d. 1.914

2. $(301 + 802) - (711 - 43) =$
   a. 349
   b. 435
   c. 1,761
   d. 1,771

3. If $A > 9$, A could equal
   a. 10
   b. 9
   c. 8
   d. 0

4. If a heart beats 27 times in 20 sec, how many times does it beat in 1 min?
   a. 108
   b. 98
   c. 81
   d. 71

5. If 1 kg equals 2.2 lb, how many kilograms will an 8.8-lb baby weigh?
   a. 19.36 kg
   b. 11 kg
   c. 6.6 kg
   d. 4 kg

6. A dieter consumed 1,550 Calories on Monday, 1,630 on Tuesday, 1,420 on Wednesday, 1,725 on Thursday, and 1,500 on Friday. What was this person's average daily caloric intake?
   a. 7,825 Cal
   b. 1,565 Cal
   c. 1,500 Cal
   d. 1,145 Cal

7. 873.65−24.344 =
   a. 630.21
   b. 849.306
   c. 849.314
   d. 859.31

8. A student spent $2.75 for lunch on Monday, $2.10 on Tuesday, and $3.25 on Wednesday. What was the average cost of lunch for the 3 days?
   a. $2.60
   b. $2.63
   c. $2.70
   d. $8.10

9. A piece of cloth is 15 ft long. If 2.3 ft at one end are damaged, how many feet of cloth remain undamaged?
   a. 12.7 ft
   b. 13.1 ft
   c. 13.7 ft
   d. 17.1 ft

10. $1\dfrac{3}{4}+2\dfrac{5}{6}=$
    a. $4\dfrac{7}{12}$
    b. 4
    c. $3\dfrac{1}{5}$
    d. $2\dfrac{7}{21}$

11. 20% of the residents of a certain area are expected to become ill this year. If 25,000 people live in this area, how many are expected to become ill?
    a. 6,250
    b. 5,000
    c. 1,250
    d. 500

12. At 8 a.m., a patient's temperature was 99.4°F. At each of the next two readings, at 12 noon and again at 4 p.m., the temperature had risen 0.4°F. What was the temperature at 4 p.m.?
    a. 98.6°F
    b. 99.8°F
    c. 100.2°F
    d. 100.6°F

13. What number is 28% of 160?
    a. 4.35
    b. 19.33

SECTION A

SECTION B

SECTION C

COMPREHENSIVE PRACTICE Test 1

COMPREHENSIVE PRACTICE Test 2

COMPREHENSIVE PRACTICE Test 3

c. 44.80
d. 517.24

14. An income tax system requires that persons having a net income between $10,000 and $16,000 pay a tax of $800 plus 24% of that part of the income in excess of $10,000. How much tax should be paid on an income of $12,500?
   a. $600
   b. $1,400
   c. $3,000
   d. $3,840

15. If a regular pentagon has a perimeter of 15 cm, how long is each side?
   a. 3 cm
   b. 3.5 cm
   c. 3.75 cm
   d. 5 cm

16. What is the maximum number of $1\frac{1}{2}$-inch strips of tape that can be cut from a 480-inch roll of tape?
   a. 160 strips
   b. 240 strips
   c. 320 strips
   d. 720 strips

17. A patient, who is supposed to get $2\frac{1}{2}$ c of low-fat milk per day, drinks $\frac{3}{4}$ c at breakfast. If the remaining amount is to be equally divided, how much will she drink at each of two meals?
   a. $\frac{7}{8}$ c
   b. 1c
   c. $1\frac{1}{2}$ c
   d. $1\frac{3}{1}$ c

18. $50.29 \div 0.47 =$
   a. 1.07
   b. 1.7
   c. 17
   d. 107

19. The ratio of substance A to substance B in a mixture is 2:3. If the mixture contains 12 mg of substance A, how much is there of substance B?
   a. 18 mg
   b. 16 mg
   c. 9 mg
   d. 8 mg

20. A jogger travels x mi each morning. Which of these equations represents the number of days she will need to jog 200 mi?
    a. $200x = $ days
    b. $200 + x = $ days
    c. $\dfrac{x}{200} = $ days
    d. $\dfrac{200}{x} = $ days

21. $7\dfrac{1}{2} - 4\dfrac{2}{3} = $
    a. 3
    b. $3\dfrac{1}{3}$
    c. $2\dfrac{1}{6}$
    d. $2\dfrac{5}{6}$

22. An acute angle is best defined as one that is
    a. less than a right angle.
    b. greater than an obtuse angle.
    c. greater than a right angle.
    d. equal to an obtuse angle.

23. A man estimates that $\dfrac{1}{5}$ of his salary is spent for taxes, $\dfrac{1}{4}$ for rent, and $\dfrac{1}{10}$ for insurance. What fraction of his salary is left for other expenses and savings?
    a. $\dfrac{9}{20}$
    b. $\dfrac{11}{20}$
    c. $\dfrac{3}{19}$
    d. $\dfrac{16}{19}$

24. What percentage of 200 is 250?
    a. 50%
    b. 80%
    c. 125%
    d. 150%

25. $2\sqrt{25} = $
    a. 7
    b. 10
    c. 25
    d. 50

26. Solve the following simultaneous equations:

$$\begin{cases} 3x - 2y = 7 \\ x + 2y = 5 \end{cases}$$

   a. $x = 4, y = 3$
   b. $x = 7, y = 9$
   c. $x = 1, y = 22$
   d. $x = 3, y = 1$

27. Nine is 30% of what number?
   a. 245
   b. 30
   c. 3
   d. 2.45

28. Which of these decimals equals 3.7%?
   a. 3.70
   b. 0.37
   c. 0.037
   d. 0.0037

29. If $\dfrac{2}{3}$ of $x = 48$, then $\dfrac{1}{2}$ of $x =$
   a. 16
   b. 24
   c. 36
   d. 72

30. If $x = 3$ and $y = 4$, then

$$\frac{5x^2 + 2y}{3(x + y)} =$$

   a. $\dfrac{233}{21}$

   b. $\dfrac{38}{21}$

   c. $\dfrac{53}{13}$

   d. $\dfrac{53}{21}$

31. Which of the following algebraic equations represents this statement: "5 less than 7 times a number (n) equals 35."
   a. $7 - 5n = 35$
   b. $7n - 5 = 35$
   c. $5(n - 7) = 35$
   d. $7n + 5 = 35$

SECTION A

SECTION B

SECTION C

COMPREHENSIVE PRACTICE Test 1

COMPREHENSIVE PRACTICE Test 2

COMPREHENSIVE PRACTICE Test 3

32. $3y^2 \times 2y^4 =$
   a. $5y^6$
   b. $6y^6$
   c. $5y^8$
   d. $6y^8$

33. Which of these decimals is approximately equal to $\frac{3}{7}$?
   a. 0.21
   b. 0.37
   c. 0.43
   d. 0.73

34. If 33% of $x = 99$, $x =$
   a. 3
   b. 32.67
   c. 33.33
   d. 300

35. $176 - (-64) =$
   a. 112
   b. 240
   c. 11,264
   d. −11,264

36. $4\frac{1}{2} \times 3\frac{5}{6} =$
   a. $12\frac{5}{12}$
   b. $12\frac{5}{8}$
   c. $13\frac{2}{3}$
   d. $17\frac{1}{4}$

37. If 75 mL of solution contains 30 mL of a specific medication, how much of that medication will be needed to provide 120 mL of the same solution?
   a. 18.75 mL
   b. 45 mL
   c. 48 mL
   d. 75 mL

38. Ben has 4 more cards than Ken. Together, they have 44 cards. If x represents the number of cards Ken has, then which of these equations represents the total number of cards?
    a. $x + 4 = 44$
    b. $2x - 4 = 44$
    c. $x + 4x = 44$
    d. $2x + 4 = 44$

39. 1f $\dfrac{3}{7} = \dfrac{5}{x}$, then $x =$

    a. $\dfrac{35}{3}$

    b. $\dfrac{15}{7}$

    c. $\dfrac{5}{21}$

    d. $\dfrac{7}{15}$

40. If the monthly expenses for a family are represented by a circle graph, how many degrees of the circle will be needed to show that 20% of the expenses are used for clothes?
    a. 20°
    b. 36°
    c. 54°
    d. 72°

SECTION A
SECTION B
SECTION C
COMPREHENSIVE PRACTICE Test 1
COMPREHENSIVE PRACTICE Test 2
COMPREHENSIVE PRACTICE Test 3

Science

45 minutes

Read each question carefully, and then select the best answer. (The correct answers and explanations are at the end of this test.)

1. Which of these organisms supplies the environment with oxygen?
   a. mammals
   b. green plants
   c. bacteria
   d. soil insects

2. According to the theory of evolution, living things that did not adapt to changes in the environment
   a. became extinct.
   b. changed to different species.
   c. changed their structure.
   d. changed their behavior.

3. If a microscope has an eyepiece of 10× and an objective of 40×, what is the total magnification?
   a. 10×
   b. 40×
   c. 50×
   d. 400×

4. The diffusion of water through a semipermeable membrane is called
   a. active transport.
   b. pinocytosis.
   c. osmosis.
   d. transpiration–tension.

5. One treatment for someone who feels faint is to have the person lie down with the feet elevated. The primary purpose is to
   a. increase the blood flow to the brain.
   b. relieve the pressure on the brain.
   c. make sure that the person does not fall.
   d. allow a faster rate of breathing.

6. Which of the following conditions may result from the heavy use of alcohol?
   a. cirrhosis
   b. emphysema

c. goiter

d. toxic shock syndrome

7. A person ingests 300 cal for breakfast, 800 cal for lunch, and 700 cal for dinner. During the same time period, the person uses 1,500 cal for metabolic energy. As a result, this person would probably

a. store the equivalent of 300 cal as body weight.

b. lose the equivalent of 300 cal in body weight.

c. neither gain nor lose weight.

d. excrete 300 cal.

8. To determine whether lower abdominal pains might be due to digestive upset and not appendicitis, a white blood cell count is taken. This is done because

a. gas in the large intestines is caused by the presence of white blood cells.

b. the number of white blood cells decreases during an infection.

c. stomach acid causes a decrease in a white blood cell count.

d. the number of white blood cells increases during infection.

Questions 9 and 10 refer to the following diagram showing several stages in the human reproductive cycle.

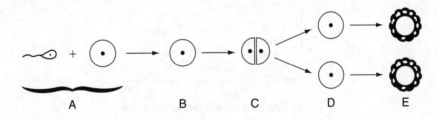

9. The structures in stage A are produced by

a. nondisjunction.

b. fertilization.

c. mitosis.

d. meiosis.

10. The structures in stage E will develop into individuals identified as

a. identical twins.

b. fraternal twins.

c. polyploid children.

d. Down's syndrome babies.

11. Which of these substances may be the end product of protein digestion?

a. cholesterol

b. lipid

c. fatty acid

d. amino acid

12. An object is traveling at a constant velocity of 100 m/sec. How far will it travel in 20 sec?

a. 5 m

b. 120 m

c. 200 m

d. 2,000 m

SECTION A

SECTION B

SECTION C

COMPREHENSIVE PRACTICE Test 1

COMPREHENSIVE PRACTICE Test 2

COMPREHENSIVE PRACTICE Test 3

13. An object of known mass and weight was taken on a flight mission to the moon. When this object was massed and weighed on the moon, it was found that
    a. the mass and weight remained the same.
    b. the mass was unchanged but the weight decreased.
    c. the weight was unchanged but the mass decreased.
    d. both the mass and weight had decreased.

14. Which of the following is *not* considered to be emitted by radioactive materials?
    a. ultraviolet rays
    b. alpha particles
    c. gamma rays
    d. beta particles

15. In the following graph, what percentage of the reactants have been converted to products when the reaction is at equilibrium?

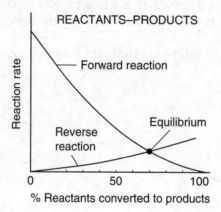

    a. 0%
    b. 50%
    c. 70%
    d. 100%

16. The correct procedure for checking the odor of a chemical substance is to
    a. inhale several shallow breaths.
    b. inhale slowly.
    c. fan air toward the nose and inhale.
    d. inhale slowly and deeply.

17. Compound A reacts with compound B to give compound C plus compounds D and E as shown by the following equation:

    A + B → C + D + E

    If 7 g of A react with 4 g of B to give 2 g C plus 3 g E, how many grams of D are produced?
    a. 5 g
    b. 6 g
    c. 11 g
    d. 16 g

Questions 18 through 20 refer to the following chart showing the vapor pressure of various substances in relation to temperature changes.

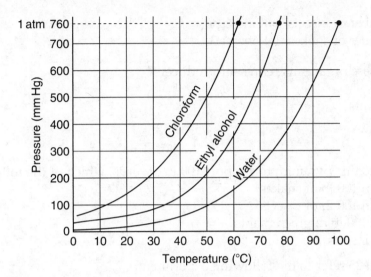

18. At 50°C, the vapor pressure of chloroform is closest to
    a. 350 mm Hg.
    b. 100 mm Hg.
    c. 200 mm Hg.
    d. 500 mm Hg.

19. The normal boiling point of ethyl alcohol is
    a. 6°C.
    b. 78°C.
    c. 80°C.
    d. 100°C.

20. As the temperature of ethyl alcohol rises from 50°C to 70°C, by approximately how many
    millimeters of mercury will its vapor pressure increase?
    a. 150 mm Hg
    b. 200 mm Hg
    c. 300 mm Hg
    d. 500 mm Hg

Questions 21 through 23 refer to the following pyramid:

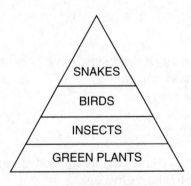

21. What first, if any, result would you expect if a disease decreases the population of birds?
    a. No change will occur.
    b. The number of green plants will increase.

    c. The number of insects will increase.

    d. The number of snakes will increase.

22. Which of these organisms represent producers?

    a. insects

    b. green plants

    c. birds

    d. snakes

23. According to this pyramid, to support 100 lb of birds, which of the following is needed?

    a. more than 100 lb of snakes

    b. more than 100 lb of insects

    c. less than 100 lb of green plants

    d. 100 lb of insects

Questions 24 and 25 refer to the following experiment:

In this study of diet and vitamin deficiency, three test groups of laboratory animals are given slightly different diets. Group I is given whole grain wheat; group II is given wheat without the outer hull; and group III is given the outer hull without the inner seed. Otherwise their diets are identical.

24. Group II develops a vitamin deficiency, and groups I and III do not. Which of the following statements provides the best explanation for this finding?

    a. Only the outer hull is needed to obtain the vitamin.

    b. Only the inner seed is needed to obtain the vitamin.

    c. The whole grain is needed to obtain the vitamin.

    d. The deficiency results from a lack of the vitamin in the rest of their diets.

25. The diet of Group II is most likely deficient in which of these vitamins?

    a. A

    b. B_1

    c. C

    d. D

26. In which of these blood diseases is the shape of red blood cells altered?

    a. sickle cell anemia

    b. hemophilia

    c. pernicious anemia

    d. leukemia

27. The genetic disease known as Down's syndrome is caused by

    a. one less chromosome than normal.

    b. an extra Y chromosome.

    c. an extra X chromosome.

    d. an extra 21st chromosome.

28. In a person who has hypoglycemia, the low blood sugar that occurs can be caused by

    a. an inability of the liver to store glucose.

    b. a deficiency of insulin.

    c. diabetes mellitus.

    d. excess insulin.

29. In which of these organs does the digestion of starch begin?
    a. large intestine
    b. small intestine
    c. mouth
    d. stomach

30. In humans, which of these blood components carries most of the oxygen?
    a. platelets
    b. white blood cells
    c. red blood cells
    d. plasma

31. An overdose of a muscle relaxant may cause a person to cease breathing because
    a. the muscles around the trachea will constrict.
    b. the lung muscles will cease to function.
    c. the diaphragm will be unable to contract.
    d. the alveoli will constrict.

32. Which of the following structures is the functional unit of the human kidney?
    a. alveolus
    b. oviduct
    c. malpighian tubule
    d. nephron

33. Which of these animals is *not* classified as a primate?
    a. man
    b. reindeer
    c. rhesus monkey
    d. gibbon

34. A walking stick is an insect that looks like the twigs of a tree in its environment. Its adaptations probably help it to
    a. compete with moths and butterflies.
    b. hide from predators.
    c. make its own food.
    d. lay many eggs.

35. Which structure in the unicellular organism pictured below is used to capture food?

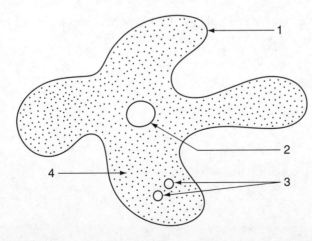

SECTION A

SECTION B

SECTION C

COMPREHENSIVE PRACTICE Test 1

COMPREHENSIVE PRACTICE Test 2

COMPREHENSIVE PRACTICE Test 3

a. 1
b. 2
c. 3
d. 4

36. The entry and exit of materials in the animal cell is regulated by which of these cell organelles?
    a. cell membrane
    b. cell wall
    c. endoplasmic reticulum
    d. nucleolus

37. The response of a plant to gravity is known as
    a. geotropism.
    b. phototropism.
    c. chemotropism.
    d. hydrotropism.

38. In a food chain, an organism that feeds on green plants is known as a
    a. producer.
    b. first-order consumer.
    c. second-order consumer.
    d. decomposer.

39. A student placed a stone in a graduated cylinder containing 30 mL of water. She then noted that the water level rose to the 55-mL mark. What is the volume of the stone?
    a. 25 mL
    b. 30 mL
    c. 55 mL
    d. 85 mL

40. Which of the following half reactions represents reduction?
    a. $C^{2+} + 2e^- \rightarrow C^0$
    b. $C^0 \rightarrow C^{4+} + 4e^-$
    c. $Na \rightarrow Na^+ + e^-$
    d. $H_2O + H^+ \rightarrow H3O^+$

41. The specific heat of water is 1 cal/g/ °C. How many calories of heat are needed to raise the temperature of 30 g of water from 25°C to 75°C?
    a. 50 cal
    b. 750 cal
    c. 1,500 cal
    d. 2,250 cal

SECTION A

SECTION B

SECTION C

COMPREHENSIVE PRACTICE Test 1

COMPREHENSIVE PRACTICE Test 2

COMPREHENSIVE PRACTICE Test 3

42. What is the volume of the water in the graduated cylinder?

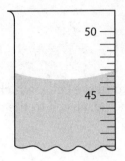

    a. 45.5 mL
    b. 45.8 mL
    c. 46.3 mL
    d. 48.5 mL

43. Which of these materials is a mixture?
    a. carbon dioxide
    b. ammonia gas
    c. oxygen
    d. air

44. Which of the following terms best describes a mixture of oil and water?
    a. saturated
    b. heterogeneous
    c. unsaturated
    d. homogeneous

45. Which of these values could be the pH of an acid rain sample?
    a. 4.0
    b. 7.0
    c. 8.0
    d. 12.0

46. When pure tall pea plants are crossed with pure short pea plants, only tall plants result. This illustrates Mendel's
    a. law of segregation.
    b. law of independent assortment.
    c. concept of unit characters.
    d. principle of dominance.

47. An atom contains 9 protons and 10 neutrons. The atomic number of this element is
    a. 1.
    b. 9.
    c. 10.
    d. 19.

48. Compounds that have different molecular structures but the same formula are called
    a. isotopes.
    b. isobars.
    c. isomers.
    d. isomorphs.

49. In the following diagram of two nerve cells, which number indicates the area where the message is transmitted from one nerve cell to the next?

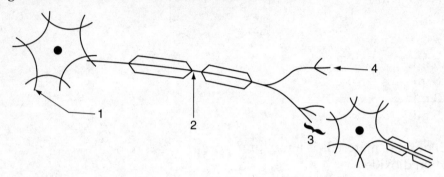

    a. 1
    b. 2
    c. 3
    d. 4

50. The part of the nervous system that enables you to understand the meaning of what you read is called the
    a. optic nerve.
    b. cerebellum.
    c. cerebrum.
    d. medulla.

51. The process by which certain human blood cells engulf bacteria is known as
    a. hemolysis.
    b. pinocytosis.
    c. phagocytosis.
    d. plasmolysis.

52. Which heart chamber pumps blood directly into the aorta?
    a. right atrium
    b. right ventricle
    c. left atrium
    d. left ventricle

53. If a person's gallbladder were removed by surgery, which of the following substances would he have the most difficulty digesting?
    a. carbohydrates
    b. nucleic acids
    c. fats
    d. proteins

54. A student wants to grow a bacterial culture. Which of these environments is best suited for growing most kinds of bacteria?
    a. an incubator at 37°C

SECTION A

SECTION B

SECTION C

COMPREHENSIVE PRACTICE Test 1

COMPREHENSIVE PRACTICE Test 2

COMPREHENSIVE PRACTICE Test 3

   b. a refrigerator at 5°C
   c. a lighted window at 72°F
   d. a dark room at 68°F

55. Which of the following parts of a compound microscope is used to adjust the amount of light?
   a. eyepiece
   b. objective lens
   c. diaphragm
   d. coarse adjustment knob

56. In the early stages of development, the embryos of birds and snakes resemble each other. This suggests that they
   a. belong to the same genus.
   b. are adapted for the same habitat.
   c. share a common ancestry.
   d. both develop in eggs.

57. In which of the following ways does an animal cell differ from a plant cell?
   a. An animal cell lacks a nucleus.
   b. An animal cell is always larger than a plant cell.
   c. An animal cell has no cell wall.
   d. An animal cell has no cell membrane.

58. Which of the following terms refers to the capacity of a microscope to distinguish between objects that lie very close to each other?
   a. staining
   b. resolving power
   c. microdissection
   d. magnifying power

Questions 59 and 60 refer to the following graph of the displacement of an object over a period of time.

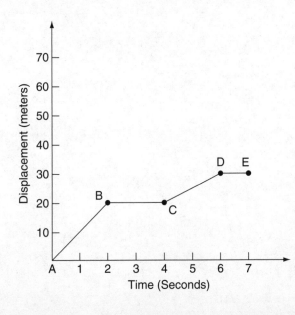

59. During the time interval BC, the velocity of the object is
    a. 0 m/sec.
    b. 5 m/sec.
    c. 10 m/sec.
    d. 20 m/sec.

60. During which time interval is the velocity greatest?
    a. DE
    b. CD
    c. BC
    d. AB

Answers to Comprehensive Practice Test 2

ANSWERS TO COMPREHENSIVE PRACTICE TEST 2: VERBAL ABILITY

1.	d	21.	c	41.	b
2.	b	22.	b	42.	b
3.	d	23.	a	43.	d
4.	a	24.	d	44.	c
5.	b	25.	b	45.	a
6.	a	26.	a	46.	a
7.	a	27.	a	47.	c
8.	a	28.	c	48.	b
9.	c	29.	a	49.	d
10.	d	30.	d	50.	b
11.	d	31.	b	51.	a
12.	b	32.	a	52.	d
13.	d	33.	d	53.	b
14.	c	34.	c	54.	c
15.	a	35.	d	55.	c
16.	d	36.	a	56.	b
17.	d	37.	c	57.	d
18.	c	38.	b	58.	a
19.	b	39.	a	59.	b
20.	c	40.	c	60.	d

ANSWERS TO COMPREHENSIVE PRACTICE TEST 2: MATHEMATICS

1. **The answer is a.**

   0.206 (3 decimals) $\times$ 6.3 (1 decimal) = 1.2978 (4 decimals)

2. **The answer is b.** Follow the order of operations to simplify this expression.

   $(301-802)-(711-43) =$
   $1,103-668 = 435$

SECTION A

SECTION B

SECTION C

COMPREHENSIVE PRACTICE Test 1

COMPREHENSIVE PRACTICE Test 2

COMPREHENSIVE PRACTICE Test 3

3.   **The answer is a.** If A > 9, it means all values of *A* are greater than 9. The only eligible choice for A is 10.

4.   **The answer is c.** You may use a proportion to solve this problem. You need to change 1 min to 60 sec. As always, make sure you align the units correctly: beats across from beats and seconds across from seconds.

$$\frac{27 \text{ beats}}{20 \text{ sec}} = \frac{x \text{ beats}}{60 \text{ sec}}$$

Rather than cross-multiply in this case, examine the two fractions closely. Notice that $20 \times 3 = 60$. Because the two fractions are equal, you may multiply 27 by 3 to obtain the missing numerator: $27 \times 3 = 81$. Therefore, $x = 81$ beats. You can also solve this problem by noticing that $20 \text{ sec} = \frac{1}{3}$ minute. Therefore, 3 times the number of beats in 20 seconds would give you the answer.

5.   **The answer is d.** You may use a proportion to solve this problem.

$$\frac{1 \text{ kg}}{2.2 \text{ lb}} = \frac{x \text{ kg}}{8.8 \text{ lb}}$$

Rather than cross-multiply in this case, examine the two fractions closely. Notice that $2.2 \times 4 = 8.8$. Because the two fractions are equal, you may multiply 1 by 4 to obtain the missing numerator: $1 \times 4 = 4$. Therefore, $x = 4$.

You may also solve this by noticing the relationship and not using a proportion.

$$\frac{8.8 \text{ lb}}{2.2 \text{ lb/kg}} = 4 \text{ kg}$$

6.   **The answer is b.** Total the five days of caloric intake: $1,550 + 1,630 + 1,420 + 1,725 + 1,500 = 7,825$. Then divide the total by 5 to find the average: $7,825 \div 5 = 1,565$.

7.   **The answer is d.** Make sure you line up the decimal points when subtracting decimals.

```
 873.650
- 24.344
---------
 849.306
```

8.   **The answer is c.** Total the amount of money spent on lunch over 3 days: $\$2.75 + \$2.10 + \$3.25 = \$8.10$. Divide this total by 3 to find the average: $\$8.10 \div 3 = \$2.70$

9.   **The answer is a.** Subtract the section of damaged cloth from the entire piece of cloth to find out how much remains undamaged.

15.0 ft (It is OK to add this 0 to the right of the decimal point.)

```
 15.0 ft
- 2.3 ft
---------
 12.7 ft
```

10. **The answer is a.** Find a common denominator and write equivalent fractions. The LCD is 12, because 4 and 6 are both factors of 12.

$$1\frac{3}{1} = 1\frac{9}{12}$$

$$2\frac{5}{6} = 2\frac{10}{12}$$

$$1\frac{9}{12} + 2\frac{10}{12} = 3\frac{19}{12} = 4\frac{7}{12}$$

11. **The answer is b.** Find 20% of 25,000 by changing 20% to a decimal and multiplying it by 25,000.

$$20\% = 0.2$$

$$0.2 \times 25,000 = 5,000 \ (20\% \text{ of } 25,000)$$

Therefore, 5,000 people are expected to become ill.

12. **The answer is c.** The patient's temperature starts out at $99.4°F$. It rises $0.4°F$ twice, for a total of an $0.8°F$ rise. To find the final temperature, add 0.8 to 99.4.

$$99.4°F + 0.8°F = 100.2°F$$

13. **The answer is c.** Turn the problem into an equation and solve for x: What number is 28% of 160? Change 28% to 0.28 (a decimal).

$$x = 28\% \times 160$$

$$x = 0.28 \times 160$$

$$x = 44.8$$

14. **The answer is b.** The tax to be paid is $800 plus 24% of $2,500 (the income in excess of $10,000). Calculate 24% of $2,500: $0.24 \times \$2,500 = \$600$. Add $600 to $800 to obtain the total taxes: $1,400.

15. **The answer is a.** A regular pentagon is a pentagon (5-sided polygon) with all its sides the same length. If the perimeter is 15 cm, then the length of each side can be calculated as follows: $15 \div 5 = 3$ cm.

16. **The answer is c.** The question is really asking, how many $1\frac{1}{2}$s are there in 480? This is a division problem. Change $1\frac{1}{2}$ to an improper fraction, invert the divisor, and multiply.

$$1\frac{1}{2} \rightarrow \frac{3}{2} \rightarrow \frac{480}{\frac{3}{2}} =$$

$$480 \times \frac{2}{3} = \frac{960}{3} = 320$$

SECTION A

SECTION B

SECTION C

COMPREHENSIVE PRACTICE Test 1

COMPREHENSIVE PRACTICE Test 2

COMPREHENSIVE PRACTICE Test 3

17. **The answer is a.** Subtract the amount of milk already drunk ($\frac{3}{4}$ c) from the total ($2\frac{1}{2}$ c) to find out how much milk remains to be drunk.

$$2\frac{1}{2} = \frac{5}{2} = \frac{10}{4}$$

$$\frac{10}{4} - \frac{3}{4} = \frac{7}{4}\,c$$

Divide $\frac{7}{4}$ c by 2 to find out how much the patient will drink at each meal.

$$\frac{7}{4} \div \frac{2}{1} = \frac{7}{4} \times \frac{1}{2} = \frac{7}{8}\,c/meal$$

18. **The answer is d.** Multiply both the dividend and the divisor by 100, and divide.

$$0.47)\overline{50.29.} \times 1$$

$$47)\overline{5,029}\;\;\frac{107}{}$$

Another way to solve this problem is by inspection. Once you have multiplied both the divisor and the dividend by 100, inspect your answer choices. Of the four answers given, only 107 makes sense for this problem; all the others are too small. It is possible to answer this problem without dividing at all.

19. **The answer is a.** You may use a proportion to solve this problem. You will need to recognize that the ratio 2:3 is the same thing as $\frac{2}{3}$. As always, be sure to align the units correctly:

$$\frac{A}{B} = \frac{A}{B}$$

$$\frac{2}{3} = \frac{12\text{ mg}}{x\text{ mg}}$$

Cross-multiply, and divide both sides by 2 to solve for x.

$$2x = 36$$

$$x = 18\text{ mg}$$

20. **The answer is d.** This is actually a rate problem: rate (r) $\times$ time (t) = distance (d). In this case, rearrange the formula:

$$t = \frac{d}{r}$$

The rate of the jogger is x mi per day, and the distance is 200 mi.

$$t = \frac{200\text{ mi}}{x\text{ mi/day}}\;\text{ or days } = \frac{200}{x}$$

21. **The answer is d.** Find a common denominator, and write equivalent fractions. The LCD is 6 because 2 and 3 are both factors of 12.

$$7\frac{1}{2} = 7\frac{3}{6} = 6\frac{9}{6}$$

$$4\frac{2}{3} = 4\frac{4}{6}$$

$$6\frac{9}{6} - 4\frac{4}{6} = 2\frac{5}{6}$$

22. **The answer is a.** An acute angle is defined as an angle less than $90°$, and a right angle is defined as angle equal to $90°$. Therefore, the best choice is a, which describes an acute angle as less than a right angle.

23. **The answer is a.** Find the lowest common denominator (LCD) for all three fractions, and then change each of the fractions to an equivalent fraction with the new denominator. Because 4, 5, and 10 are all factors of 20, 20 is the LCD. Then add them.

$$\frac{1}{4} = \frac{5}{20}$$

$$\frac{1}{5} = \frac{4}{20}$$

$$\frac{1}{10} = \frac{2}{20}$$

$$\frac{5}{20} + \frac{4}{20} + \frac{2}{20} = \frac{11}{20}$$

If $\frac{11}{20}$ of the man's salary is spent already, then $\frac{9}{20}$ must remain.

24. **The answer is c.** This is one of three types of common percentage problems: finding the percentage when you know the base and the percent. Convert the question to an equation, substituting $x\%$ for "what percentage." (Deal with x being a percentage at the end of the problem.)

What percentage of 200 is 250?

$$x\% \times 200 = 250$$

$$200x = 250$$

Divide both sides by 200, and change 1.25 to a percentage by multiplying by 100.

$$x = 1.25 \times 100 = 125\%$$

25. **The answer is b.**

$$2\sqrt{25} =$$

$$2 \times 5 = 10$$

SECTION A

SECTION B

SECTION C

COMPREHENSIVE PRACTICE Test 1

COMPREHENSIVE PRACTICE Test 2

COMPREHENSIVE PRACTICE Test 3

26. **The answer is d.** Solve this problem by substituting the values in the equations. The only values that work are $x = 3, y = 1$.

$3(3) - 2(1) = 7$

$3 + 2(1) = 5$

Another method is to add the two equations and solve for x, and then y.

$$\begin{array}{l} 3x - 2y = 7 \\ \underline{x + 2y = 5} \\ 4x = 12 \\ x = 3 \end{array}$$

27. **The answer is b.** Turn the problem into an equation and solve for x, and change 30% to a decimal by dividing 30% by 100.

Nine is 30% of what number?

$9 = 30\% \times x$

$9 = \left(\dfrac{30\%}{100} \right) \times x$

$9 = 0.30x$

Divide both sides by 0.30 to solve for x.

$30 = x$

28. **The answer is c.** To change a percentage to a decimal, divide the percentage by 100 and drop the percentage symbol (%). When you divide by 100, move the decimal point two places to the left.

$3.7\% \div 100 = 0.037$

29. **The answer is c.** You are given:

$\dfrac{2}{3} x = 48$

Multiply both sides by $\dfrac{3}{2}$.

$x = 48 \times \dfrac{3}{2} = 72$

To find $\dfrac{1}{2}x$, divide 72 by 2.

$$\frac{72}{2} = 36$$

30. **The answer is d.**

$$\frac{5x^2 + 2y}{3(x + y)} = \frac{5(3^2) + 2 \times 4}{3(3 + 4)}$$

$$\frac{5(9) + 8}{3 \times 7} = \frac{45 + 8}{21} = \frac{53}{21}$$

31. **The answer is b.** You need to be familiar with certain words and how they translate from word problems to equations. Here is the problem again: "5 less than 7 times a number (n) equals 35."

    • "5 less than" means –5.
    • "7 times a number (n)" means $7n$.
    • "equals 35" means = 35.
    • Put this all together, and you get: $7n - 5 = 35$.

32. **The answer is b.** Recall the rules for multiplying powers with similar bases: add the exponents. Therefore

$$3y^2 \times 2y^4 = 6y^{2+4} = 6y^6$$

33. **The answer is c.** To convert to a decimal, divide 7 into 3:

$$\frac{0.428}{7)3.000} \approx 0.43$$

34. **The answer is d.** This is one of three types of common percentage problems: finding the base when you know the percent and the percentage. The problem again: If 33% of x is 99, what is x?

    $0.33x = 99$

    Divide both sides by 0.33 to solve for x.

    $x = 300$

35. **The answer is b.** Recall the rules for subtracting negative numbers: Subtracting a negative is like adding a positive. Therefore

$$176 - (-64) = 176 + 64 = 240$$

36. **The answer is d.** Change each mixed number to an improper fraction, cross-cancel between the 9 and the 6 (cancel a 3), and multiply.

SECTION A

SECTION B

SECTION C

COMPREHENSIVE PRACTICE **Test 1**

COMPREHENSIVE PRACTICE **Test 2**

COMPREHENSIVE PRACTICE **Test 3**

$$4\frac{1}{2} \times 3\frac{5}{6} =$$

$$\frac{9}{2} \times \frac{23}{6} =$$

$$\frac{3}{2} \times \frac{23}{2} =$$

$$\frac{69}{4} = 17\frac{1}{4}$$

37. **The answer is c.** You may set up a proportion to solve this problem. As always, be sure to align the units correctly: milliliters of solution across from milliliters of solution and milliliters of medication across from milliliters of medication.

$$\frac{75 \text{ mL of solution}}{30 \text{ mL of medication}} = \frac{120 \text{ mL of solution}}{x \text{ mL of medication}}$$

Cross-multiply, and divide both sides by 75 to solve for x.

$$75x = 3600$$

$$x = 48 \text{ mL}$$

38. **The answer is d.** Ken's cards = x. If Ben has 4 more cards than Ken, then Ben has $x + 4$ cards. If their total number of cards is 44, then $x + x + 4 = 44$.

$$2x + 4 = 44$$

39. **The answer is a.** By now, you are no doubt comfortable with the familiar setup of a proportion.

$$\frac{3}{7} = \frac{5}{x}$$

Cross-multiply, and divide both sides by 3 to solve for x.

$$3x = 35$$

$$x = \frac{35}{3}$$

40. **The answer is d.** Recall that there are 360° in a circle. Once you know this, calculate 20% of 360°: $0.2 \times 360° = 72°$ (20% of the whole circle).

ANSWERS TO COMPREHENSIVE PRACTICE TEST 2: SCIENCE

1. **The answer is b.** Green plants undergo a process called photosynthesis. During this process, light energy captured by the pigment chlorophyll fuels the conversion of carbon dioxide and water to glucose and oxygen.

2. **The answer is a.** This statement is in accordance with the theory of natural selection, which states that organisms with features that allow them to deal with changes in the environment are more successful and have a greater chance of surviving to a reproductive age. Thus a species without these features could become extinct.

3. **The answer is d.** The total magnification is a product of the magnifications of the objective used and the eyepiece.

4. **The answer is c.** Osmosis is the diffusion of water across a semipermeable membrane.

5. **The answer is a.** Often people who feel faint have experienced a drop in blood pressure. Having the person lie down with the feet elevated increases the blood flow to the brain.

6. **The answer is a.** Alcohol abuse can lead to cirrhosis of the liver.

7. **The answer is a.** Excess calories are stored as body weight. The intake was 1,800 Cal and the expenditure of energy was 1,500 Cal. The difference (300 Cal) is the excess.

8. **The answer is d.** Infection, not gastric upset, increases the white blood cell count.

9. **The answer is d.** Gametes (sperm and egg) are produced by meiosis, resulting in monoploid gametes.

10. **The answer is a.** The division of a fertilized egg into two parts results in identical twins. If two separate eggs were fertilized at the same time, the resultant twins would be fraternal.

11. **The answer is d.** Proteins are made up of amino acids.

12. **The answer is d.** Use the following formula: distance = velocity × time.

    distance = 20 m × 100 m/sec = 2,000 m

13. **The answer is b.** Mass is a property of an object and remains the same on earth as on the moon. However, weight results from the force exerted by gravity, and it changes when going from earth to the moon because the earth and moon have different masses.

14. **The answer is a.** Alpha and beta particles and gamma rays are all types of radiation. Ultraviolet rays are light rays, which the human eye cannot detect, but they are not radioactive.

15. **The answer is c.** According to this graph, 70% of the reactants have been converted to products when the reaction reaches equilibrium.

SECTION A

SECTION B

SECTION C

COMPREHENSIVE PRACTICE Test 1

COMPREHENSIVE PRACTICE Test 2

COMPREHENSIVE PRACTICE Test 3

16. **The answer is c.** This procedure prevents inhalation of a dangerous amount of a substance.

17. **The answer is b.** The law of conservation of mass states that mass is neither created nor destroyed in a chemical reaction. The sum of the masses of the reactants must equal the sum of the masses of the products.

   A + B = 7g + 4 g = 11g

   C + E = 2 g + 3 g = 5 g

   Compound D must equal the difference between sum of the reactants and the masses of C and E.

   11g−5g = 6g of D

18. **The answer is d.** According to this chart, the vapor pressure of chloroform is closest to 500 mm Hg.

19. **The answer is c.** The normal boiling point of a liquid is the temperature at which the vapor pressure of the liquid is equal to the atmospheric pressure. Atmospheric pressure at sea level is taken to be 1 atm (1 atmosphere or 760mm Hg). Thus, ethyl alcohol's vapor pressure is 1 atm at approximately 80°C.

20. **The answer is c.** At 50° the pressure of ethyl alcohol is 200 mm Hg. At 70° the pressure is 500 mm Hg, for a difference of 300 mm Hg.

21. **The answer is c.** The diagram shows a food chain in which birds feed on insects. If the number of birds declines, then the number of insects would increase.

22. **The answer is b.** Green plants are producers because they produce food by means of photosynthesis.

23. **The answer is b.** The diagram increases in size in the direction of birds to insects, indicating that more insects are required to support a certain amount of birds. Thus, 100 pounds of birds consume an amount of insects exceeding 100 pounds.

24. **The answer is a.** Group II is the only group that did not receive the outer hull.

25. **The answer is b.** Vitamin B_1 (thiamin) is the only one of the choices that is found in nuts and whole grains (outer husk).

26. **The answer is a.** Anemia is any condition that impairs the oxygen-carrying capacity of red blood cells. A specific type, sickle cell anemia, is a disorder in which abnormal hemoglobin becomes spiky when the hemoglobin is delivering or picking up oxygen. This can cause the red blood cells to rupture (and take on the appearance of a sickle) and produce clots in small blood vessels.

27. **The answer is d.** Some genetic diseases are caused by additional or too few copies of certain chromosomes. Down's syndrome is caused by non-disjunction resulting in an additional copy of chromosome 21.

28. **The answer is d.** Hypoglycemia, or low blood sugar, can be caused by the presence of excess insulin. Insulin is a hormone that is necessary to bring blood glucose into the liver for storage. If too much insulin is present, the glucose levels in the blood decrease.

29. **The answer is c.** The saliva contains an enzyme called salivary amylase, which begins the process of starch digestion.

30. **The answer is c.** Red blood cells contain hemoglobin, which is an oxygen carrier. Each hemoglobin molecule can bind up to four molecules of oxygen, and there are over 200,000 hemoglobin molecules per red blood cell. When the blood reaches the tissue that needs oxygen, hemoglobin releases the oxygen.

31. **The answer is c.** The diaphragm is a muscle beneath the lungs. As it contracts and relaxes, the volume and pressure in the chest cavity change. These changes are involved in the processes of inhalation and exhalation. A muscle relaxant interferes with breathing because of its effect on the diaphragm.

32. **The answer is d.** The alveoli are the functional units of the lung; malpighian tubules are excretory structures found in insects; oviducts are the part of the female reproductive structure where fertilization occurs. The nephron is the functional unit of the kidney where urine is formed.

33. **The answer is b.** A reindeer is not classified as a primate.

34. **The answer is b.** An adaptation or group of adaptations such as found in the walking stick help camouflage it, thus hiding it from predators.

35. **The answer is a.** The organism surrounds a food particle and ingests it via the process of phagocytosis.

36. **The answer is a.** The cell membrane contains pores and channels that regulate the substances that can enter into or exit from the cell.

37. **The answer is a.** Geotropism is a plant's response toward or away from gravity.

38. **The answer is b.** Producers are green plants, which herbivores or omnivores (first-order consumers) feed on. Second-order consumers are carnivores or omnivores, and they feed on herbivores. Decomposers, such as bacteria, convert dead matter in the soil to organic matter that can be utilized by the producers.

39. **The answer is a.** If the reading on the graduated cylinder rose from 30 mL to 55 mL, the volume of the solid must equal 25 mL on the graduated cylinder scale because the increase is due to the displacement of water by the stone.

40. **The answer is a.** Reduction is the gain of electrons, which occurs only in equation a.

41. **The answer is c.** The specific heat of a substance is the heat needed in Calories to change the temperature of 1 g of substance by 1°C. To heat 1 g of water from 25°C to 75°C, it takes 50 Cal. To do this for 30 g, it takes 1,500 Calories (50 Cal × 30 g). The formula for specific heat capacity is:

specific heat capacity = heat (mass × change in temperature)

42. **The answer is c.** When making volume measurements, the reading must be taken at the bottom of the meniscus. The meniscus is the natural curvature found at the surface of water in a tube due to the clinging of the water to the sides of the container.

43. **The answer is d.** Air is made up of many types of gases, such as nitrogen, oxygen, and hydrogen. The amounts of the gases that make up air are not constant, meaning that the air in New York City probably contains less oxygen than the air in the middle of Vermont.

44. **The answer is b.** Oil and water do not mix, making it a heterogeneous mixture.

45. **The answer is a.** Acids have pHs below 7.

46. **The answer is d.** Since all of the offspring are tall, the trait of being tall must be dominant over the trait of being short, which is recessive.

47. **The answer is b.** The atomic number of an element is equal to the number of protons in the nucleus of the atom. Mass number is the sum of protons and neutrons.

48. **The answer is c.** An isomer of a compound has a different molecular structure but the same molecular formula as the compound.

49. **The answer is c.** As a message is transmitted down the axon, it reaches the terminus. At the terminus, chemicals are released that travel across the synapse to the next neuron. In this manner, a message is transmitted from one neuron to another.

50. **The answer is c.** The cerebellum is responsible for coordinating movement, and the medulla controls involuntary actions such as breathing and swallowing. The optic nerve is involved with vision.

51. **The answer is c.** This process involves the engulfment of bacteria by the plasma membrane. This encloses the bacteria in a sac that is then released into the cell, where enzymes usually break it down.

52. **The answer is d.** The left ventricle pumps blood via the aorta to the body, and the right ventricle pumps blood via the pulmonary arteries to the lungs. Both atria are receiving chambers.

53. **The answer is c.** The gallbladder stores bile, which helps to break down fats.

54. **The answer is a.** Bacteria grow best at $37°C$, which is close to body temperature.

55. **The answer is c.** The diaphragm of a microscope is used to adjust the amount of light.

56. **The answer is c.** Comparative embryology indicates a common ancestry among vertebrates.

57. **The answer is c.** Animal cells do not have cell walls.

58. **The answer is b.** Resolving power is defined as the ability of a microscope to distinguish between two objects that lie very close to each other.

59. **The answer is a.** Displacement is the change in an object's position. During the interval BC on the graph, the object remains at 20 m; there is no displacement. Velocity is the rate at which an object's position changes and to the direction of the change. There is no change in the object's position during the BC time interval. Therefore, its velocity is zero.

60. **The answer is d.** Velocity is the time rate of change of displacement. During the time interval AB, the object's displacement is 20 m in 2 sec. During the BC and the DE time intervals, there is no displacement of the object. The CD time interval indicates a displacement of 10 m in 2 sec. Therefore, the AB time interval has the greatest velocity.

SECTION A

SECTION B

SECTION C

COMPREHENSIVE PRACTICE Test 1

COMPREHENSIVE PRACTICE Test 2

COMPREHENSIVE PRACTICE Test 3

Comprehensive Practice Test 3

Verbal Ability

Word Knowledge and Reading Comprehension

45 Minutes

WORD KNOWLEDGE: Read each sentence carefully. Then, on the basis of what is stated in the sentence, select the correct answer to the incomplete statement. (The correct answers are at the end of this test.)

1. The worker manipulated the tools with ease.
   Manipulated means
   a. manufactured.
   b. handled.
   c. stored.
   d. selected.

2. Their names were omitted from the guest list. They were
   a. included.
   b. excluded.
   c. underlined.
   d. italicized

3. The medication was sprayed into the patient's nasal passage.
   Nasal refers to the
   a. spine.
   b. ears.
   c. nose.
   d. eyes.

4. The odor was so obnoxious that no one wanted to stay in the room.
   Obnoxious means
   a. prevalent.
   b. strong.
   c. acrid.
   d. repulsive.

5. The ancient burial ground was found under a knoll near the lake.
   Knoll means
   a. ditch.
   b. mound.
   c. grove.
   d. glade.

6. The lawyer succeeded in having the client's charge reduced by proving that the client acted under
   a. deference.
   b. embellishment.
   c. duress.
   d. ignorance.

7. Much of the monetary policy is set by the national government.
   Monetary refers to
   a. diplomacy.
   b. insurance.
   c. money.
   d. defense.

8. Frank refused to listen to reason; he was just being perverse.
   Perverse means
   a. ignorant.
   b. contrary.
   c. silly.
   d. obtuse.

9. The relationship eroded quickly when Helen went back to her old job.
   Eroded means
   a. ended.
   b. grew.
   c. deepened.
   d. diminished.

10. After three years of work, we were successful in bringing our dream to
    a. dissidence.
    b. trepidation.
    c. gratuity.
    d. fruition.

11. The suspect implicated the young lawyer with his statement.
    Implicated means
    a. involved.
    b. convicted.
    c. shocked.
    d. charged.

12. The apathy during the campaign cost the politician the election.
    Apathy means
    a. corruption.
    b. indifference.
    c. resentment.
    d. obstacle.

13. The novel about the eighteenth century referred to highwaymen as
    a. resisters.
    b. troopers.
    c. characters.
    d. marauders.

14. The differences between the two research study results were so small they were
    a. momentary.
    b. negligible.
    c. fragmented.
    d. critical.

15. I knew I could trust my friend with the secret because he had always been
    a. ingenious.
    b. trusting.
    c. discreet.
    d. callous.

16. A person who is difficult to please is said to be
    a. indignant.
    b. marked.
    c. notorious.
    d. fastidious.

17. The dealer suspected that the painting was bogus. He said that the painter's signature was clearly
    a. copied.
    b. original.
    c. reproduced.
    d. forged.

18. Sandstone is a rock with tiny spaces that permit water to pass through it. We can say that it is
    a. impervious.
    b. porous.
    c. homogeneous.
    d. opaque.

19. The chemist fabricated a new polymer.
    Fabricated means
    a. fermented.
    b. created.
    c. incurred.
    d. decomposed.

SECTION A

SECTION B

SECTION C

COMPREHENSIVE PRACTICE Test 1

COMPREHENSIVE PRACTICE Test 2

COMPREHENSIVE PRACTICE Test 3

20. With all of the sudden changes in the methods of childrearing, society is definitely in a state of
    a. indiscretion.
    b. heresy.
    c. flux.
    d. secession.

21. The stream was a very unreliable divider for the property because of its tendency to
    a. freeze.
    b. trickle.
    c. stagnate.
    d. meander.

22. The soldiers made a foray into enemy territory.
    Foray means
    a. make a raid.
    b. take a chance.
    c. have a battle.
    d. carry a message.

23. The application of butter to the burnt flesh will exacerbate the wound.
    Exacerbate means
    a. aggravate.
    b. soothe.
    c. protect.
    d. inflame.

24. The contestant looked askance at his opponent. He looked
    a. admiringly.
    b. hopefully.
    c. scornfully.
    d. fearfully.

25. The strident quality of the bird's call made it very easy to identify.
    Strident means
    a. harsh.
    b. monotonous.
    c. melodious.
    d. staccato.

26. The juvenile was behaving so defiantly that he could only be described as
    a. recalcitrant.
    b. taciturn.
    c. notorious.
    d. prohibitive.

27. The monarch issued several edicts before beginning the evening's entertainment.
    Edict means
    a. proposal.
    b. command.
    c. restriction.
    d. retreat.

28. The stand upon which a coffin rests is called a
    a. bier.
    b. pall.
    c. chalice.
    d. sepulcher.

29. The young man's provincial attitude kept him from getting the job.
    Provincial means
    a. superior.
    b. belligerent.
    c. narrow.
    d. snobbish.

30. The schism between the two families seemed irreparable.
    Schism means
    a. feud.
    b. separation.
    c. disagreement.
    d. relationship.

READING COMPREHENSION: There are five reading passages in this section. Read each passage carefully. Then, on the basis of what you have read in the passage, select the best answer for each question.

I

Zoologists have studied how cold-blooded insects go about their business all through winter, just as they have questioned how cold-blooded fish manage in the subfreezing water around Antarctica. Down to a certain temperature, winter insects can make do by absorbing sunlight; many are dark-colored so they can absorb as much heat as possible from the sun. Others absorb heat by basking on dark surfaces. Heavy layers of hair or scales slow the loss of heat generated or absorbed. Insects also beat their wings while at rest to warm themselves.

Many insect species adapt their behavior to cold. Southern or warm-climate species of black flies, for example, mate in the air, and females fly long distances for the blood meal necessary for the eggs to mature. But Arctic black files mate on the ground when they are too cold to fly, and eggs are presupplied with nutrients.

Keeping active in the cold season is important; keeping alive—and unfrozen—is essential. When living tissue freezes, expanding ice crystals destroy cell membranes, causing irreversible and fatal damage. Death comes even before freezing is complete, when there is no longer enough liquid in the cell for the enzyme activity essential to life.

Insects survive subfreezing temperatures by supercooling, lowering the freezing point of their body fluids, and either by slowing ice formation or by being able to function even when their extracellular fluids have been frozen. Both groups use "antifreezes": the polyhydric alcohols sorbitol and glycerol (chemically similar to the glycerol used in automobiles) and the disaccharide trehalose.

Insects in the first group manage by reducing the chance that ice will form in their circulatory fluids. Ice tends to form rapidly around a nucleator, a tiny ice crystal or speck of dust that offers a solid frame for other molecules to attach themselves to. These insects purge their bodies of potential nucleators, principally by emptying their guts, and produce antifreezes, which lower the freezing point by raising the concentration of solutes in the body fluids (salt water has a lower freezing point than fresh water, for example). The antifreezes have multiple hydroxyl radicals in their molecules, which tend to bond with the hydrogen in the water molecules, thus greatly reducing their tendency to aggregate into ice crystals.

(Excerpted by permission of *Science 83* magazine. Copyright © the American Association for the Advancement of Science.)

31. Based on this article, we can surmise that one means by which some insects lessen the likelihood of their body fluids freezing is
    a. drinking salt water.
    b. beating their wings.
    c. flying long distances.
    d. eliminating body wastes.

32. The passage states that some insects slow their loss of heat by
    a. basking on dark surfaces.
    b. having hair and scales.
    c. increasing the number of nucleators.
    d. eating meals of blood.

33. The eggs of Arctic black flies contain
    a. trehalose.
    b. stored food.
    c. antifreeze.
    d. sorbitol.

34. Which of these substances most likely reduces the ice formation in the insects' body fluids?
    a. proteins
    b. acid
    c. polyhydric alcohols
    d. saturated lipids

35. According to the passage, when living tissue freezes,
    a. the cells lose fluid.
    b. the metabolic processes speed up.
    c. the cell membrane is destroyed.
    d. the concentration of solutes increases.

36. The tiny specks of dust in an insect's body fluids are referred to as
    a. antifreezes.
    b. glycols.
    c. trehaloses.
    d. nucleators.

Verbal Ability

359

SECTION A

SECTION B

SECTION C

COMPREHENSIVE PRACTICE Test 1

COMPREHENSIVE PRACTICE Test 2

COMPREHENSIVE PRACTICE Test 3

II

For the Jivaro Indians in the headwaters of the Amazon, beer is a greater necessity than solid food. Adult males drink from three to four gallons of it a day, adult females from one to two gallons, and a nine-year-old child will down half a gallon. Even though almost all of the protein in their diet must be obtained by going out to hunt, Jivaro hunters will often abandon the pursuit of prey and return to the settlement because the supply of beer is about to run out. Since women produce the beer, a man finds it desirable to acquire at least two wives so as to be able to entertain many guests and thus become known for his generosity. The Bemba also regard beer as equivalent to our notion of solid food; on days when beer is drunk, very little other food is eaten. The Bemba's high regard for beer as a major food is justified, because the sorghum from which it is made provides a number of B vitamins in which the rest of the diet is deficient, as well as a number of important minerals. A foreigner who sees Africans drinking beer, knowing that they are short of food, will usually condemn it—not realizing that beer is both a nutritional and a social necessity. If a man cannot give a beer party, even a small one, from time to time, he loses standing in his society. For the Bemba, providing beer is the most important way to repay social obligations, to honor kin, or to offer tribute to a chief. It rewards people who have given aid, and it is offered to deities. Tribal councils, marriages, and initiation ceremonies cannot take place without it. No wonder that the Bemba work hard at cultivating the land needed to produce enough grain for brewing.

Beer is similarly important in many modern societies; a pint of even a weak European beer provides nearly a tenth of the calcium and phosphorus needed daily, and about a fifth of the B vitamins, in addition to carbohydrates and several other vitamins and minerals—in effect serving as a liquid bread. In British villages and city neighborhoods, the pub is the focus for social life. It has long been the place for exchanging gossip, for the public airing and settlement of disputes, and for the reinforcement of friendships. A small village that loses its only pub loses much of what held the community together.

37. Which of the following titles is best for this passage?
    a. "Beer: A Multipurpose Drink"
    b. "The Nutritional Significance of Beer"
    c. "Beer: An International Drink"
    d. "The Social influence of Beer"

38. The Bemba brew a beer from
    a. sorghum.
    b. corn.
    c. barley.
    d. malt.

39. The authors compare beer nutritionally to
    a. milk.
    b. soup.
    c. bread.
    d. protein.

40. A foreign visitor to the Bemba tribe is likely to regard their beer consumption as
    a. frivolous.
    b. ceremonial.
    c. obligatory.
    d. nutritious.

41. According to the passage, the Jivaro men are likely to stop which of the following activities when there is little beer left to drink?
    a. hunting for meat
    b. performing tribal ceremonies
    c. offering tribute to a chief
    d. tending the fields

42. According to the passage, which of the following uses of beer in modern American society parallels a use of beer in the Bemba tribe?
    a. toasting friends at the local pub
    b. adding flavor to a sauce
    c. marking the end of the working day
    d. shampooing one's hair

III

The United States was born in Philadelphia on July 4, 1776, with approval of the Declaration of Independence, and squalled to life in September 1787 with the drafting of the Constitution. Though Independence Hall was the nursery for the foundling, the seed was implanted by William Penn a century earlier.

Penn, a socially prominent convert to the persecuted Society of Friends (Quakers), early resolved to provide an atmosphere in which all beliefs could flourish. His opportunity arrived when he requested the king to repay a crown debt to his father with a land grant in the colonies. Charles II, delighted with the prospect of easy payment while ridding the land of an embarrassing rebel, happily complied.

Penn's vision was simple but revolutionary—men of all faiths living in harmony and freedom. Even in the colonies, many of which were founded to foster religious tolerance, freedom of worship was limited to the majority sect. Penn guaranteed personal freedoms by allowing every taxpayer a vote, a prisoner the right to be heard, each man a trial by jury, and taxation only by law.

For his town, Philadelphia, Penn chose a site on the bluffs overlooking the Schuylkill . . . and Delaware Rivers, 70 miles up the broad Delaware from the Atlantic. Penn's utopia was the first city in the colonies to benefit from city planning. In laying out his "Greene Countrie Towne," Penn provided a geometric grid of straight streets, with provisions for five city parks—one in each quadrant and one in the center. Except for Center Square, which was usurped by City Hall, these original havens of green survive.

Halfway between the northern and southern colonies, Philadelphia provided a link between the sometimes divergent cultures. The atmosphere of personal freedom and intellectual stimulation attracted leading artists, statesmen, writers and politicians. (One such newcomer was 17-year-old Benjamin Franklin, who arrived in 1723 with hope in his heart and hardly a shilling in his pocket.) Within a century, Philadelphia had become the colonial center for art, science, education, politics, and commerce, and was the second largest English-speaking city in the world.

(Basic text reproduced by permission of the American Automobile Association, copyright owner.)

43. A good title for the passage would be
    a. "The Geography of Philadelphia."
    b. "William Penn's Biography."
    c. "Philadelphia's Beginnings."
    d. "The Society of Friends."

44. Penn was interested in building a city in which
    a. religious freedom was practiced.
    b. political activism was common.
    c. architectural design was advanced.
    d. monetary policy was set by the King.

45. It can be inferred from the passage that City Hall is located
    a. beside the Schuylkill River.
    b. along the Delaware River.
    c. in the northwest quadrant.
    d. in the center of the city.

46. According to the passage, the layout of the original streets most likely resembled
    a. concentric circles.
    b. wheel spokes.
    c. graph paper.
    d. parallel curves.

47. It can be inferred from the passage that Benjamin Franklin went to Philadelphia hoping for
    a. diplomatic training.
    b. intellectual development.
    c. economic improvement.
    d. religious freedom.

48. According to the passage, Philadelphia served as a
    a. gathering place for religious fanatics.
    b. haven for paupers.
    c. gateway to the other colonies.
    d. tie between two different societies.

IV

Using microcomputers, high-speed movie cameras, and a technique called synchronized electromyography, a Michigan University professor and a colleague disproved an old hypothesis that the tongues of frogs work like a crossbow when they feed on insects. The tongue of the common frog *Bufo marinus* works like a catapult, they reported in June 1982.

SECTION A

SECTION B

SECTION C

COMPREHENSIVE PRACTICE Test 1

COMPREHENSIVE PRACTICE Test 2

COMPREHENSIVE PRACTICE Test 3

To discover this, the researchers connected various muscle groups in the frog's throat by hair-like wires to machines that measured tiny increases in electrical voltage. Changes in voltage occurred when muscle fibers were stimulated by a signal from the frog's brain. By synchronizing these measurements with a 400-frames-a-second camera focused on the tongue, the researchers were able to isolate the major muscle groups involved in each action of the tongue.

Since this was pure research—the pursuit of knowledge for its own sake—the question arises: Does it have any practical use? One of the researchers, Dr. Carl Gans, responds that "first of all, my mother, who is 83 years old, was very pleased" when she read about it.

In a more serious vein, the 60-year-old biologist continues: "There certainly is a practical application for understanding how muscles move bone and how nerves control them. There's certainly a practical application for these fine-wire electrode techniques that I use. I teach a course in these techniques right now, and about half the people in the course are dentists."

Dentists are interested in using the techniques, he says, in the treatment of muscle and bone abnormalities of the human mouth.

Dr. Gans says he has since studied the tongues of three other frog species, and "they all work differently." One of the more interesting species, he says, is the *Rhinophrinus* of Mexico. Its tongue, he says, works "like a kind of artillery piece on a rolling carriage—the kind you used to have on ships of war back in the pirate days."

(Copyright © 1983 by The New York Times Company. Reprinted by permission.)

49. The method used to make this discovery included the
    a. measuring of nerve impulses.
    b. stimulation of muscle groups.
    c. constraint of tongue motion.
    d. confirmation of a recognized hypothesis.

50. It can be inferred from the passage that electromyography most likely means
    a. isolating muscle groups according to tongue action.
    b. implanting wires into muscle tissue.
    c. measuring electrical voltage associated with muscle movement.
    d. dissecting frog tissue with laser equipment.

51. It can be inferred from the passage that Dr. Gans recognized
    a. the possible rejection of his research by the medical community.
    b. his mother's lack of understanding of his work.
    c. the potential for criticism of his type of research.
    d. the reaction to his remark about his family.

52. It can be inferred that the research technique may be applied to
    a. deadening pain.
    b. correcting physical defects.
    c. controling caries.
    d. improving academic courses.

53. It can be inferred from the passage that Dr. Gans's hobby may be a study of
    a. economics.
    b. military art.
    c. naval history.
    d. cartography.

54. It can be inferred from the passage that tongue action in frogs
    a. has adapted to environmental needs.
    b. is similar in all species Gans has studied.
    c. cannot be analyzed using the special technique in most cases.
    d. does not require many impulses from the brain.

V

An electro-mechanical artificial leg that accepts subconscious signals from the wearer has been developed at the Moss Rehabilitation Hospital for use by people with amputations above the knee.

Howard Hillstrom, senior research scientist for the project, said Thursday that the prosthesis was set in motion when the wearer consciously or subconsciously sent signals to remaining muscles about the knee and hip.

The hospital says research on the project began three years ago, under the direction of Dr. Gordon D. Moskowitz, after studies showed that muscles remained active after a limb was removed.

By analyzing muscular activity at the hip and thigh, the team of researchers determined a reliable pattern that upper leg muscles follow when the knee is willed to flex or extend, the hospital said.

Additional research revealed that a portion of the energy dissipated by the muscles could be recovered and used to create motion.

The research team then created a prototype of the electro-mechanical leg that has been successfully tested on an amputee, the hospital reported.

The prosthesis is controlled by an external minicomputer that receives impulses, causing the leg to react, Mr. Hillstrom said.

"It's feasible that the minicomputer will be contained within the leg as research on the project continues," he said.

Through subconscious signals, the wearer may walk with minimal effort while conscious signals permit him or her to avoid obstacles and stumbling, Mr. Hillstrom said.

The research team says it hopes to have a clinical model of the device, called the Drexel-Moss knee, ready in three to five years.

An ultralight plastic prosthetic material, also developed at the hospital, will provide a natural-looking enclosure for the knee, the researchers said.

Other principal researchers on the project are Donald Meyers of the National Bureau of Standards in Washington, and Ronald Triolo, a research scientist at the hospital's rehabilitation engineering center.

SECTION A

SECTION B

SECTION C

COMPREHENSIVE PRACTICE Test 1

COMPREHENSIVE PRACTICE Test 2

COMPREHENSIVE PRACTICE Test 3

55. The main topic of this passage is the
    a. flow of brain waves to amputated limbs.
    b. research in muscle movement.
    c. energy produced by muscles.
    d. development of an amputee's device.

56. According to the passage, the preliminary research discovered that
    a. the knee is the focus of movement in the leg.
    b. muscles continue to function after surgery.
    c. a prosthesis can be fitted better to a stump above the knee.
    d. subconscious impulses can be relayed to minicomputers.

57. The result of the analysis of muscular activity was the discovery of
    a. the relationship between the hip and the thigh.
    b. the energy released after a movement.
    c. a specific routine of the muscles.
    d. a means to attach the prosthesis.

58. According to the passage, the development of the prosthesis has reached the
    a. implementation stage.
    b. production stage.
    c. design stage.
    d. pilot stage.

59. Currently, the minicomputer is located
    a. outside the body.
    b. inside the artificial leg.
    c. inside the amputee's stump.
    d. inside the amputee's head.

60. Research at the hospital has included work on artificial
    a. cartilage.
    b. ligaments.
    c. skin.
    d. nerves.

Mathematics

45 Minutes

Work each problem carefully. Use scrap paper to do your calculations. (The correct answers are at the end of this test.)

1. On a certain day, 85% of a school's student body is in attendance. Which of the following statements can be made with certainty?
   a. 85% of each class is present.
   b. 15% of the student body is absent.
   c. 85% attendance rate is normal for the student body.
   d. 15% of most classes is absent.

2. $2,652 \div 13 =$
   a. 24
   b. 204
   c. 240
   d. 2,040

3. $1\frac{4}{5} + 2\frac{1}{3} =$

   a. $3\frac{5}{8}$

   b. $3\frac{5}{12}$

   c. $3\frac{1}{5}$

   d. $4\frac{2}{15}$

4. A patient's caloric intake is 1,595 on Monday, 1,385 on Tuesday, 1,335 on Wednesday, and 1,725 on Thursday. What is that patient's average daily caloric intake over the 4 days?
   a. 1,205 Cal
   b. 1,507 Cal
   c. 1,510 Cal
   d. 6,040 Cal

5. A dieter lost an average of 0.5 lb per day over a 2-week period. If the dieter's weight was 135 lb initially, what was it at the end of these 2 weeks?
   a. 134 lb
   b. 128 lb
   c. 127.5 lb
   d. 125 lb

SECTION A

SECTION B

SECTION C

COMPREHENSIVE PRACTICE Test 1

COMPREHENSIVE PRACTICE Test 2

COMPREHENSIVE PRACTICE Test 3

6. $(14.3)(2.4) =$
   a. 5.958
   b. 16.7
   c. 29.2
   d. 34.32

7. What is the arithmetic average of 7, 9, 21, 1, and 2?
   a. 5
   b. 8
   c. 21
   d. 40

8. How many liters are in 2,750 mL?
   a. 275,000 L
   b. 2,750 L
   c. 2.75 L
   d. 0.00275 L

9. Round off 6,845.0793 to the nearest hundredth.
   a. 6,845.079
   b. 6,800.079
   c. 6,845.08
   d. 6,845.07

10. A child's temperature dropped an average of 0.2°F/hr over a 12-hr period. If the initial temperature was 102.4°F at 10 a.m., what was the reading at 10 p.m.?
    a. 102.2°F
    b. 101°F
    c. 100.2°F
    d. 100°F

11. $3 + 6(7) =$
    a. 16
    b. 45
    c. 63
    d. 126

12. To get 1 as an answer, you must multiply $\frac{7}{8}$ by
    a. $\frac{7}{8}$
    b. 1
    c. $\frac{8}{7}$
    d. $1\frac{1}{8}$

SECTION A

SECTION B

SECTION C

COMPREHENSIVE PRACTICE Test 1

COMPREHENSIVE PRACTICE Test 2

COMPREHENSIVE PRACTICE Test 3

13. Young's rule states that the drug dose for a child is determined by the following formula:

$$\text{child's dose} = \frac{C}{C + 12} \times \text{adult dose}$$

where C = the child's age in years.

If the adult dose of medication is 6 mg, how much of the medication should you give a 6-year-old child?

a. 1 mg
b. 2 mg
c. 3 mg
d. 6 mg

14. An antibiotic solution contains 180,000 units per 1 mL of solution. How many milliliters are needed to provide 540,000 units?

a. $\frac{1}{3}$ mL

b. $\frac{1}{4}$ mL

c. $1\frac{1}{3}$ mL

d. 3 mL

15. $48.41 \div 0.47 =$
a. 103
b. 13.0
c. 10.3
d. 1.03

16. May Smith went into labor at 10:35 p.m. Her labor lasted 11 hr 45 min. At what time was her baby born?
a. 9:55 a.m.
b. 10:10 a.m.
c. 10:20 a.m.
d. 11:15 a.m.

17. The daily cost of a bed in a certain hospital is $225. If the cost rises 12%, what will the daily cost be?
a. $237
b. $252
c. $260
d. $270

18. If $4x + 3 = 7x - 12$, then $x =$
a. 12
b. 5
c. -5
d. $\frac{12}{7}$

19. $\frac{1}{2}$ of $\left(\frac{1}{3} + \frac{1}{6}\right) =$

   a. $\frac{1}{4}$

   b. 1

   c. $\frac{4}{6}$

   d. $\frac{1}{9}$

20. Before starting a diet, a person consumed an average of 3,000 Cal/day. While dieting, that person consumed an average of 1,800 Cal/day. By what percentage did the calories consumed decrease?

   a. 16.6%
   b. 40%
   c. 60%
   d. 66%

21. The following formula can be used to convert temperature from Fahrenheit to Centigrade. How many degrees Fahrenheit are equivalent to 40°C?

   $$C = \frac{5}{9}(°F - 32)$$

   a. −9.8°F
   b. 8°F
   c. 14.4°F
   d. 104.0°F

22. A jogger averages $\frac{4}{5}$ mi in 9 min. If this speed is maintained, how many miles can the jogger run per hour?

   a. $5\frac{1}{3}$ mi

   b. $7\frac{1}{5}$ mi

   c. $8\frac{1}{5}$ mi

   d. $8\frac{1}{3}$ mi

23. In a health club, the ratio of joggers to swimmers is 7:2. For every 40 swimmers, how many joggers would we expect to find in this club?

   a. 280 joggers
   b. 140 joggers
   c. 129 joggers
   d. 11 joggers

24. Which of these fractions is the equivalent of 0.45?

    a. $\dfrac{1}{45}$

    b. $\dfrac{9}{20}$

    c. $\dfrac{4}{5}$

    d. $\dfrac{5}{9}$

25. On a scale drawing of a room, 1 in represents 3 ft. How many feet are represented by $5\dfrac{3}{4}$ in?

    a. $15\dfrac{3}{4}$ ft

    b. 18 ft

    c. $17\dfrac{1}{4}$ ft

    d. 19 ft

26. If $\dfrac{1}{3}$ of $x = 40$, then $\dfrac{3}{8}$ of $x =$

    a. 15

    b. 45

    c. 106.67

    d. 120

27. 4.6% of 150 =

    a. 690

    b. 32.6

    c. 6.9

    d. 3.26

28. If $\dfrac{2}{3}$ c of coleslaw provides 60 Cal, how many calories are provided by $\dfrac{1}{2}$ c of coleslaw?

    a. 20 Cal

    b. 30 Cal

    c. 40 Cal

    d. 45 Cal

29. What is the maximum number of $\dfrac{3}{4}$-lb bags of nuts that can be made from 48 lb?

    a. 16 bags

    b. 36 bags

    c. 60 bags

    d. 64 bags

SECTION A

SECTION B

SECTION C

COMPREHENSIVE PRACTICE Test 1

COMPREHENSIVE PRACTICE Test 2

COMPREHENSIVE PRACTICE Test 3

30. A shopper bought 6.3 lb of potatoes for $4.41 and 4.9 lb of tomatoes for $3.92. Which vegetable costs less per pound and by how much?
    a. Potatoes cost 18¢/lb less.
    b. Tomatoes cost 10¢/lb less.
    c. Tomatoes cost 18¢/lb less.
    d. Potatoes cost 10¢/lb less.

31. 125% of what number = 80?
    a. 0.64
    b. 60
    c. 64
    d. 100

32. What is the perimeter of a rectangle that is 15 cm long and 6 cm high?
    a. 21 cm
    b. 42 cm
    c. 90 cm
    d. 180 cm

33. A rectangle has a perimeter of 50 cm. If this rectangle is 10 cm wide, how many centimeters long is it?
    a. 5 cm
    b. 15 cm
    c. 30 cm
    d. 40 cm

34. Which of these percentages is another way of expressing $5.15x$?
    a. 515% of x
    b. 51.5% of x
    c. 5.15% of x
    d. 0.0515% of x

35. What percentage of 125 is 375?
    a. 33.33%
    b. 250%
    c. 300%
    d. 468.75%

36. A multivitamin that contains 0.5 mg of vitamin B_6 supplies 23% of the U.S. Recommended Daily Allowance (USRDA) of that vitamin for adults. Find, to the nearest tenth of a milligram, the USRDA of vitamin B_6 for adults.
    a. 2.2 mg
    b. 2.0 mg
    c. 0.2 mg
    d. 0.5 mg

37. Factor completely: $x^2 - 81$.
    a. $(x + 9)(x - 9)$
    b. $2x^3 - 81$
    c. $(x - 9)^2$
    d. $x(x - 81)$

38. A patient's room measures 10 ft wide by 15 ft long. By how much would the area of this room increase if the room were 1 ft longer and 1 ft wider?
    a. 10 ft^2
    b. 15 ft^2
    c. 25 ft^2
    d. 26 ft^2

39. $2(x + 3y) + 3(x + 2y) =$
    a. $5(2x + 5y)$
    b. $5x + 5y$
    c. $5x + 10y$
    d. $5x + 12y$

40. A discount pharmacy takes $1 off prescription medicines that cost between $20 and $40. Which of these statements best describes the rate of discount for prescriptions in this price range?
    a. The same discount rate is applied to all prescriptions.
    b. The average discount rate is 3.75%.
    c. The discount rate is higher for the less expensive prescriptions.
    d. The discount rate is higher for the more expensive prescriptions.

SECTION A

SECTION B

SECTION C

COMPREHENSIVE PRACTICE Test 1

COMPREHENSIVE PRACTICE Test 2

COMPREHENSIVE PRACTICE Test 3

Science

45 Minutes

Read each question carefully, and then select the correct answer. (The correct answers are at the end of this test.)

1. Which of these chemicals is often added to drinking water to help prevent cavities?
   a. calcium carbonate
   b. tin (II) fluoride
   c. potassium phosphate
   d. zinc chloride

2. What would be a likely result if all the bees and butterflies in an area were destroyed?
   a. Birds would have more food.
   b. More plant seeds would be produced.
   c. More flowers would bloom.
   d. Fewer plant seeds would be produced.

3. Most carbon dioxide leaves the blood through the capillaries of the
   a. kidney.
   b. heart.
   c. lung.
   d. liver.

4. Alcohol can be classified in which of the following drug categories?
   a. depressants
   b. stimulants
   c. barbiturates
   d. amphetamines

5. The following diagram shows a lever with a heavy box on one end. The arrows show the location and direction of four possible forces applied to the lever. Which one will require the least effort to lift the box if the force is in the direction and at the point shown by the arrow?

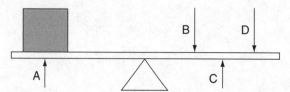

   a. A
   b. B
   c. C
   d. D

6. Which of the arrows in the following graph represents the wavelength of the wave shown?

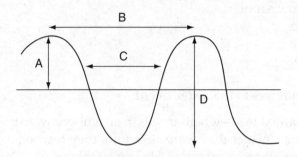

a. A
b. B
c. C
d. D

7. Which of the following is given to provide immunity to an infectious disease?
   a. an antibiotic
   b. a barbiturate
   c. an antiseptic
   d. a vaccine

8. Missing links are important to the study of
   a. evolution.
   b. budding yeast.
   c. food webs.
   d. chemical bonds.

9. What is the temperature reading on the thermometer? (It is calibrated in degrees Fahrenheit.)

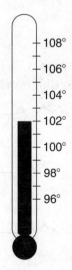

a. 100.7°F
b. 101.2°F
c. 101.4°F
d. 102.0°F

SECTION **A**

SECTION **B**

SECTION **C**

COMPREHENSIVE PRACTICE **Test 1**

COMPREHENSIVE PRACTICE **Test 2**

COMPREHENSIVE PRACTICE **Test 3**

10. A closed container of hydrogen gas is warmed from 20°C to 25°C. If the volume remains the same, what will happen to the pressure inside the container?
    a. It will remain the same.
    b. It will decrease.
    c. It will fluctuate.
    d. It will increase.

The next question refers to this experiment:

Hans Spemann wanted to see whether cells in an embryo were different from the time they started to divide or whether they were alike until they reached a certain stage. He worked with very young salamander embryos. He knew which part normally develops into nerve cells and which into skin cells. He cut these parts out and reversed their positions. They grew into cells like the areas around them: Skin became nerve and nerve became skin. Then he tried the experiment again with older embryos. This time each patch of skin or nerve stayed what it had been before.

11. These results support which of the following conclusions?
    a. Very young salamander embryo cells are all alike and can develop into any tissue.
    b. Young salamander embryo cells are specialized from the beginning.
    c. Very young salamander embryo cells all resemble nerve cells.
    d. Older salamander embryo nerve cells can become skin cells.

12. Which of these particles is always electrically charged?
    a. an ion
    b. a molecule
    c. an atom
    d. a neutron

13. A nucleotide that contains uracil would most likely be found in the compound
    a. NADH.
    b. ATP.
    c. RNA.
    d. DNA.

14. Which type of circuit is shown in the diagram?

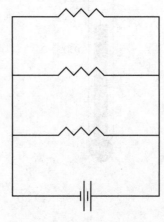

a. open
b. complex
c. series
d. parallel

15. The device shown in the following circuit diagram consists of copper wire wrapped around an iron rod and connected to a switch and a battery.

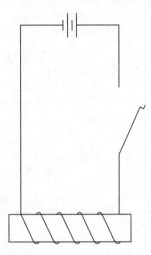

When the switch is closed, the device could serve as
a. a transformer.
b. an electromagnet.
c. a motor.
d. a generator.

16. Two forces act on an object as shown in the diagram.

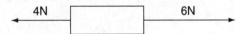

The magnitude of the net force on the object, in newtons, is
a. 2 N.
b. 6 N.
c. 10 N.
d. 24 N.

17. Most fungi differ from green plants in that fungi lack
a. cellulose.
b. cytoplasm.
c. chlorophyll.
d. enzymes.

18. Which structure in the brain is responsible for regulating the heartbeat?
a. medulla
b. cerebellum
c. cerebrum
d. dura mater

SECTION A

SECTION B

SECTION C

COMPREHENSIVE PRACTICE Test 1

COMPREHENSIVE PRACTICE Test 2

COMPREHENSIVE PRACTICE Test 3

19. Which of these gases causes eye irritation?
    a. nitrogen
    b. helium
    c. carbon dioxide
    d. sulfur oxide

20. Which of the following graphs best indicates the relationship between time and the velocity of a freely falling object?

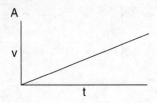
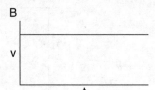

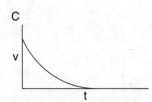
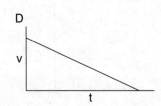

    a. A
    b. B
    c. C
    d. D

21. The code of a gene is delivered to the ribosome by
    a. a DNA molecule.
    b. a hormone.
    c. a messenger RNA molecule.
    d. an enzyme.

22. All organisms (autotrophs and heterotrophs) use the chemical process of respiration to make
    a. glucose.
    b. ATP.
    c. RNA.
    d. oxygen.

23. Which of these diagrams correctly shows a water wave passing through a small opening in a barrier?

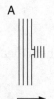
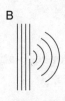

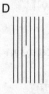

a. A
b. B
c. C
d. D

24. In which organ does the blood lose urea and reabsorb glucose?
    a. spleen
    b. kidney
    c. liver
    d. lymph nodes

Questions 25 through 27 refer to this chart showing approximate energy expenditure in a variety of activities:

Activity	Time (hr)	Men Rate (cal/min)	Total	Women Rate (cal/min)	Total
Sleeping	8	1.1	530	1.0	480
Sitting, driving a car, bench work	6	1.5	540	1.1	400
Standing or limited walking	6	2.5	900	1.5	540
Walking, purposeful, outdoors	2	3.0	360	2.5	300
Occupational activities involving light physical work, weekend swimming	2	4.5	540	3.0	360
	24		2,870		2,080

(Chart adapted from *Recommended Dietary Allowances*, 6th ed. *Report of Food and Nutrition Board* [Public 1146], National Academy of Sciences—National Research Council, Washington, D.C., 1964.)

25. In which of the following activities do men expend energy most rapidly?
    a. bench work
    b. limited walking
    c. walking outdoors
    d. light physical work

26. In which of the following activities do women use the highest number of calories over a 24-hour period?
    a. sleeping
    b. sitting, driving a car, bench work
    c. standing or limited walking
    d. light physical work and sports

SECTION A
SECTION B
SECTION C
COMPREHENSIVE PRACTICE Test 1
COMPREHENSIVE PRACTICE Test 2
COMPREHENSIVE PRACTICE Test 3

27. Based on the data, which of these conclusions can be drawn?
    a. The numbers of calories used by men and women are the most similar for purposeful walking activities.
    b. Men use calories as rapidly sitting as women do walking outdoors.
    c. Women use calories more quickly than men do when driving a car.
    d. Women burn calories more slowly than men do in all activities listed.

28. An equal arm balance is balanced when 20 washers are on one side and 10 bolts are on the other. Four bolts are added to one side. How many washers must be added to the other side to maintain balance?
    a. 14 washers
    b. 8 washers
    c. 4 washers
    d. 2 washers

Questions 29 and 30 refer to the following chart.

Solubility in water

	carbonate	chloride	hydroxide	iodide	nitrate	sulfate
Aluminum	n	s	i	s	s	s
Ammonium	s	s	s	s	s	s
Barium	i	s	i	s	s	i
Calcium	i	s	ss	s	s	ss
Copper II	i	s	i	d	s	ss
Iron III	n	s	i	n	s	ss
Lead	i	ss	i	ss	s	i
Potassium	s	s	s	s	s	s
Silver	i	i	n	i	s	ss
Sodium	s	s	s	s	s	s
Zinc	i	s	i	s	s	s

KEY

d	decomposes
i	insoluble
n	not isolated
s	soluble
ss	slightly soluble

29. Which of these compounds is the most soluble?
    a. lead chloride
    b. lead hydroxide
    c. lead iodide
    d. lead nitrate

30. Which of these compounds reacts with water?
    a. aluminum carbonate
    b. barium hydroxide
    c. copper II iodide
    d. lead chloride

31. Bones have several functions. Which of the following pairs of bones contain bones whose principal function is protection of organs?
    a. radius and ulna
    b. cranium and rib cage
    c. patella and humerus
    d. pelvis and femur

32. The following table shows the melting and boiling points for four substances.

Substance	Melting Point	Boiling Point
W	240°F	105°F
X	10°F	80°F
Y	105°F	1,600°F
Z	115°F	280°F

Which of these substances is a liquid over the smallest temperature range?
    a. W
    b. X
    c. Y
    d. Z

33. A solution of sodium hydroxide is being added, drop by drop, to a solution of hydrochloric acid. Which of these chemical processes is likely to occur?
    a. hydrogenation
    b. oxidation
    c. reduction
    d. neutralization

34. The bond in sodium chloride is
    a. covalent.
    b. dipole.
    c. ionic.
    d. nuclear.

35. What type of immunity is present when the body develops antibodies after illness?
    a. active
    b. inborn
    c. passive
    d. artificial

SECTION A

SECTION B

SECTION C

COMPREHENSIVE PRACTICE Test 1

COMPREHENSIVE PRACTICE Test 2

COMPREHENSIVE PRACTICE Test 3

Questions 36 and 37 refer to this diagram of the human eye:

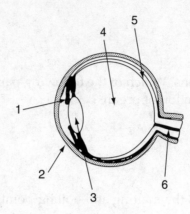

36. Rods and cones are found in the structure labeled
    a. 1.
    b. 2.
    c. 5.
    d. 6.

37. Light entering the eye is normally finely focused for near vision by the action of the structure numbered
    a. 2.
    b. 3.
    c. 4.
    d. 6.

38. Which of these microscopes is used to study the structure of a virus?
    a. interference
    b. phase-contrast
    c. compound light
    d. electron

39. Many people believe that the reason maple trees drop their leaves in the late fall is that the temperature is near freezing. Which of the following statements would *least* support this idea?
    a. Maple trees in South Florida drop their leaves in late fall.
    b. Maple trees growing near city lights stay green longer than those far from the lights.
    c. Maple trees in northern Minnesota drop their leaves in late fall.
    d. Maple trees pass through a time of near freezing before they bud.

40. A student wanted to test the effects different sugars have on the growth of a certain mold. The sugars to be tested were glucose, fructose, and sucrose. One gram of each sugar was placed in a tube of 10 mL of water, and a bit of the mold was put in each of the three solutions. To add a control to the experiment, the student should also have
    a. made two setups of each of the three sugars.
    b. made one setup of just water and mold.
    c. tested ribose and galactose sugars.
    d. kept the three setups in the light.

SECTION A

SECTION B

SECTION C

COMPREHENSIVE PRACTICE Test 1

COMPREHENSIVE PRACTICE Test 2

COMPREHENSIVE PRACTICE Test 3

41. Which of these substances is associated with the process of cell respiration?
    a. ATP
    b. RNA
    c. DNA
    d. Rh factor

42. The following sequence of activities occurs during sexual reproduction:
    formation of egg and sperm − x − rapid cell division − new organism
    Which activity is represented by x?
    a. meiosis
    b. fertilization
    c. protein synthesis
    d. cleavage

43. In which way do white blood cells differ from red blood cells?
    a. The body produces more white blood cells.
    b. White blood cells contain hemoglobin.
    c. Some white blood cells are capable of amoebalike movement.
    d. White blood cells carry oxygen.

44. Blue litmus paper turns red when placed in a solution having which of the following pH values?
    a. 14
    b. 12
    c. 7
    d. 3

45. The speed of sound in air is approximately
    a. 1,100 ft/sec.
    b. 1,100 ft/min.
    c. 4,400 ft/min.
    d. 186,000 ft/sec.

46. As the temperature of a solvent increases, the solubility of a solid solute generally
    a. increases.
    b. decreases.
    c. remains the same.
    d. depends on pressure.

47. Which of these diagrams correctly shows the shape of the magnetic field in the vicinity of two magnets whose north poles are facing each other?

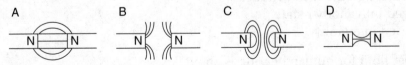

    a. A
    b. B
    c. C
    d. D

48. There are 5 g of salt dissolved in 25 mL of water solution. What percentage solution is it?
    a. 5%
    b. 12.5%
    c. 20%
    d. 25%

49. What kind of electrical charge does an electron have?
    a. negative
    b. neutral
    c. magnetic
    d. positive

50. In this diagram of a bean seed, which letter represents stored food for the growing embryo?

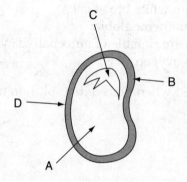

    a. A
    b. B
    c. C
    d. D

51. In plants, the opening and closing of stomates is controlled by
    a. sieve cells.
    b. root hairs.
    c. transpiration.
    d. guard cells.

52. Many chemical reactions occur more rapidly with platinum as a catalyst. At the end of such reactions, the platinum is found to be
    a. unchanged in weight.
    b. combined into the final product.
    c. changed into another state.
    d. increased in quantity.

53. The upper limit for human hearing is about
    a. 400 vibrations per second.
    b. 2,000 vibrations per second.
    c. 20,000 vibrations per second.
    d. 40,000 vibrations per second.

54. Which of the following substances is consumed during cell respiration?
    a. water
    b. amylase
    c. urea
    d. glucose

55. If a plain soda cracker is chewed slowly, after a while it begins to taste more
    a. bland.
    b. bitter.
    c. sweet.
    d. salty.

56. An example of asexual reproduction in plants is
    a. the fusion of gametes.
    b. pollination by a bee.
    c. an onion bulb.
    d. a fruit.

57. Which of these structures secretes a substance that controls the rate of beard growth and the deepening of the voice in men as they mature?
    a. thymus
    b. adrenal glands
    c. testes
    d. parathyroid glands

58. Two atoms are isotopes if they have the same atomic number but a different number of
    a. neutrons.
    b. mesons.
    c. electrons.
    d. protons.

59. How much of 12 g of a radioactive isotope with a half-life of 20 years will be left after 40 years?
    a. 0 g
    b. 3 g
    c. 6 g
    d. 8 g

60. A ball is moving with *no* forces acting on it. The ball will
    a. accelerate.
    b. slow down and stop.
    c. slow down but not stop.
    d. maintain its velocity.

SECTION A

SECTION B

SECTION C

COMPREHENSIVE PRACTICE Test 1

COMPREHENSIVE PRACTICE Test 2

COMPREHENSIVE PRACTICE Test 3

Answers to Comprehensive Practice Test 3

ANSWERS TO COMPREHENSIVE PRACTICE TEST 3: VERBAL ABILITY

1.	b	21.	d	41.	a
2.	b	22.	a	42.	a
3.	c	23.	a	43.	c
4.	d	24.	c	44.	a
5.	b	25.	a	45.	d
6.	c	26.	a	46.	c
7.	c	27.	b	47.	c
8.	b	28.	a	48.	d
9.	d	29.	c	49.	b
10.	d	30.	b	50.	c
11.	a	31.	d	51.	c
12.	b	32.	b	52.	b
13.	d	33.	b	53.	c
14.	b	34.	c	54.	a
15.	c	35.	c	55.	d
16.	d	36.	d	56.	b
17.	d	37.	a	57.	c
18.	b	38.	a	58.	d
19.	b	39.	c	59.	a
20.	c	40.	a	60.	c

ANSWERS TO COMPREHENSIVE PRACTICE TEST 3: MATHEMATICS

1. **The answer is b.** If 85% of the student body is present, then 15% of the same group—the student body—must be absent, because the two percentages must total 100% (the entire student body). Choices a, c, and d cannot be inferred from this information. We do not know about individual classes or normal rates.

2. **The answer is b.** This problem requires long division.

$$\frac{204}{13)\overline{2,652}}$$

You can check your answer by multiplying 13 by 204. If you have divided correctly, the product of 13 and 204 will be 2,652.

3.   **The answer is d.** First, find a common denominator for $\frac{4}{5}$ and $\frac{2}{3}$, and then write equivalent fractions. The LCD (lowest common denominator) is 15, because 3 and 5 are factors of 15.

$$1\frac{4}{5} = 1\frac{12}{15}$$

$$2\frac{1}{3} = 2\frac{5}{15}$$

$$1\frac{12}{15} + 2\frac{5}{15} = 3\frac{17}{15} = 4\frac{2}{15}$$

You cannot leave an improper fraction in your answer; so convert $\frac{7}{15}$ into 1 whole ($\frac{15}{15}$), and add this whole to 3. This gives you 4, with $\frac{2}{15}$ left over.

4.   **The answer is c.** Add the four daily totals: $1{,}595 + 1{,}385 + 1{,}335 + 1{,}725 = 6{,}040$. Now divide this total by 4 to find the daily average.

$$\frac{1{,}510}{4\overline{)6{,}040}}$$

5.   **The answer is b.** First calculate how much weight the dieter lost over the 2-week period. To do this, multiply the average daily weight loss by the number of days in 2 weeks (14). $.0.5 \text{ lb/day} \times 14 \text{ days} = 7 \text{ lb}$

Now subtract 7 from the dieter's initial weight of 135 lb to find out how much the dieter weighed at the end of the 2-week period: $135 \text{ lb} - 7 \text{ lb} = 128 \text{ lb}$.

6.   **The answer is d.** Remember, to multiply decimals, you may ignore the decimal points until the very end of the problem. When you finish multiplying, total the decimal points in the numbers you are multiplying, and, starting from the rightmost digit, count to the left the same number of places.

     14.3 1 decimal point
    × 2.4 1 decimal point

     572
    + 2860

     34.32 2 decimal points

7.   **The answer is b.** To find the arithmetic average, add the numbers: $7 + 9 + 21 + 1 + 2 = 40$. Then divide this sum by the numbers you have added up: $40 \div 5 = 8$.

SECTION A

SECTION B

SECTION C

COMPREHENSIVE PRACTICE Test 1

COMPREHENSIVE PRACTICE Test 2

COMPREHENSIVE PRACTICE Test 3

8. **The answer is c.** You must recall that there are 1,000 mL in 1 L. To change milliliters to liters, you divide by 1,000, that is, move the decimal point 3 places to the left.

$$\frac{2,750 \text{ mL}}{1,000 \text{ mL/L}} = 2.75 \text{ L}$$

9. **The answer is c.** To round off to the nearest hundredth, you must examine the digit in the thousandths place; if it is 5 or bigger, round the hundredths digit up 1. If it is less than 5, the hundredths digit remains the same. In the given number, 6,845.0793, the digit in the thousandths place (9) is larger than 5. Therefore, you round the digit in the hundredths place up 1, from 7 to 8.

10. **The answer is d.** To find the total drop in temperature, multiply the average hourly drop of 0.2°F by the total number of hours, 12.
$0.2°\text{F/hr} \times 12 \text{ hr} = 2.4°\text{F drop}$
Now subtract this from the initial temperature of 102.4°F to find the reading 12 hours later.
$102.4°\text{F} - 2.4°\text{F} = 100°\text{F}$

11. **The answer is b.** Follow the order of operations to solve this problem. Multiply 6 and 7 first, and then add 3 to the product:
$3 + (6)7 =$
$3 + 42 = 45$

12. **The answer is c.** The reciprocal of $\frac{7}{8}$ is $\frac{8}{7}$, which is defined as the number needed to multiply by in order to obtain a product of 1. The reciprocal of $\frac{7}{8}$ is just what we need in this case.

$$\frac{7}{8} \times \frac{8}{7} = \frac{56}{56} = 1$$

13. **The answer is b.** To solve this problem, substitute the known amounts into the formula.

$$\text{child's dose} = \frac{C}{C + 12} \times \text{adult dose}$$

$$\text{child's dose} = \frac{6}{6 + 12} \times 6 \text{ mg}$$

Simplify.

$$\frac{6}{18} \times \frac{6}{1} = \frac{36}{18} = 2 \text{ mg}$$

14. **The answer is d.** You may set up a proportion to solve this problem. Be sure to align the units correctly: milliliters across from milliliters and units across from units.

$$\frac{180,000 \text{ units}}{1 \text{ mL}} = \frac{540,000 \text{ units}}{x \text{ mL}}$$

Cross-multiply, and divide both sides by 450,000 to solve for x.
$1,800,000\ x = 540,000$

$$x = \frac{54}{18} = 3\ \text{mL}$$

You can also solve this by noting that

$$\frac{540,000\ \text{units}}{180,000\ \text{units/mL}} = 3\ \text{mL}$$

15. **The answer is a.** To divide decimals, you must make sure the divisor (the number outside the box) is a whole number. In this case, move the decimal 2 places to the right to change 0.47 to 47. You must move the decimal 2 places to the right in the dividend as well.

$$48.41 \div 0.47 = 0.47\overline{)48.41} = 47\overline{)4{,}841}\ \ (= 103)$$

16. **The answer is c.** If May Smith's labor had lasted a full 12 hr, her baby would have been delivered at 10:35 a.m. However, her labor was 15 min less than 12 hr; so subtract 15 min from 10:35 a.m. to arrive at her delivery time of 10:20 a.m.

17. **The answer is b.** This problem involves percentage increase. Solve this problem in three steps. First, turn 12% into a decimal by dividing by 100.

$12\% \div 100 = 0.12$
Calculate 12% of $225 by multiplying.

$$\begin{array}{r} 225 \\ \times\ 0.12 \\ \hline 27.00 \end{array}$$

Finally, add this amount to the original price to find the new price.
$225 + $27 = $252
You can also solve this problem by finding 112% of $225.

18. **The answer is b.** Subtract 3 from both sides, subtract $7x$ from both sides, and then divide both sides by -3 to solve for x.
$$\begin{array}{r} 4x + 3 = 7x - 12 \\ -3 \qquad\qquad -3 \\ \hline 4x = 7x - 15 \\ -7x - 7x \\ \hline -3x = -15 \\ x = 5 \end{array}$$

19. **The answer is a.** Add the fractions in the parentheses first (you will need to find a common denominator), and then multiply that sum by $\frac{1}{2}$. Remember to reduce your answer.

$$\frac{1}{2} \times \left(\frac{1}{3} + \frac{1}{6}\right) = \frac{1}{2} \times \left(\frac{2}{6} + \frac{1}{6}\right) = \frac{1}{2} \times \frac{3}{6} = \frac{3}{12} = \frac{1}{4}$$

SECTION A

SECTION B

SECTION C

COMPREHENSIVE PRACTICE Test 1

COMPREHENSIVE PRACTICE Test 2

COMPREHENSIVE PRACTICE Test 3

20. **The answer is b.** This problem involves percentage decrease. Solve this problem in two steps. First, calculate the drop in average daily calorie consumption.

3,000 Cal/day − 1,800 Cal/day = 1,200 Cal/day

Second, calculate what percentage 1,200 (the drop) is of 3,000 (the original total).

$$\frac{1,200}{3,000} = \frac{12}{30} = \frac{2}{5}$$

Convert the fraction into a decimal: 2 ÷ 5 = 0.4. Multiply 0.4 by 100 to find the percentage: 0.4 × 100 = 40%.

21. **The answer is d.** Substitute 40° for C in the formula, and then solve for °F.

$$C = \frac{5}{9}\,(^\circ F - 32)$$

$$40 = \frac{5}{9}\,(^\circ F - 32)$$

Multiply both sides of the equation by $\frac{9}{5}$, simplify, and add 32 to both sides.

$$\frac{40}{1} \times \frac{9}{5} = \frac{5}{9} \times \frac{9}{5}\,(^\circ F - 32)$$

$$\frac{360}{5} = (^\circ F - 32)$$

$$72 = (^\circ F - 32)$$
$$F = 104^\circ$$

22. **The answer is a.** You may set up a proportion to solve this problem. As always, make sure you align the units properly: miles across from miles and minutes across from minutes.

$$\frac{\frac{4}{5}\,\text{mi}}{9\,\text{min}} = \frac{x\,\text{mi}}{60\,\text{min}}$$

Cross-multiply, simplify, and divide both sides by 9 to solve for x.

$$9x = 60 \times \frac{4}{5}$$

$$9x = \frac{240}{5}$$

$$9x = 48$$

$$x = \frac{48}{9} = 5\frac{3}{9} = 5\frac{1}{3}$$

23. **The answer is b.** You may set up a proportion to solve this problem. As always, make sure you align the units correctly: joggers across from joggers and swimmers across from swimmers.

$$\frac{7\,\text{joggers}}{2\,\text{swimmers}} = \frac{x\,\text{joggers}}{40\,\text{swimmers}}$$

Cross-multiply, and divide both sides by 2 to solve for x.

$$2x = 280$$
$$x = 140\,\text{joggers}$$

SECTION A

SECTION B

SECTION C

COMPREHENSIVE PRACTICE Test 1

COMPREHENSIVE PRACTICE Test 2

COMPREHENSIVE PRACTICE Test 3

24. **The answer is b.** Because 0.45 ends in the hundredths place, change it to a fraction by placing 45 over 100 and reducing the fraction by dividing by 5.

$$0.45 = \frac{45}{100} = \frac{9}{20}$$

25. **The answer is c.** You may set up a proportion to solve this problem. As always, make sure you align the units correctly: inches across from inches, and feet across from feet.

$$\frac{1 \text{ in}}{3 \text{ ft}} = \frac{5\frac{3}{4} \text{ in}}{x \text{ ft}}$$

Cross-multiply to solve for x, and change $5\frac{3}{4}$ to an improper fraction.

$$x = 3 \times 5\frac{3}{4}$$

$$x = \frac{3}{1} \times \frac{23}{4} = \frac{69}{4} = 17\frac{1}{4} \text{ ft}$$

You can also solve this problem by multiplying $5\frac{3}{4}$ in by 3 ft/in

$$5\frac{3}{4} \text{ in} \times 3 \text{ ft/in} = 17\frac{1}{4} \text{ in}$$

26. **The answer is b.** First, solve for x by multiplying both sides by 3. Then substitute 120 for x, and multiply by $\frac{3}{8}$.

$$\frac{1}{3}x = 10$$

$$3 \times \frac{1}{3}x = 40 \times 3$$

$$x = 120$$

$$\frac{3}{8} \times 120 = \frac{360}{8} = 45$$

27. **The answer is c.** Change 4.6% to a decimal by dividing by 100: $4.6\% \div 100 = 0.046$. Then multiply 0.046 by 150 to find your answer.
$0.046 \times 150 = 6.900 = 6.9$

28. **The answer is d.** You may set up a proportion to solve this problem. As usual, make sure you align the units correctly: cups across from cups and calories across from calories.

$$\frac{\frac{2}{3} c}{60 \text{ cal}} = \frac{\frac{1}{2} c}{x \text{ cal}}$$

Cross-multiply, simplify, and multiply both sides by $\frac{3}{2}$ to solve for x.

$$\frac{2}{3}x = \frac{1}{2}60$$

$$\frac{2}{3}x = 30$$

$$x = \frac{3}{2}30$$

$$x = \frac{90}{2} = 45 \text{ cal}$$

You can also solve this problem by realizing that, if $\frac{2}{3}$ c provides 60 cal, then 1 c provides 90 cal and $\frac{1}{2} \times 90 = 45$ cal.

29. **The answer is d.** This question is really asking how many groups of $\frac{3}{4}$ s there are in 48. This is division:

$$48 \text{ lb} \div \frac{3}{4} \text{ lb} =$$

Invert the divisor and multiply.

$$\frac{48}{1} \times \frac{4}{3} =$$

$$\frac{192}{3} = 64 \text{ bags}$$

30. **The answer is d.** To find out how much each pound of potatoes cost, divide the total cost by the total number of pounds. Do the same for the tomatoes. Then compare the results.

$$\frac{\$4.41}{6.3 \text{ lbs}} = \$0.70/\text{lb potatoes}$$

$$\frac{\$3.92}{4.9 \text{ lbs}} = \$0.80/\text{lb tomatoes}$$

$0.80 \text{ (tomatoes)} - \$0.70 \text{ (potatoes)} = \$0.10$

The potatoes cost 10¢/lb less

31. **The answer is c.** Turn the problem into an equation and solve for x.

125% of what number = 80?
$1.25 \times x = 80$
$1.25x = 80$
Divide both sides by 1.25 to solve for x.
$x = 64$

32. **The answer is b.** Use this formula to find the perimeter (P) of a rectangle:
$P = 2w \times 2l$
where w = width and l = length. Substitute 15 cm for length and 6 cm for width:
$P = 2(15) + 2(6) = 30 + 12 = 42$ cm

33. **The answer is b.** Use the perimeter (P) formula to find the length.
$P = 2w \times 2l$
where w = width and l = length. Substitute 50 cm for perimeter and 10 cm for width, subtract 20 from both sides, and divide both sides by 2 to solve for l.
$50 = 2(10) + 2l$
$50 = 20 + 2l$
$\underline{-20 \quad -20}$
$30 = 2l$

$\quad \div 2 \qquad \div 2$

$l = 15$

34. **The answer is a.** To convert 5.15 into a percentage, multiply by 100, and tack on a percentage (%) sign.
$5.15 \times 100 = 515\%$
$\quad 5.15x = 515\%$ of x

35. **The answer is c.** This is one of three types of common percentage problems: finding the percentage when you know the base and the percent. First convert the word problem into an equation.
What percentage of 125 is 375?
$x\% \times 125 = 375$
Deal with x being a percentage at the end of the problem. Divide both sides by 125, and change the result to a percentage.
$125x = 375$
$x = 3 \times 100 = 300\%$
You may also solve this problem by setting up a fraction:
$$\frac{375}{125} = 3.$$
To change 3 to a percentage, multiply by 100: $3 \times 100 = 300\%$.

36. **The answer is a.** The problem states that 0.5 mg is equal to 23% of the USDRA of vitamin B_6 for adults. Restate this fact as an equation.
$0.5 = 23\%$ of x
$0.5 = 0.23x$
where x is the total USDRA of vitamin B_6.
Divide both sides by 0.23 to solve for x.
$$x = \frac{0.5}{0.23} = 2.17 \text{ mg}$$
The problem asks for the answer to the nearest tenth, so you must round off to the nearest tenth. Because the digit in the hundredths place is 5 or bigger, round the tenths digit up 1.
$2.17 \text{ mg} \approx 2.2 \text{ mg}$

SECTION A

SECTION B

SECTION C

COMPREHENSIVE PRACTICE Test 1

COMPREHENSIVE PRACTICE Test 2

COMPREHENSIVE PRACTICE Test 3

37. **The answer is a.** The product $x^2 - 81$ is known as a difference of two squares, because both the first and last terms are perfect squares and they are being subtracted from one another. There is a shortcut for factoring such a product. Knowing that your answer will be two binomials, you may assume the first term of each will be the square root of x^2, that the second term will be the square root of 81, and that the second terms will be opposite in sign. The signs must be opposite so that, when multiplied, their terms will cancel each other out.
$(x + 9)(x - 9) = x^2 + 9x - 9x + 81 = x^2 - 81$

38. **The answer is d.** First, find the area (A) of the original room, using this formula:
$A = lw$
where l = length and w = width.
$A = 10 \text{ ft} \times 15 \text{ ft}$
$A = 150 \text{ ft}^2$
If the room's dimensions were increased by 1 ft, the new formula would be:
$A = 11 \text{ ft} \times 16 \text{ ft}$
$A = 176 \text{ ft}^2$
The new area exceeds the original area by 26 ft^2: $176 - 150$.

39. **The answer is d.** Distribute the 2 and the 3 over their respective sums, and combine like terms.
$2(x + 3y) + 3(x + 2y)$
$2x + 6y + 3x + 6y$
$5x + 12y$

40. **The answer is c.** The question asks you to consider prescriptions in the $20-to-$40 price range. A discount of $1 is 5% of $20 and 2.5% of $40. Therefore, the less expensive prescription receives a higher discount rate.

ANSWERS TO COMPREHENSIVE PRACTICE TEST 1: SCIENCE

1. **The answer is b.** Fluorides are added to drinking water in many communities to prevent cavities.

2. **The answer is d.** Bees and butterflies are necessary for pollination. Thus, fewer plant seeds would be produced if bees and butterflies were destroyed.

3. **The answer is c.** At the alveoli, the functional units of the lung, gas exchange occurs between the capillaries and these thin sacs full of oxygen. Carbon dioxide is released into the alveoli to be exhaled, and oxygen diffuses into the capillaries to be transported to the body.

4. **The answer is a.** Alcohol has a depressant effect on the central nervous system.

5. **The answer is d.** The force applied by the lever is proportional to the force itself and to the distance away from the balance. The force applied at D is the greatest distance away, so less effort will be needed here.

6. **The answer is b.** The wavelength of a wave is defined as the distance between crests of the wave.

7. **The answer is d.** A vaccine introduces a portion of a specific virus to a person to stimulate the body's immune system to create antibodies to the virus.

8. **The answer is a.** Scientists are continually searching for missing links in evolution.

9. **The answer is d.** The correct reading is 102.0°F.

10. **The answer is d.** According to Gay-Lussac's law, as temperature is increased at a constant volume, pressure increases proportionally.

11. **The answer is a.** In Spemann's first experiment, it was clear that the cells were all alike and had not specialized yet. In his second experiment, he found that cells from the older embryos had become specialized for nerve and skin functions.

12. **The answer is a.** An ion is an atom whose number of electrons and number of protons are not equal. An ion has an extra or a missing electron. If it is missing an electron, it has a net positive charge. If it gains an electron, it has a net negative charge.

13. **The answer is c.** Nucleotides are components of nucleic acids (DNA and RNA). Uracil is found in RNA and is replaced by thymine in DNA. ATP and NADH are not nucleic acids.

14. **The answer is d.** Any circuit with the same voltage across all resistors is a parallel circuit.

15. **The answer is b.** Whenever a wire is wrapped around a rod and connected across a power source like a battery, the device will act as an electromagnet.

16. **The answer is a.** Since the forces are in the opposite directions, they are not added. The smaller force is subtracted from the stronger force, and the resultant force is in the same direction as the stronger one.

SECTION A

SECTION B

SECTION C

COMPREHENSIVE PRACTICE Test 1

COMPREHENSIVE PRACTICE Test 2

COMPREHENSIVE PRACTICE Test 3

17. **The answer is c.** Fungi are heterotrophic and do not photosynthesize. Thus, they do not contain chlorophyll.

18. **The answer is a.** The medulla is responsible for regulating involuntary functions, such as heart rate and breathing.

19. **The answer is d.** Sulfur oxide causes lung and eye irritation.

20. **The answer is a.** A freely falling object falls at a constant acceleration: $g = 9.8 \text{ m/sec}^2$. The graph that shows velocity increasing at a constant rate is A.

21. **The answer is c.** The m-RNA molecule takes information from the DNA in the nucleus and brings it to the ribosome, where it directs the production of proteins according to the code it received from the DNA.

22. **The answer is b.** ATP is the product of respiration (aerobic or anaerobic) in all organisms.

23. **The answer is b.** When a wave passes through a small opening in a barrier, it spreads at the same rate in all directions. The only diagram that fits this description is choice b.

24. **The answer is b.** As the blood is filtered in the kidney, glucose is reabsorbed by the body, and urea is excreted in the urine as waste.

25. **The answer is d.** Light physical work requires the greatest number of calories per minute according to the data chart.

26. **The answer is c.** Of the activities noted in the choices, women used the most Calories, 540 in 24 hr, standing or doing limited walking outdoors. Choice a used 480 Cal. Choice b used 400 Cal. Choice d used 360 Cal.

27. **The answer is d.** The rate of calorie expenditure is greater for men than for women in all the listed activities. None of the other choices is supported by the data on the chart.

28. **The answer is b.** Two washers are equivalent in mass to 1 bolt. Thus, 4 bolts are equivalent in mass to 8 washers. The equal arm balance is balanced at a ratio of 2 washers to 1 bolt; if 4 bolts are added to one side, 8 washers are needed to balance it.

29. **The answer is d.** According to the table, lead chloride and lead iodide are slightly soluble (slightly able to dissolve in water), whereas lead hydroxide is insoluble. Lead nitrate, on the other hand, is completely soluble in water.

30. **The answer is c.** According to the key, d represents a substance that decomposes in water. Decomposition is a reaction in which one reactant produces more than one product. Of the four choices, only copper II iodide decomposes in water.

31. **The answer is b.** The cranium protects the brain, and the rib cage protects the heart and lungs. The femur, humerus, radius, and ulna are involved in movement.

32. **The answer is b.** The melting point is the temperature at which a substance changes from a solid to a liquid, and the boiling point refers to the temperature at which the substance changes from a liquid to a gas. The chart indicates that substance X is a liquid over the

shortest range; it turns into a liquid at 10°F and becomes a gas at 80°F. Thus, it remains a liquid for a span of 70°, unlike the other substances that remain in this phase for much longer periods.

33. **The answer is d.** When a strong base is added to a strong acid, a salt and water are produced. This is termed a neutralization reaction.

34. **The answer is c.** Sodium ions and chloride ions are attracted to each other due to their opposite charges. The result of their union is an ionic bond, and the formation of a compound called sodium chloride.

35. **The answer is a.** It is rare for someone to be infected with the chicken pox virus more than once. This is an example of the presence of active immunity. After the first infection, the body retains some of the antibodies to the virus, which prevents reinfection.

36. **The answer is c.** Number 5 points to the retina, which contains the rods and cones, structures that respond to light and send messages to the brain, resulting in vision.

37. **The answer is b.** Number 3 points to the lens, which focuses light on the retina.

38. **The answer is d.** The electron microscope allows the observation of much smaller particles than phase-contrast or compound light microscopes.

39. **The answer is a.** In South Florida the temperature is not near freezing in late fall.

40. **The answer is b.** A control represents normal conditions and can be used as a baseline for comparison. This control also shows that sugars are a factor in the experiment.

41. **The answer is a.** In cellular respiration, glucose is broken down in the cell, and energy in the form of ATP is produced. Through this process, food becomes energy at the cellular level.

42. **The answer is b.** x represents fertilization, which occurs between the formation of gametes and cleavage.

43. **The answer is c.** White blood cells are drawn to areas of tissue damage by chemicals released at the site of the injury. They move to the tissues with amoebalike movement and help defend the body against infection. Red blood cells contain hemoglobin for the transport of oxygen.

44. **The answer is d.** Blue litmus paper turns red in the presence of an acid. Acids have pHs that are lower than 7.

45. **The answer is a.** The speed of sound in air is 332 m/s, or 1,100ft/sec.

46. **The answer is a.** As a general rule, the solubility of a solid in water increases with increasing temperature. The solubility of a gas increases with decreasing temperature.

47. **The answer is b.** Magnetic field lines must point away from the nearest north pole. Like poles repel each other; unlike attract.

SECTION A

SECTION B

SECTION C

COMPREHENSIVE PRACTICE Test 1

COMPREHENSIVE PRACTICE Test 2

COMPREHENSIVE PRACTICE Test 3

48. **The answer is c.** The assumption is that 1 mL of water has a mass of 1 g.

$$\frac{5\,g}{25\,mL} \times 100 = 20\%$$

49. **The answer is a.** An electron carries a negative charge, a proton carries a positive charge, and a neutron carries no charge.

50. **The answer is a.** A points to the endosperm, which provides the growing embryo with nutrients.

51. **The answer is d.** Guard cells surround the stomata and regulate their opening and closing.

52. **The answer is a.** Catalysts increase the rate of a reaction but are neither changed nor consumed in the course of the reaction.

53. **The answer is c.** The frequency of sound waves heard by the human ear ranges from 20 to 20,000 Hz (vibrations per second).

54. **The answer is d.** Glucose is broken down during cellular respiration, and energy in the form of ATP is formed.

55. **The answer is c.** Saliva contains the enzyme amylase, which breaks down starches, such as crackers, into sugars.

56. **The answer is c.** The bulb is an example of vegetative propagation, a form of asexual reproduction.

57. **The answer is c.** The testes produce the hormone testosterone, which is responsible for the development of many of the male maturation steps.

58. **The answer is a.** Isotopes have the same atomic number (number of protons) but a different mass number (sum of protons and neutrons). Thus, an isotope has the same number of protons and a different number of neutrons.

59. **The answer is b.** Half-life refers to the time it takes half of the mass of a radioactive substance to decay. After 20 years, 6 g of the substance would be left. After 20 more years, 3 g of the substance would remain.

60. **The answer is d.** Newton's law, $F = ma$, states that with no force acting on an object, there will be no acceleration; therefore, the ball will maintain its velocity.

NOTES

NOTES

NOTES

NOTES